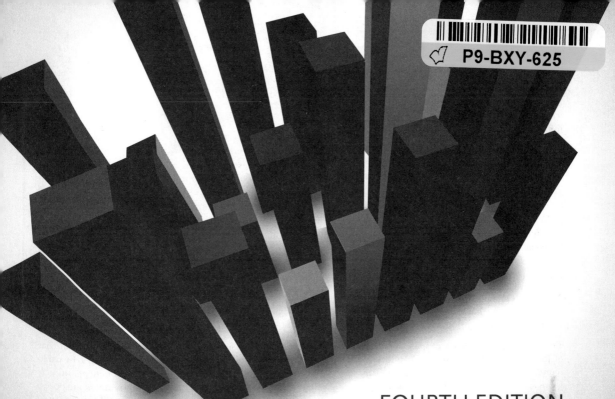

FOURTH EDITION

HEALTH CARE
FINANCE

Basic Tools For Nonfinancial Managers

JUDITH J. BAKER, PhD, CPA
and
R. W. BAKER, JD
Dallas, Texas

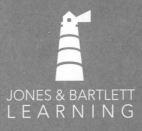

JONES & BARTLETT
LEARNING

World Headquarters
Jones & Bartlett Learning
5 Wall Street
Burlington, MA 01803
978-443-5000
info@jblearning.com
www.jblearning.com

Jones & Bartlett Learning books and products are available through most bookstores and online booksellers. To contact Jones & Bartlett Learning directly, call 800-832-0034, fax 978-443-8000, or visit our website, www.jblearning.com.

Production Credits

Executive Publisher: William Brottmiller
Publisher: Michael Brown
Editorial Assistant: Chloe Falivene
Associate Production Editor: Rebekah Linga
Senior Marketing Manager: Sophie Fleck Teague
Manufacturing and Inventory Control Supervisor: Amy Bacus
Composition: Laserwords Private Limited, Chennai, India
Cover and Title Page Design: Kristin E. Parker
Cover and Title Page Image: © andkuch/ShutterStock, Inc.
Printing and Binding: Edwards Brothers Malloy
Cover Printing: Edwards Brothers Malloy

To order this product, use ISBN: 978-1-284-02986-4

Library of Congress Cataloging-in-Publication Data
Baker, Judith J., author.
  Health care finance : basic tools for nonfinancial managers / Judith J. Baker and R.W. Baker.—Fourth edition.
      p. ; cm.
  Includes bibliographical references and index.
  ISBN 978-1-4496-8727-4 (pbk.)—ISBN 1-4496-8727-X (pbk.)
  I. Baker, R. W., author. II. Title.
  [DNLM: 1. Financial Management—United States. 2. Health Facilities—economics—United States. 3. Health Facility Administration—United States. W 80]
  RA971.3
  362.1068'1—dc23
                                                                                              2013010480

6048
Printed in the United States of America
17 16 15 14 13   10 9 8 7 6 5 4 3 2 1

Table of Contents

New to This Edition

THE FOURTH EDITION

The *Fourth Edition* continues to provide practical information with examples taken from real life in the healthcare finance world. For example, we have added the following:

A new chapter about "Strategic Planning and the Healthcare Financial Manager." This subject was suggested to us as a valuable addition to the book, and we took the suggestion. The chapter contains details about the planning process; examples of mission, vision, and value statements; and a governmental strategic planning cycle example. A new appendix contains "Sample SWOT Worksheets and Question Guides."

A new case study about "Strategic Financial Planning in Long-Term Care." The case study was written for us by Dr. Neil Dworkin. Dr. Dworkin is Emeritus Associate Professor of Management at Western Connecticut State University, where he taught strategic management, finance, marketing, health policy, and health delivery systems.

Two new and updated chapters about information systems, electronic health records (EHR), and their financial management. Substantial financial incentives and penalties are involved with the adoption or nonadoption of electronic health records. Multiple initiatives and staggered transition periods will affect facilities and eligible professionals over the next several years. These two chapters help managers understand what is at stake and how their roles fit within the transition.

A new chapter about "Electronic Health Records Framework: Incentives, Standards, Measures, and Meaningful Use." This chapter explains how a major EHR incentive program in force today actually works. Many managers are thrown into working intensively with some aspect of these requirements. This chapter explains the program's inner workings and provides examples.

New visuals, examples, multiple updates, and supplemental materials have been added throughout.

We have restructured the Metropolis Health System (MHS) case study information into a comprehensive suite of information. This section now includes the major case study followed by an appendix containing an MHS financial statement and excerpts from notes. A second appendix shows how an MHS hospital was turned around using comparative analysis. Then a mini-case study describes a proposal to add a retail pharmacy to an MHS hospital. The restructuring now provides an interactive suite of case study material.

New website links. The Fourth Edition website now provides website links for those who want to take a deeper look at some subjects. (The links can also be used as a springboard for additional assignments.)

In short, we have continued to work to reveal the basic tools of healthcare finance and make them usable.

Preface

Our world of work is divided into three parts: the healthcare consultant, the instructor, and the writer. Over the years, we have taught managers in seminars, academic settings, and corporate conference rooms. Most of the managers were midcareer adults, working in all types of healthcare disciplines. We taught them and they taught us. One of the things they taught us was this: a nonfinancial manager pushed into dealing with the world of finance often feels a dislocation and a change of perspective, and that experience can be both difficult and exciting. We have listened to their questions and concerns as these managers grapple with this new world. This book is the result of their experiences, and ours.

The book is designed for use by a manager (or future manager) who does not have an educational background in financial management. It has long been our philosophy that if you can truly understand how a thing works—whatever it is—then you own it. This book is created around that philosophy. In other words, we intend to make financial management transparent by showing how it works and how a manager can use it.

USING THE BOOK

Users will find examples and exercises covering many types of healthcare settings and providers included. The case study of Metropolis Hospital System is woven throughout the book. Three mini-case studies are provided to give an even broader view of the subjects covered. "Progress Notes" set out learning objectives at the beginning of each chapter. An "Information Checkpoint" segment at the end of each chapter tells the user three things: information needed, where this information can be obtained, and how this information can be used. A "Key Terms" section follows the "Information Checkpoint." Each of these features displays its own quick-reference icon.

Access to the website is shown in Appendix B, "Web-Based and Software Learning Tools." For users who prefer a calculator, Appendix B provides guidance on where to obtain information on using a business analyst calculator. And for those users who choose neither a computer nor a calculator, instructions are set out so problems can also be worked by hand, with paper and pencil.

Acknowledgments

This book originated during the course of our activity-based costing seminars for Irwin Professional Seminars, when class members kept inserting finance questions into the sessions. The original concept for the book was clarified when Cleo Boulter, then Associate Professor at the University of Texas at Houston Center on Aging, recruited us to teach intensive finance sessions to her midcareer students, an arrangement that continued over a period of years. The needs of these students and their reaction to the material provided the core of the book's First Edition content.

The *Fourth Edition* has evolved with the help of numerous instructors and students who give us feedback; we listen. In particular we thank Dr. Neil Dworkin, Emeritus Associate Professor of Management at Western Connecticut State University, who has provided input and an excellent new case study. We wish to acknowledge the continuing support of Janet Feldman, PhD, RN, Vice President, Qualitas Associates, Downers Grove, Illinois, along with certain technical support provided by Colleene McMurphy, CPA, of McMurphy and Associates, Winnsboro, Texas.

The input from finance sessions we taught as Adjunct Faculty at Texas Womans' University in Dallas also contributed to shaping the content of the *Fourth Edition*. Our continued gratitude goes to Craig Sheagren, Senior Vice President/CFO, McDonough District Hospital, Macomb, Illinois, and Nancy M. Borkowski, PhD, Professor, Department. of Professional Management/Health Management, St. Thomas University, Miami, Florida, for their encouragement, information, suggestions, and assistance with the original concept of the book. We also thank John Brocketti, Chief Financial Officer, SUMA Health System, Akron, Ohio; Christine Pierce, Partner, The Resource Group, Cleveland, Ohio; and Dr. Frank Welsh, Cincinnati, Ohio, for their ongoing information and suggestions.

Many others also contributed suggestions, recommendations, and information to help shape and refine the initial concept. We continue to acknowledge these individuals, listed below, including their original affiliations:

Ian G. Worden, CPA, Regional Vice President of Finance/CFO, PeaceHealth, Eugene, Oregon
Carol A. Robinson, Medical Records Director, Titus Regional Medical Center, Mt. Pleasant, Texas
John Congelli, Vice President of Finance, Genesee Memorial Hospital, Batavia, New York
Charles A. Keil, Cost Accountant, Genesee Memorial Hospital, Batavia, New York
George O. Kimbro, CPA, CFO, Hunt Memorial Hospital District, Greenville, Texas
Bob Gault, Laboratory Director, Hunt Memorial Hospital District, Greenville, Texas
Ted J. Stuart, Jr., MD, MBA, Northwest Family Physicians, Glendale, Arizona
Mark Potter, EMS Director, Hopkins County Memorial Hospital, Sulphur Springs, Texas
and
Leonard H. Friedman, PhD, Assistant Professor, Coordinator, Health Care Administration Program, Oregon State University, Corvallis, Oregon
Patricia Chiverton, EdD, RN, Dean, University of Rochester School of Nursing, Rochester, New York
Donna M. Tortoretti, RNC, Chief Operating Officer, Community Nursing Center, University of Rochester School of Nursing, Rochester, New York
Billie Ann Brotman, PhD, Professor of Finance, Department. of Economics and Finance, Kennesaw State University, Kennesaw, Georgia

About the Authors

Judith J. Baker, PhD, CPA, is Executive Director of Resource Group, Ltd., a Dallas-based health care consulting firm. She earned her Bachelor of Science degree in Business Administration at the University of Missouri, Columbia and her Master of Liberal Studies with a concentration in Business Management at the University of Oklahoma, Norman. She earned her Master of Arts and Doctorate in Human and Organizational Systems, with a concentration in costing systems, at the Fielding Institute, Santa Barbara, California. She is an adjunct faculty member at the Case Western Reserve University Frances Payne Bolton School of Nursing.

Judith has over thirty years experience in health care and consults on numerous health care systems and costing problems. She has worked with health care systems, costing, and reimbursement throughout her career. As a CMS contractor she has assisted in validation of costs for new programs and for rate setting and consults on cost report design.

Judith has written over 40 articles, manuals, and books. She served as Consulting Editor for Aspen Publishers, Inc. Her books include *Activity-Based Costing and Activity-Based Management for Health Care, Prospective Payment for Long-Term Care: An Annual Guide,* and *Prospective Payment for Home Health Agencies.* She is editor emeritus of the quarterly *Journal of Healthcare Finance.*

R.W. Baker, JD, is Managing Partner of Resource Group, Ltd., a Dallas-based health care consulting firm. He has more than 30 years of experience in health care and has designed, directed, and administered numerous financial impact studies for health care providers. His recent studies have centered around facility-specific MDS data collection and analysis. He and his firm subcontracted to the HCFA/CMS Nursing Home Case Mix and Quality Demonstration for over nine years.

R.W. is the editor of continuing professional education seminar manuals and training manuals for facility personnel and for research staff members. He served as a Consulting Editor with Aspen Publishers, Inc. and is co-author of *A Step-by-Step Guide to the Minimum Data Set* (Aspen Publishers, Inc.).

About the Contributor

Neil R. Dworkin, PhD, is Emeritus Associate Professor of Management at Western Connecticut State University, where he was Coordinator of the Masters in Health Administration Program and where he taught Strategic Management, Finance, Marketing, Health Policy, and Health Delivery Systems. Dr. Dworkin is also a licensed nursing home administrator in Connecticut and New York.

Healthcare Finance Overview

Introduction to Healthcare Finance

THE HISTORY

Financial management has a long and distinguished history. Consider, for example, that Socrates wrote about the universal function of management in human endeavors in 400 B.C. and that Plato developed the concept of specialization for efficiency in 350 B.C. Evidence of sophisticated financial management exists from much earlier times: the Chinese produced a planning and control system in 1100 B.C., a minimum-wage system was developed by Hammurabi in 1800 B.C., and the Egyptians and Sumerians developed planning and record-keeping systems in 4000 B.C.[1]

Many managers in early history discovered and rediscovered managerial principles while attempting to reach their goals. Because the idea of management thought as a discipline had not yet evolved, they formulated principles of management because certain goals had to be accomplished. As management thought became codified over time, however, the building of techniques for management became more organized. Management as a discipline for educational purposes began in the United States in 1881. In that year, Joseph Wharton created the Wharton School, offering college courses in business management at the University of Pennsylvania. It was the only such school until 1898, when the Universities of Chicago and California established their business schools. Thirteen years later, in 1911, 30 such schools were in operation in the United States.[2]

Over the long span of history, managers have all sought how to make organizations work more effectively. Financial management is a vital part of organizational

After completing this chapter, you should be able to

1. Discuss the three viewpoints of managers in organizations.
2. Identify the four elements of financial management.
3. Understand the differences between the two types of accounting.
4. Identify the types of organizations.
5. Understand the composition and purpose of an organization chart.

effectiveness. This text's goal is to provide the keys to unlock the secrets of financial management for nonfinancial managers.

THE CONCEPT

A Method of Getting Money in and out of the Business

One of our colleagues, a nurse, talks about the area of healthcare finance as "a method of getting money in and out of the business." It is not a bad description. As we shall see, revenues represent inflow and expenses represent outflow. Thus, "getting money in" represents the inflow (revenues), whereas "getting money out" (expenses) represents the outflow. The successful manager, through planning, organizing, controlling, and decision making, is able to adjust the inflow and outflow to achieve the most beneficial outcome for the organization.

HOW DOES FINANCE WORK IN THE HEALTHCARE BUSINESS?

The purpose of this text is to show how the various elements of finance fit together: in other words, how finance works in the healthcare business. The real key to understanding finance is understanding the various pieces and their relationship to each other. If you, the manager, truly see how the elements work, then they are yours. They become your tools to achieve management success.

The healthcare industry is a service industry. It is not in the business of manufacturing, say, widgets. Instead, its essential business is the delivery of healthcare services. It may have inventories of medical supplies and drugs, but those inventories are necessary to service delivery, not to manufacturing functions. Because the business of health care is service, the explanations and illustrations within this book focus on the practice of financial management in the service industries.

VIEWPOINTS

The managers within a healthcare organization will generally have one of three views: (1) financial, (2) process, or (3) clinical. The way they manage will be influenced by which view they hold.

1. The financial view. These managers generally work with finance on a daily basis. The reporting function is part of their responsibility. They usually perform much of the strategic planning for the organization.
2. The process view. These managers generally work with the system of the organization. They may be responsible for data accumulation. They are often affiliated with the information system hierarchy in the organization.
3. The clinical view. These managers generally are responsible for service delivery. They have direct interaction with the patients and are responsible for clinical outcomes of the organization.

Managers must, of necessity, interact with one another. Thus, managers holding different views will be required to work together. Their concerns will intersect to some degree, as illustrated by **Figure 1–1**. The nonfinancial manager who understands healthcare finance will be able to interpret and negotiate successfully such interactions between and among viewpoints.

In summary, financial management is a discipline with a long and respected history. Healthcare service delivery is a business, and the concept of financial management assists in balancing the inflows and outflows that are a part of the business.

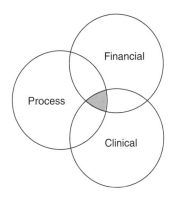

Figure 1–1 Three Views of Management Within an Organization.

WHY MANAGE?

Business does not run itself. It requires a variety of management activities in order to operate properly.

THE ELEMENTS OF FINANCIAL MANAGEMENT

There are four recognized elements of financial management: (1) planning, (2) controlling, (3) organizing and directing, and (4) decision making. The four divisions are based on the purpose of each task. Some authorities stress only three elements (planning, controlling, and decision making) and consider organizing and directing as a part of the controlling element. This text recognizes organizing and directing as a separate element of financial management, primarily because such a large proportion of a manager's time is taken up with performing these duties.

1. Planning. The financial manager identifies the steps that must be taken to accomplish the organization's objectives. Thus, the purpose is to identify objectives and then to identify the steps required for accomplishing these objectives.
2. Controlling. The financial manager makes sure that each area of the organization is following the plans that have been established. One way to do this is to study current reports and compare them with reports from earlier periods. This comparison often shows where the organization may need attention because that area is not effective. The reports that the manager uses for this purpose are often called feedback. The purpose of controlling is to ensure that plans are being followed.
3. Organizing and directing. When organizing, the financial manager decides how to use the resources of the organization to most effectively carry out the plans that have been established. When directing, the manager works on a day-to-day basis to keep the results of the organizing running efficiently. The purpose is to ensure effective resource use and provide daily supervision.

4. Decision making. The financial manager makes choices among available alternatives. Decision making actually occurs parallel to planning, organizing, and controlling. All types of decision making rely on information, and the primary tasks are analysis and evaluation. Thus, the purpose is to make informed choices.

THE ORGANIZATION'S STRUCTURE

The structure of an organization is an important factor in management.

Organization Types

Organizations fall into one of two basic types: profit oriented or nonprofit oriented. In the United States, these designations follow the taxable status of the organizations. The profit-oriented entities, also known as proprietary organizations, are responsible for paying income taxes. Proprietary subgroups include individuals, partnerships, and corporations. The nonprofit organizations do not pay income taxes.

There are two subgroups of nonprofit entities: voluntary and government. Voluntary nonprofits have sought tax-exempt status. In general, voluntary nonprofits are associated with churches, private schools, or foundations. Government nonprofits, on the other hand, do not pay taxes because they are government entities. Government nonprofits can be (1) federal, (2) state, (3) county, (4) city, (5) a combination of city and county, (6) a hospital taxing district (with the power to raise revenues through taxes), or (7) a state university (perhaps with a teaching hospital affiliated with the university). The organization's type may affect its structure. **Exhibit 1–1** summarizes the subgroups of both proprietary and nonprofit organizations.

Exhibit 1–1 Types of Organizations

Profit Oriented—Proprietary
Individual
Partnership
Corporation
Other
Nonprofit—Voluntary
Church Associated
Private School Associated
Foundation Associated
Other
Nonprofit—Government
Federal
State
County
City
City-County
Hospital District
State University
Other

Organization Charts

In a small organization, top management will be able to see what is happening. Extensive measures and indicators are not necessary because management can view overall operations. But in a large organization, top management must use the management control system to understand what is going on. In other words, to view operations, management must use measures and indicators because he or she cannot get a firsthand overall picture of the total organization.

As a rule of thumb, an informal management control system is acceptable only if the manager can stay in close contact with all aspects of the operation. Otherwise, a formal system is required. In the context of health care, therefore, a one-physician practice (**Figure 1–2**) could use an informal method, but a hospital system (**Figure 1–3**) must use a formal method of management control.

The structure of the organization will affect its financial management. Organization charts are often used to illustrate the structure of the organization. Each box on an organization chart represents a particular area of management responsibility. The lines between the boxes are lines of authority.

In the health system organization chart illustrated in Figure 1–3, the president/chief executive officer oversees seven senior vice presidents. Each senior vice president has vice presidents reporting to him or her in each particular area of responsibility designated on the chart. These vice presidents, in turn, have an array of other managers reporting to them at varying levels of managerial responsibility.

The organization chart also shows the degree of decentralization within the organization. Decentralization indicates the delegating of authority for decision making. The chart thus illustrates the pattern of how managers are allowed—or required—to make key decisions within the particular organization.

The purpose of an organization chart, then, is to indicate how responsibility is assigned to managers and to indicate the formal lines of communication and reporting.

TWO TYPES OF ACCOUNTING

Financial

Financial accounting is generally for outside, or third party, use. Thus, financial accounting emphasizes external reporting. External reporting to third parties in health care includes, for example, government entities (Medicare, Medicaid, and other government programs) and health plan payers. In addition, proprietary organizations may have to report to stockholders, taxing district hospitals have to report to taxpayers, and so on.

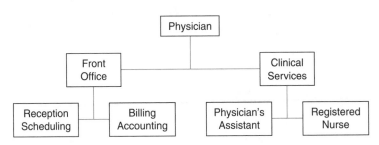

Figure 1–2 Physician's Office Organization Chart.
Courtesy of Resource Group, Ltd., Dallas, Texas.

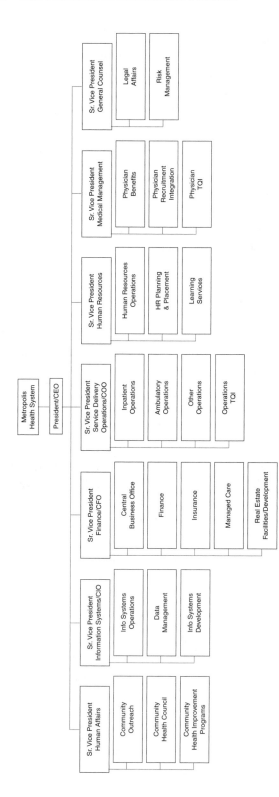

Figure 1–3 Health System Organization Chart.
Courtesy of Resource Group, Ltd., Dallas, Texas.

Financial reporting for external purposes must be in accordance with generally accepted accounting principles. Financial reporting is usually concerned with transactions that have already occurred: that is, it is retrospective.

Managerial

Managerial accounting is generally for inside, or internal, use. Managerial accounting, as its title implies, is used by managers. The planning and control of operations and related performance measures are common day-by-day uses of managerial accounting. Likewise, the reporting of profitability of services and the pricing of services are other common ongoing uses of managerial accounting. Strategic planning and other intermediate and long-term decision making represent an additional use of managerial accounting.[3]

Managerial accounting intended for internal use is not bound by generally accepted accounting principles. Managerial accounting deals with transactions that have already occurred, but it is also concerned with the future, in the form of projecting outcomes and preparing budgets. Thus, managerial accounting is prospective as well as retrospective.

 INFORMATION CHECKPOINT

What is needed?	Reports for management purposes.
Where is it found?	With your supervisor.
How is it used?	To manage better.
What is needed?	Organization chart.
Where is it found?	With your supervisor or in the administrative offices.
How is it used?	To better understand the structure and lines of authority in your organization.

 KEY TERMS

Controlling
Decision Making
Financial Accounting
Managerial Accounting
Nonprofit Organization (also see Voluntary Organization)
Organization Chart
Organizing
Planning
Proprietary Organization (also see Profit-Oriented Organization)

DISCUSSION QUESTIONS

1. What element of financial management do you perform most often in your job?
2. Do you perform all four elements? If not, why not?
3. Of the organization types described in this chapter, what type is the one you work for?
4. Have you ever seen your company's organization chart? If so, how decentralized is it?
5. If you receive reports in the course of your work, do you believe that they are prepared for outside (third party) use or for internal (management) use? What leads you to believe this?

NOTES

1. C. S. George, Jr., *The History of Management Thought,* 2nd ed. (Englewood Cliffs, NJ: Prentice Hall, 1972), 1–27.
2. Ibid., 87.
3. S. Williamson et al., *Fundamentals of Strategic Planning for Healthcare Organizations* (New York: The Haworth Press, 1997).

Four Things the Healthcare Manager Needs to Know About Financial Management Systems

WHAT DOES THE MANAGER NEED TO KNOW?

Financial management is both an art and a science. You, as a manager, need to perceive the structure and reasoning that underlies management actions. To do so, you need to be able to answer the following four questions:

1. What are the four segments that make a financial management system work?
2. How does the information flow?
3. What are the basic system elements?
4. What is the annual management cycle for reporting results?

This chapter provides answers to each of these four questions. It also discusses how to communicate financial information to others. This ability is a valuable skill for a successful manager.

HOW THE SYSTEM WORKS IN HEALTH CARE

The information that you, as a manager, work with is only one part of an overall system. To understand financial management, it is essential to recognize the overall system in which your organization operates. An order exists within the system, and it is generally up to you to find that order. Watch for how the information fits together. The four segments that make a healthcare financial system work are (1) the original records, (2) the information system, (3) the accounting system, (4) and the reporting system. Generally speaking, the original records provide evidence that some event has occurred; the information system gathers this evidence; the accounting system records the evidence, and the reporting system produces reports of the effect. The healthcare manager needs to know that these separate elements exist and that they work together for an end result.

THE INFORMATION FLOW

Structure of the Information System

Information systems can be simplistic or highly complex. They can be fully automated or semiautomated. Occasionally—even today—they can still be generated by hand and not by computer. (This last instance is becoming rare and can happen today only in certain small and relatively isolated healthcare organizations that are not yet required to electronically submit their billings.)

We will examine a particular information system and point out the basics that a manager should be able to recognize. **Figure 2–1** shows information system components for an ambulatory care setting. This complex system uses a clinical and financial data repository; in other words, both clinical and financial data are fed into the same system. An automated medical record is also linked to the system. These are basic facts that a manager should recognize about this ambulatory information system.

In addition, the financial information, both outpatient and any relevant inpatient, is fed into the data repository. Scheduling-system data also enter the data repository, along with any relevant inpatient care plan and nursing information. Again, all of these are basic facts that a manager should recognize about this ambulatory care information system.

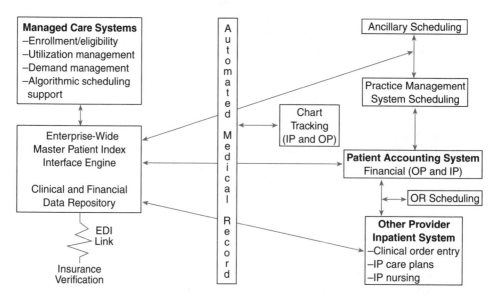

Figure 2–1 Information System Components for an Ambulatory Care Setting. OP, Outpatient; IP, Inpatient; OR, Operating Room.

These items have all been inputs. One output from the clinical and financial data repository (also shown in Figure 2–1) is insurance verification for patients through an electronic data information (EDI) link to insurance company databases. Insurance verification is daily operating information. Another output is decision-making information for managed care strategic planning, including support for demand, utilization, enrollment, and eligibility, plus some statistical support. The manager does not have to understand the specifics of all the inputs and outputs of this complex system, but he or she should recognize that these outputs occur when this ambulatory system is activated.

Function of Flowsheets

Flowsheets illustrate, as in this case, the flow of activities that capture information.[1] Flowsheets are useful because they portray who is responsible for what piece of information as it enters the system. The manager needs to realize the significance of such information. We give, as an example, obtaining confirmation of a patient's correct address. The manager should know that a correct address for a patient is vital to the smooth operation of the system. An incorrect address will, for example, cause the billing to be rejected. Understanding this connection between deficient data (e.g., a bad address) and the consequences (the bill will be rejected by the payer and thus not be paid) illustrates the essence of good financial management knowledge.

We can examine two examples of patient information flows. The first, shown in **Figure 2–2**, is a physician's office flowsheet for address confirmation. Four different personnel are

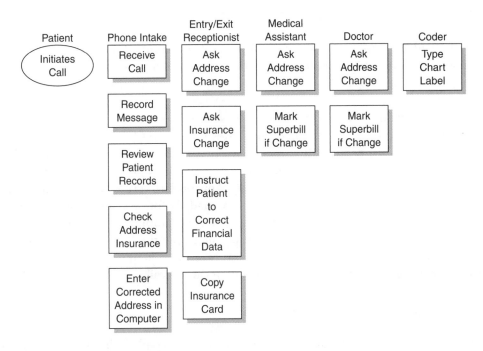

Figure 2–2 Physician's Office Flowsheet for Address Confirmation.

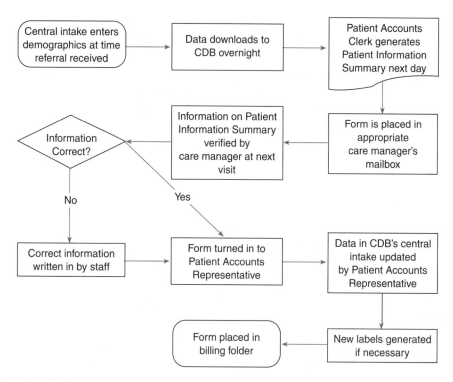

Figure 2–3 Health System Flowsheet for Verification of Patient Information.

involved, in addition to the patient. This physician has computed the cost of a bad address as $12.30 to track down each address correction. He pays close attention to the handling of this information because he knows there is a direct financial management consequence in his operation.

The second example, shown in **Figure 2–3**, is a health system flowsheet for verification of patient information. This flowsheet illustrates the process for a home care system. In this case, the flow begins not with a receptionist, as in the physician office example, but with a central database. This central database downloads the information and generates a summary report to be reviewed the next day. Appropriate verification is then made in a series of steps, and any necessary corrections are made before the form goes to the billing department. The object of the flow is the same in both examples: that is, the billing department must have a correct address to receive payment. But the flow is different within two different systems. A manager must understand how the system works to understand the consequences—then good financial management can prevail.

BASIC SYSTEM ELEMENTS

To understand financial management, it is essential to decipher the reports provided to the manager. To comprehend these reports, it is helpful to understand certain basic system elements that are used to create the information contained in the reports.

Chart of Accounts—The Map

The chart of accounts is a map. It outlines the elements of your company in an organized manner. The chart of accounts maps out account titles with a method of numeric coding. It is designed to compile financial data in a uniform manner that the user can decode.

The groupings of accounts in the chart of accounts should match the groupings of the organization. In other words, the classification on the organization chart (as discussed in the previous chapter) should be compatible with the groupings on the chart of accounts. Thus, if there is a human resources department on your facility's organization chart, and if expenses are grouped by department in your facility, then we would expect to find a human resources grouping in the chart of accounts.

The manager who is working with financial data needs to be able to read and comprehend how the dollars are laid out and how they are gathered together, or assembled. This assembly happens through the guidance of the chart of accounts. That is why we compare it to a map.

Basic guidance for healthcare charts of accounts is set out in publications such as that of Seawell's *Chart of Accounts for Hospitals.*[2] However, generic guides are just that—generic. Every organization exhibits differences in its own chart of accounts that express the unique aspects of its structure. We examine three examples to illustrate these differences. Remember, we are spending time on the chart of accounts because your comprehension of detailed financial data may well depend on whether you can decipher your facility's own chart of accounts mapping in the information forwarded for your use.

The first format, shown in **Exhibit 2–1**, is a basic use, probably for a smaller organization. The exhibit is in two horizontal segments, "Structure" and "Example." There are three

---

Exhibit 2–1 Chart of Accounts, Format I

Structure		
X	XX	XX
Financial Statement Element	Primary Subclassification	Secondary Subclassification

Example		
1	10	11
Asset	Current Asset	Petty Cash— Front Office
(Financial Statement Element)	(Primary Subclassification)	(Secondary Subclassification)

Exhibit 2–2 Chart of Accounts, Format II

Structure				
XX	XX	X	XXXX	XX
Entity Designator	Fund Designator	Financial Statement Element	Primary Subclassification	Secondary Subclassification

Example				
10	10	4	3125	03
Hospital A	General Fund	Revenue	Lab—Microbiology	Payer: XYZ HMO
10	10	6	3125	10
Hospital A	General Fund	Expense	Lab—Microbiology	Clerical Salaries
(Entity Designator)	(Fund Designator)	(Financial Statement Element)	(Primary Subclassification)	(Secondary Subclassification)

parts to the account number. The first part is one digit and indicates the financial statement element. Thus, our example shows "1," which is for "Asset." The second part is two digits and is the primary subclassification. Our example shows "10," which stands for "Current Asset" in this case. The third and final part is also two digits and is the secondary subclassification. Our example shows "11," which stands for "Petty Cash—Front Office" in this case. On a report, this account number would probably appear as 1-10-11.

The second format, shown in **Exhibit 2–2**, is full use and would be for a large organization. The exhibit is again in two horizontal segments, "Structure" and "Example," and there are now two line items appearing in the Example section. This full-use example has five parts to the account number. The first part is two digits and indicates the entity designator number. Thus, we conclude that there is more than one entity within this system. Our example shows "10," which stands for "Hospital A." The second part is two digits and indicates the fund designator number. Thus, we conclude that there is more than one fund within this system. Our example shows "10," which stands for "General Fund."

The third part of Exhibit 2–2 is one digit and indicates the financial statement element. Thus, the first line of our example shows "4," which is for "Revenue," and the second line of our example shows "6," which is for "Expense." (The third part of this example is the first part of the simpler example shown in Exhibit 2–1.) The fourth part is four digits and is the primary subclassification. Our example shows 3125, which stands for "Lab—Microbiology." The number 3125 appears on both lines of this example, indicating that both the revenue and the expense belong to Lab—Microbiology. (The fourth part of this example is the second part of the simpler example shown in Exhibit 2–1. The simpler example used only two digits for this part, but this full-use example uses four digits.) The fifth and final part is two digits and is the secondary subclassification. Our example shows "03" on the first line, the revenue line, which stands for "Payer: XYZ HMO" and indicates the source of the revenue. On the second line, the expense line, our example shows "10," which stands for "Clerical Salaries." Therefore, we understand that these are the clerical salaries belonging to Lab—Microbiology in Hospital A. (The fifth part of this example is the third and final part of the simpler example shown in Exhibit 2–1.) On a report, these account numbers might appear as 10-10-4-3125-03 and 10-10-6-3125-10. Another optional use that is easier to read at a glance is 10104-3125-03 and 10106-3125-10.

Because every organization is unique and because the chart of accounts reflects that uniqueness, the third format, shown in **Exhibit 2–3**, illustrates a customized use of the chart of accounts. This example is adapted from a large hospital system. There are four parts to its chart of accounts number. The first part is an entity designator and designates a company within the hospital system. The fund designator two-digit part, as traditionally used (see Exhibit 2–2), is missing here. The financial statement element one-digit part, as traditionally used (see Exhibit 2–2), is also missing here. Instead, the second part of Exhibit 2–3 represents the primary classification, which is shown as an expense category ("Payroll") in the example line. The third part of Exhibit 2–3 is the secondary subclassification, representing a labor subaccount expense designation ("Regular per-Visit RN"). The fourth and final part of Exhibit 2–3 is another subclassification that indicates the department within the company ("Home Health"). On a report for this organization, therefore, the account

---

Exhibit 2–3 Chart of Accounts, Format III

Structure			
XX	XXXX	XXXX	XXXX
Company Category	Expense	Subaccount	Department
(Entity Designator)	(Primary Classification)	(Secondary Subclassification)	(Additional Subclassification)

Example			
21	7000	2200	7151
Home Care Services	Payroll	Regular per-Visit RN	Home Health
(Company)	(Expense Category)	(Subaccount)	(Department)

number 21-7000-2200-7151 would indicate the home care services company's payroll for regular per-visit registered nurses (RNs) in the home health department. Finally, remember that time spent understanding your own facility's chart of accounts will be time well spent.

Books and Records—Capture Transactions

The books and records of the financial information system for the organization serve to capture transactions. **Figure 2–4** illustrates the relationship of the books and records to each other. As a single transaction occurs, the process begins. The individual transaction is recorded in the appropriate subsidiary journal. Similar such transactions are then grouped and balanced within the subsidiary journal. At periodic intervals, the groups of transactions are gathered, summarized, and entered in the general ledger. Within the general ledger, the transaction groups are reviewed and adjusted. After such review and adjustment, the transactions for the period within the general ledger are balanced. A document known as the trial balance is used for this purpose. The final step in the process is to create statements that reflect the transactions for the period. The trial balance is used to produce the statements.

All transactions for the period reside in the general ledger. The subsidiary journals are so named because they are "subsidiary" to the general ledger: in other words, they serve to

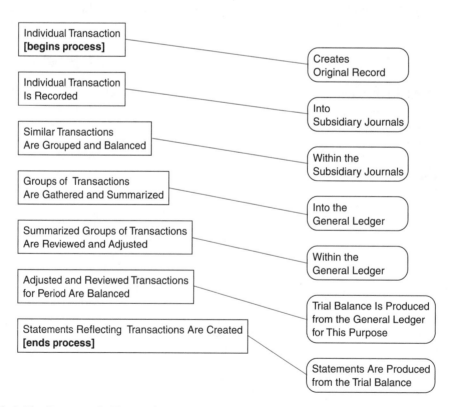

Figure 2–4 The Progress of a Transaction.
Courtesy of Resource Group, Ltd., Dallas, Texas.

THE BOOKS

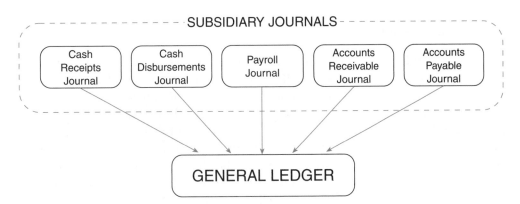

Figure 2–5 Recording Information: Relationship of Subsidiary Journals to the General Ledger.
Courtesy of Resource Group, Ltd., Dallas, Texas.

support the general ledger. **Figure 2–5** illustrates this concept. Another way to think of the subsidiary journals is to picture them as feeding the general ledger. The important point here is to understand the source and the flow of information as it is recorded.

Reports—The Product

Reports are more fully treated in a subsequent chapter of this text (see Chapter 10). It is sufficient at this point to recognize that reports are the final product of a process that commences with an original transaction.

THE ANNUAL MANAGEMENT CYCLE

The annual management cycle affects the type and status of information that the manager is expected to use. Some operating information is "raw"—that is, unadjusted. When the same information has passed further through the system and has been verified, adjusted, and balanced, it will usually vary from the initial raw data. These differences are a part of the process just described.

Daily and Weekly Operating Reports

The daily and weekly operating reports generally contain raw data, as discussed in the preceding paragraph. The purpose of such daily and weekly reports is to provide immediate operating information to use for day-to-day management purposes.

Quarterly Reports and Statistics

The quarterly reports and statistics generally have been verified, adjusted, and balanced. They are called interim reports because they have been generated some time during the reporting period of the organization and not at the end of that period. Managers often use quarterly reports as milestones. A common milestone is the quarterly budget review.

Annual Year-End Reports

Most organizations have a 12-month reporting period known as a fiscal year. A fiscal year, therefore, covers a period from the first day of a particular month (e.g., January 1) through the last day of a month that is one year, or 12 months, in the future (e.g., December 31). If we see a heading that reads, "For the year ended June 30," we know that the fiscal year began on July 1 of the previous year. Anything less than a full 12-month year is called a "stub period" and is fully spelled out in the heading. If, therefore, a company is reporting for a three-month stub period ending on December 31, the heading on the report will read, "For the three-month period ended December 31." An alternative treatment uses a heading that reads, "For the period October 1 to December 31."

Annual year-end reports cover the full 12-month reporting period or the fiscal year. Such annual year-end reports are not primarily intended for managers' use. Their primary purpose is for reporting the operations of the organization for the period to outsiders, or third parties.

Annual year-end reports represent the closing out of the information system for a specific reporting period. The recording and reporting of operations will now begin a new cycle with a new year.

COMMUNICATING FINANCIAL INFORMATION TO OTHERS

The ability to communicate financial information effectively to others is a valuable skill. It is important to

- Create a report as your method of communication.
- Use accepted terminology.
- Use standard formats that are accepted in the accounting profession.
- Begin with an executive summary.
- Organize the body of the report in a logical flow.
- Place extensive detail into an appendix.

The rest of this book will help you learn how to create such a report. Our book will also sharpen your communication skills by helping you better understand how heathcare finance works.

 INFORMATION CHECKPOINT

What is needed?	An explanation of how the information flow works in your unit.
Where is it found?	Probably with the information system staff; perhaps in the administrative offices.
How is it used?	Study the flow and relate it to the paperwork that you handle.

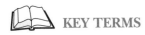 **KEY TERMS**

Accounting System
Chart of Accounts
General Ledger
Information System
Original Records
Reporting System
Subsidiary Journals
Trial Balance

 DISCUSSION QUESTIONS

1. Have you ever been informed of the information flow in your unit or division?
2. If so, did you receive the information in a formal seminar or in an informal manner, one-on-one with another individual? Do you think this was the best way? Why?
3. Do you know about the chart of accounts in your organization as it pertains to information you receive?
4. If so, is it similar to one of the three formats illustrated in this chapter? If not, how is it different?
5. Do you work with daily or weekly operating reports? With quarterly reports and statistics?
6. If so, do these reports give you useful information? How do you think they could be improved?

NOTES

1. J. J. Baker, *Activity-Based Costing and Activity-Based Management for Health Care* (Gaithersburg, MD: Aspen Publishers, Inc., 1998).
2. L. V. Seawell, *Chart of Accounts for Hospitals* (Chicago: Probus Publishing Company, 1994).

Record Financial Operations

Assets, Liabilities, and Net Worth

OVERVIEW

Assets, liabilities, and net worth are part of the language of finance. As such, it is important to understand both their composition and how they fit together. Short definitions appear below, followed by examples.

Assets

Assets are economic resources that have expected future benefits to the business. In other words, assets are what the organization owns and/or controls.

Liabilities

Liabilities are "outsider claims" consisting of economic obligations, or debts, payable to outsiders. Thus, liabilities are what the organization owes, and the outsiders to whom the debts are due are creditors of the business.

Net Worth

"Insider claims" are also known as owner's equity, or net worth. These are claims held by the owners of the business. An owner has a claim to the entity's assets because he or she has invested in the business. No matter what term is used, the sum of these claims reflects what the business is worth, net of liabilities—thus "net worth."

The Three-Part Equation

An accounting equation reflects a relationship among assets, liabilities, and net worth as follows: assets equal

Progress Notes

After completing this chapter, you should be able to

1. Recognize typical assets.
2. Recognize typical liabilities.
3. Understand net worth terminology.
4. See how assets, liabilities, and net worth fit together.

liabilities plus net worth. The three pieces must always balance among themselves because this is how they fit together. The equation is as follows:

$$Assets = Liabilities + Net\ Worth$$

WHAT ARE EXAMPLES OF ASSETS?

All of the following are typical business assets.

Examples of Assets

Cash, accounts receivable, notes receivable, and inventory are all assets. If the Great Lakes Home Health Agency (HHA) has cash in its bank account, that is an economic resource—an asset. The HHA is owed money for services rendered; these accounts receivable are also an economic resource—an asset. If certain patients have signed a formal agreement to pay the HHA, then these notes receivable are likewise economic resources—assets. All types of business receivables are assets. The Great Lakes HHA also has an inventory of medical supplies (dressings, syringes, IV tubing, etc.) that are used in its day-to-day operations. This inventory on hand is an economic resource—an asset. Land, buildings, and equipment are also assets. **Exhibit 3–1** summarizes asset examples.

Short-Term Versus Long-Term Assets

Assets are often labeled either "current" or "long-term" assets. Current is another word for "short-term." If an asset can be turned into cash within a 12-month period, it is current, or short term. If, on the other hand, an asset cannot be converted into cash within a 12-month period, it is considered long term. In our Great Lakes HHA example, accounts receivable should be collected within 1 year and thus should be current assets. Likewise, the inventory should be converted to business use within 1 year; thus, it too is considered short term.

Classification of the note receivable depends on the length of time that payment is promised. If the entire note receivable will be paid within 1 year, it is a short-term asset. Consider, however, what would happen if the note is to be paid over 3 years. A portion of the note—that amount to be paid in the coming 12 months—will be classified as short-term, or current, and the rest of the note—that amount to be paid further in the future—will be classified as long-term.

The land, building, and equipment will generally be classified as long-term because these assets will not be converted into cash in the coming 12 months. Buildings and equipment are also generally stated at a net

Exhibit 3–1 Asset Examples

Cash
Accounts receivable
Notes receivable
Inventory
Land
Buildings
Equipment

figure called book value, which reduces their historical cost by any accumulated deprecia-tion. (The concept of depreciation is discussed in Chapter 8.)

WHAT ARE EXAMPLES OF LIABILITIES?

All of the following are typical business liabilities.

Examples of Liabilities

Accounts payable, payroll taxes due, notes payable, and mortgages payable are all liabilities. The Great Lakes HHA owes vendors for medical supplies it has purchased. The amount owed to the vendors is recognized as accounts payable. When the HHA paid its employees, it withheld payroll taxes, as required by the government. The payroll taxes withheld are due to be paid to the government and thus are also a liability. The HHA has borrowed money and signed a formal agreement and thus the amount due is a liability. The HHA also has a mortgage on its building. This mortgage is likewise a liability. In other words, debts are liabilities. **Exhibit 3–2** summarizes liability examples.

Short-Term Versus Long-Term Liabilities

Liabilities are also usually labeled as either "current" (short-term) or "long-term" liabilities. In this case, if a liability is expected to be paid within a 12-month period, it is current, or short-term. If, however, the liability cannot reasonably be expected to be paid within a 12-month period, it is considered long-term. In our Great Lakes HHA example, accounts payable and payroll taxes due should be paid within 1 year and thus should be labeled as current liabilities.

Classification of the note payable depends on the length of time that payment is prom-ised. If the HHA is going to pay the entire note payable within 1 year, it is a short-term liability. But consider what would happen if the note is to be paid over 3 years. A por-tion of the note—that amount to be paid in the coming 12 months—will be classified as short-term, or current, and the rest of the note—that amount to be paid further in the future—will be classified as long-term. The mortgage will be treated slightly differently. That portion to be paid within the coming 12 months will be classified as a short-term liability, while the remaining mortgage balance will be labeled as long-term.

WHAT ARE THE DIFFERENT FORMS OF NET WORTH?

Net worth—the third part of the accounting equation—is labeled differently, depend-ing on the type of organization. For-profit organizations will have equity accounts with which to report their net worth. (Equity is the ownership right in property or the

Exhibit 3–2 Liability Examples

| Accounts payable |
| Payroll taxes due |
| Notes payable |
| Mortgage payable |
| Bonds payable |

money value of property.) For example, a sole proprietorship or a partnership's net worth may simply be labeled as "Owners' Equity." A corporation, on the other hand, will generally report two types of equity accounts: "Capital Stock" and "Retained Earnings." Capital stock represents the owners' investment in the company, indicated by their purchase of stock. Retained earnings, as the name implies, represents undistributed company income that has been left in the business.

Not-for-profit organizations will generally use a different term such as "Fund Balance" to report the difference between assets and liabilities in their report. This is presumably because nonprofits should not, by definition, have equity. Governmental entities in the United States may also use the term "Fund Balance" in their reports. **Exhibit 3–3** summarizes terminology examples for net worth as just discussed.

Exhibit 3–3 Net Worth Terminology Examples

For-profit sole proprietors or partnerships:
　　Owners' Equity
For-profit corporations:
　　Capital Stock
　　Retained Earnings
Not-for-profit (nonprofit) companies:
　　Fund Balance

 INFORMATION CHECKPOINT

What is needed?	A report that shows the balance sheet for your organization.
Where is it found?	Probably with your supervisor.
How is it used?	Study the balance sheet to find the assets and liabilities. Check the equity section to see whether equity is listed as net worth or as fund balance.

 KEY TERMS

Assets
Equity
Fund Balance
Liabilities
Net Worth

 DISCUSSION QUESTIONS

1. Do you ever work with balance sheets in your current position?
2. If so, is the balance sheet you receive for your department only or for the entire organization? Do you know why this reporting method (departmental versus entire organization) was chosen by management?

3. If you receive a copy of the balance sheet, is one distributed to you once a month, once a year, or on some other more irregular basis? What are you supposed to do with it upon receipt?
4. Do you think the balance sheet report you receive gives you useful information? How do you think it could be improved?

Revenues (Inflow)

OVERVIEW

Revenue represents amounts earned by an organization: that is, actual or expected cash inflows due to the organization's major business. In the case of health care, revenue is mostly earned by rendering services to patients. Revenue flows into the organization and is sometimes referred to as the revenue stream.

Revenue is generally defined as the value of services rendered, expressed at the facility's full established rates. For example, hospital A's full established rate for a certain procedure is $100, but Giant Health Plan has negotiated a managed care contract whereby the plan pays only $90 for that procedure. The revenue figure— the full established rate—is $100. Revenues can be received in the form of cash or credit. Most, but not all, healthcare revenues are received in the form of credit.

RECEIVING REVENUE FOR SERVICES

One way that revenue is classified is by whether payment is received before or after the service is delivered. The amount of revenue received for services is often influenced by this classification.

Payment after Service Is Delivered

The traditional payment method in health care is that of payment after service is delivered. Two basic types of payment after service is delivered are discussed in this section: fee for service and discounted fee for service. One evolved from the other.

Progress Notes

After completing this chapter, you should be able to

1. Understand how receiving revenue for services is a revenue stream.
2. Recognize contractual allowances and discounts and their impact on revenue.
3. Understand the differences in sources of healthcare revenue.
4. See how to group revenue for planning and control.

1. Fee for service. The truly traditional U.S. method of receiving revenue for services is fee for service. The provider of services is paid according to the service performed. Before the 1970s, with very few exceptions, fee for service was the dominant method of payment for health services in the United States.[1]
2. Discounted fee for service. In this variation on the original fee for service, a contracted discount is agreed upon. The organization providing the services then receives a payment that is discounted in accordance with the contract. Sometimes the contract contains fee schedules. A large provider of services can have many different contracts, all with different discounted contractual arrangements. Many variations are therefore possible.

Payment before Service Is Delivered

Traditional payment methods in the United States have begun to give way to payment before service is delivered. There are multiple names and definitions for such payment. We have chosen to use a general descriptive term for payment received before service is delivered: predetermined per-person payment. The payment method itself and its rate-setting variations are discussed in this section.

1. Predetermined per-person payment. Payment received before service is delivered is generally at an agreed-upon predetermined rate. Payment, therefore, consists of the predetermined rate for each person covered under the agreement. Thus, the amount received is a per-head or per-person count at a particular point in time.
2. Rate-setting differences. Different agreements can use varying assumptions about the group to be served, and these variations will affect the rate-setting process. Numerous variations are therefore possible.

Contractual Allowances and Other Deductions from Revenue

Revenues are recorded at the organization's full established rates, as previously discussed. Those amounts estimated to be uncollectible are considered to be deductions from revenues and are recorded as such on the books of the organization. (For purposes of the external financial statements released for third-party use, reported revenue must represent the amounts that payers [or patients] are obligated to pay. Therefore, the terms gross revenue and deductions from revenue will not be seen on external statements. The discussion that follows, however, pertains to the books and records that are used for internal management, where these classifications will be used.)

Contractual allowances are the difference between the full established rate and the agreed-upon contractual rate that will be paid. Contractual allowances are often for composite services. Take the case of hospital A as an example. As discussed in the overview to this chapter, hospital A's full established rate for a certain procedure is $100, but Giant Health Plan has negotiated a managed care contract whereby the plan pays only $90 for that procedure. The $10 difference between the revenue figure ($100) and the contracted amount that the plan pays ($90) represents the contractual allowance.

It is not uncommon for different plans to pay different contractual rates for the same service. This practice is illustrated in **Table 4–1**, which shows contractual rates to be paid for visit codes 99213 and 99214 for 10 different health plans. Note the variations in rates.

The second major deduction from revenue classification is an allowance for bad debts, also known as a provision for doubtful accounts. (Again, for purposes of the external financial statements released for third-party use, the provision for doubtful reports must be reported separately as an expense item. The discussion that follows, however, still pertains to the books and records that are used for internal management, where the classification of deductions from revenue will be used.) The allowance for bad debts is charged with the amount of services received on credit (recorded as accounts receivable) that are estimated to result in credit losses.

Beyond contractual allowances and a provision for bad debts, the third major deduction from revenue classification is charity service. Charity service is generally defined as services provided to financially indigent patients.

Table 4–1 Variations in Physician Office Revenue for Two Visit Codes

| | Visit Codes | |
Payer	99213	99214
FHP	$25.35	$35.70
HPHP	42.45	58.85
MC	39.05	54.90
UND	39.90	60.40
CCN	44.00	70.20
MAYO	45.75	70.75
CGN	10.00	10.00
PRU	39.05	54.90
PHCS	45.00	50.00
ANA	38.25	45.00

Rates for illustration only.

SOURCES OF HEALTHCARE REVENUE

Healthcare revenue in the United States comes from a variety of public programs (governmental sources) and private payers. The sources of healthcare revenue are generally termed payers. Payer mix—the proportion of revenues realized from the different types of payers—is a measure that is often included in the profile of a healthcare organization. For example, "Hospital A has a payer mix that includes 40% Medicare and 33% Medicaid" might be part of the profile.

Governmental Sources

The Medicare Program

Title XVIII of the Social Security Act is commonly known as Medicare. Actually entitled "Health Insurance for the Aged and Disabled," Medicare legislation established a health insurance program for the aged in 1965. The program was intended to complement other benefits (such as retirement, survivors', and disability insurance benefits) under other titles within the Social Security Act.

The Medicare program currently has four parts. The first part, known as Part A, is hospital insurance (HI) and is funded primarily by a mandatory payroll tax. The second part, known as Part B, is called supplementary medical insurance (SMI). SMI is voluntary and is funded primarily by insurance premiums (usually deducted from monthly Social Security benefit checks of those enrolled) supplemented by federal general revenue funds. Guidelines determine both the services to be covered and the eligibility of the individual to receive the services under the Medicare program. Medicare claims (billings) are processed by fiscal agents who act on behalf of the federal government. These fiscal agents, known as Medicare Administrative Contractors (MACs), process both Part A (HI) and Part B (SMI) Medicare claims.

Medicare's third part, Part C, is known as "Medicare Advantage." Medicare Advantage consists of managed care plans, private fee-for-service plans, preferred provider organization plans, and specialty plans. Although Medicare Advantage is offered as an alternative to traditional Medicare, coverage must never be less than what Part A and Part B (traditional Medicare) would offer the beneficiary.

Medicare's fourth part, Part D, is the prescription drug benefit, effective as of January 1, 2006. The prescription drug benefit represents expanded coverage. It is a voluntary program that requires payment of a separate premium and contains cost-sharing provisions.

The Medicare program covers approximately 95% of the U.S. aged population along with certain eligible individuals receiving Social Security disability benefits.[2] Medicare is an important source of healthcare revenue to most healthcare organizations.

The Medicaid Program

Title XIX of the Social Security Act is commonly known as Medicaid. Medicaid legislation established a federal and state matching entitlement program in 1965. The program was intended to provide medical assistance to eligible needy individuals and families.

The Medicaid program is state specific. The federal government has established broad national guidelines. Each state has the power to set eligibility, service restrictions, and payment rates for services within that state. In doing so, each state is bound only by the broad national guidelines. Medicaid policies are complex, and considerable variation exists among states. The federal government is responsible for a certain percentage of each state's Medicaid expenditures; the specific amount due is calculated by an annual formula. The state pays the providers of Medicaid services directly. Thus, the source of Medicaid revenue to a healthcare organization is considered to be the state government's Medicaid program representative.

The Medicaid program is the largest U.S. government program providing funds for medical and health-related services for the poor.[3] Therefore, although the proportion of Medicaid services within the payer mix may vary, Medicaid is a source of healthcare revenue in almost every healthcare organization.

Other Programs

There are numerous other sources of federal, state, and local revenues for healthcare organizations. Generally speaking, for most organizations, none of the other revenue sources will exceed the Title XVIII and Title XIX programs just discussed. Other programs include the Department of Veterans' Affairs health programs, workers' compensation programs, and state-only general assistance programs (versus the federal-and-state jointly funded Medicaid program). Still other public programs are school health programs, public health clinics, maternal and child health services, migrant healthcare services, certain mental health and drug and alcohol services, and special programs such as Native American healthcare services.

Managed Care Sources

In the 1970s, managed care began to appear in healthcare models in the United States. An all-purpose definition of managed care is: managed care is a means of providing health-care services within a network of healthcare providers. The responsibility to manage and provide high-quality and cost-effective health care is delegated to this defined network of providers.[4] A central concept of managed care is the coordination of all healthcare services for an individual. In general, managed care plans receive a predetermined amount per member in premiums.

Types of Plans

The most prevalent type of managed care plan today is the health maintenance organization (HMO). Members enroll in the HMO. They prepay a fixed monthly amount; in return, they receive comprehensive health services. The members must use the providers who are designated by the HMO; if they go outside the designated providers, they must pay all or a large part of the cost themselves. The designated providers of services in turn contract with the HMO to provide services at agreed-upon rates. Several different forms of HMOs have evolved over time.

The preferred provider organization (PPO) is a type of plan found across the United States. It consists of a group of providers called a panel. The panel members are an approved group of various types of providers, including hospitals and physicians. The panel is limited in size and generally has utilization review powers. If the patients in a PPO use health providers who are not within the PPO itself, they must pay a higher amount in deductibles and coinsurance.

Types of Contracts

In the case of an HMO, the designated providers of health services contract with the HMO to provide services at agreed-upon rates. The different types of HMOs—including the staff model, the group model, the network model, the point-of-service model, and the individual practice association (IPA) model—have various methods of arriving at these rates. A PPO contracts with its selected group, who are all participating payers, to buy services for its eligible beneficiaries on the basis of discounted fee for service. A large healthcare facility will have one or more individuals responsible for managed care contracting.[5]

Other Revenue Sources

A considerable amount of healthcare revenue is still realized from sources other than Title XVIII, Title XIX, and managed care:

- Commercial insurers. Generally speaking, conventional indemnity insurers, or commercial insurers, simply pay for the eligible health services used by those individuals who pay premiums for healthcare insurance. They do not tend to have a say in how those health services are administered.
- Private pay. This is payment by patients themselves or by the families of patients. Private pay is more prevalent in nursing facilities and in assisted-living facilities than in hospital settings. Physicians' offices also receive a certain amount of private pay revenue.

Table 4–2 Sample Monthly Statement of Revenue by Source

Summary	Year to Date	%
Private revenue	$100,000	2.9
HMO revenue	560,000	16.7
Medicare revenue	1,420,000	42.4
Medicaid revenue	820,000	24.5
Commercial revenue	400,000	12.0
Other revenue	50,000	1.5
Total	$3,350,000	100.0%

- Other. Additional sources of revenue for healthcare facilities include donations received by voluntary nonprofit organization, tax revenues levied by governmental nonprofit organizations, and grant funding.

Healthcare revenue is often reported to managers by source of the revenue. **Table 4–2** presents such a revenue summary. This example covers all types of sources discussed in this section. Both dollar totals and proportionate percentages by source are reported.

GROUPING REVENUE FOR PLANNING AND CONTROL

Grouping revenue by different classifications is an effective method for managers to use the information to plan and to control. In the preceding paragraphs, we have seen revenue reported by source. Other classification examples are now discussed.

Revenue Centers

A revenue center classification is one form of a responsibility center. In a responsibility center, the manager is responsible, as the name implies, for a particular set of activities. In the case of a revenue center, a particular unit of the organization is given responsibility for generating revenues to meet a certain target. Actually, the responsibility in the healthcare setting is more for generating volume than for generating a specific revenue dollar amount. (The implication is that the volume will, in turn, generate the dollars.) Revenue centers tend to occur most often in special programs where volume is critical to survival of the program.

Care Settings

Grouping revenue by care setting recognizes the different sites at which services are delivered. The most basic grouping by care settings is inpatient versus ambulatory services. **Exhibit 4–1**, however, illustrates a six-way classification of care setting revenues within a health system. In this case, hospital inpatient, hospital outpatient, off-site clinic, skilled

Exhibit 4–1 Revenues by Care Setting

42% Hospital Inpatient	38% Hospital Outpatient	4% Off-Site Clinic
8% Skilled Nursing Facility	6% Home Health Agency	2% Hospice

nursing facility, home health agency, and hospice are all accounted for. A percentage is shown for each. This type of classification is useful for a brochure or a report that profiles the different types of healthcare services offered by the organization.

Service Lines

In traditional cost accounting circles, a product line is a grouping of similar products.[6] In the healthcare field, many organizations opt instead for "service line" terminology. A service line is a grouping of similar services. Strategic planning sometimes sets out service lines.

Hospitals

A number of hospitals have adopted the major diagnostic categories (MDCs) as service lines. One advantage of MDCs is that they are a universal designation in the United States. MDCs also have the advantage of possessing a standard definition. In another approach to service line classification, a hospital recently updated its strategic plan and settled on five service lines: (1) medical, (2) surgical, (3) women and children, (4) mental health, and (5) rehabilitation (neuro-ortho rehab) (**Figure 4–1**).[7]

Long-Term Care

A continuing care retirement community (CCRC) can use its various levels of care as a starting point. Thus, the CCRC usually has four service lines, listed in the descending order of resident acuity: (1) skilled nursing facility, (2) nursing facility, (3) assisted living, and (4) independent living. The skilled nursing facility provides services for the highest level of resident acuity, and the independent living provides services for the

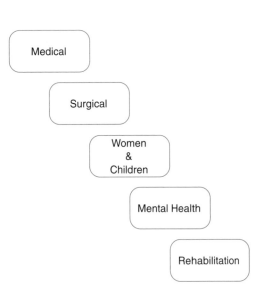

Figure 4–1 Hospital Service Lines.
Courtesy of Resource Group, Ltd., Dallas, Texas.

lowest level of resident acuity. One adjustment to this approach includes isolating subacute services from the remainder of skilled nursing facility services. Another adjustment involves splitting independent living into two categories, one for Housing and Urban Development (HUD)–subsidized independent housing and the other for private-pay independent housing. **Figure 4–2** illustrates CCRC service lines by acuity level.

Home Care

Numerous categories of service delivery can be considered "home care." A practical approach was taken by one home care entity—part of a health system—that defined its "key functions." Key functions can in turn be converted to service lines (**Figure 4–3**).

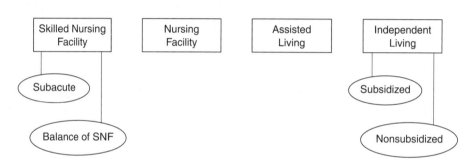

Figure 4–2 Long-Term Care Service Lines.
Courtesy of Resource Group, Ltd., Dallas, Texas.

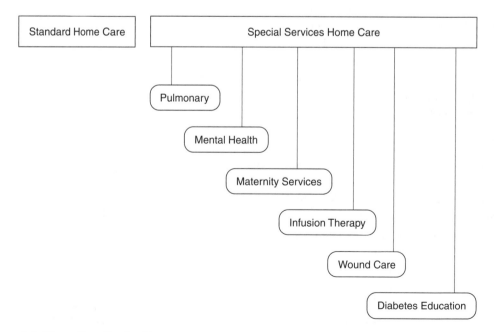

Figure 4–3 Home Care Service Lines.
Courtesy of Resource Group, Ltd., Dallas, Texas.

Physician Groups

Service delivery for physician groups will vary, of course, with the nature of the group itself. A generic set of service lines is presented in **Figure 4–4**.

Other Service Designations

Other classifications may meet the needs of particular organizations. Columbia/HCA is now reported to classify its services in a disease management approach. The classification consists of eight disease management areas: (1) cancer, (2) cardiology, (3) diabetes, (4) behavioral health, (5) workers' compensation, (6) women's services, (7) senior care, and (8) emergency services.[8]

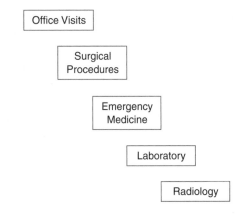

Figure 4–4 Physician's Group Service Lines. Courtesy of Resource Group, Ltd., Dallas, Texas.

Other Types of Revenue Groupings

Other healthcare organizations may have revenue groupings that are not service lines. An entity that provides services is able to choose service lines as a method of grouping its revenue. But if the entity sells or makes a product (rather than providing services), its revenue will have to be classified differently. Two examples within the healthcare industry follow: a retail pharmacy and a pharmaceutical manufacturer.

Retail Pharmacy

A retail pharmacy's revenue primarily comes from sales. A typical retail pharmacy may group revenues into three major categories of sales: Prescription Drugs, Nonprescription (Over-the-Counter, or OTC) Drugs, and Other Merchandise. (The major category of "Other Merchandise" would then have subcategories such as Cosmetics, Greeting Cards, Gifts, etc.)

Pharmaceutical Manufacturer

A pharmaceutical manufacturer's revenue groupings would likewise be specific to its type of healthcare business. These organizations are producing a product rather than providing a service. Its major categories of revenues will probably be by type of drug manufactured. The next subcategory might then either be national versus international revenues, or perhaps a classification of revenues by U.S. geographic region.

In summary, the entity's revenue classification system, whatever it may be, must be consistent with the current structure and purpose of the organization.

 INFORMATION CHECKPOINT

What is needed?	A report that shows revenue in your organization.
Where is it found?	With your supervisor.

How is it used?   Examine the report to find various revenue sources; look for how the contractual allowances and discounts are handled on the report.

What is needed?   A report that groups revenue by some type of classification.

Where is it found?   With your supervisor, or in the information services division.

How is it used?   Examine the report to discover the methods that are used for grouping. You will probably find that these groupings are used for performance measures. They can also be used for control and planning.

 KEY TERMS

Discounted Fee for Service
Fee for Service
Managed Care
Medicaid Program
Medicare Program
Payer Mix
Revenue

 DISCUSSION QUESTIONS

1. Does your organization receive revenue mainly in the form of payment after service is delivered or payment before service is delivered?
2. Why do you think this is so?
3. What do you believe the proportion of revenues from different sources is for your organization?
4. Do you believe that this proportion (payer mix) will change in the future? Why?
5. What grouping of revenue do you believe your organization uses (revenue centers, care settings, service lines, other)?
6. From your perspective, would there be a better grouping possible? If so, why do you think it is not used?

NOTES

1. Texas Medical Association, American Medical Association, Texas Medical Foundation, and Texas Osteopathic Medical Association, *A Guide to Forming Physician-Directed Managed Care Networks* (Austin, TX: Texas Medical Association, 1994), 3.
2. Health Care Financing Administration, *Health Care Financing Review: Medicare and Medicaid Statistical Supplement* (Baltimore, MD: U.S. Department of Health and Human Services, 1997), 8.

3. Ibid., 9.

4. D. I. Samuels, *Capitation: New Opportunities in Healthcare Delivery* (Chicago: Irwin Professional Publishing, 1996), 20–21.

5. D. E. Goldstein, *Alliances: Strategies for Building Integrated Delivery Systems* (Gaithersburg, MD: Aspen Publishers, Inc., 1995), 283; and Texas Medical Association, American Medical Association, Texas Medical Foundation, and Texas Osteopathic Medical Association, *A Guide to Forming Physician-Directed Managed Care Networks* (Austin, TX: Texas Medical Association, 1994), 4–6.

6. C. Horngren et al., *Cost Accounting: A Managerial Emphasis*, 9th ed. (Englewood Cliffs, NJ: Prentice Hall, 1998), 116.

7. When ICD-10 is fully implemented, it is possible that the term "major diagnostic categories" (MDCs) may have to be replaced with some other universal designation. Whether these hospitals will change the names of their service line designations to match the new titles is unknown at this point. We do know it will take time to decide upon such a change and then additional time to implement the change.

8. A. Sharpe and G. Jaffe, "Columbia/HCA Plans for More Big Changes in Health-Care World," *Wall Street Journal*, 28 May, 1997, A8.

Expenses (Outflow)

OVERVIEW

Expenses are the costs that relate to the earning of revenue. Another way to think of expenses is as the costs of doing business. Just as revenues represent the inflow into the organization, so do expenses represent the outflow—a stream of expenditures flowing out of the organization. Examples of expenses include salary expense for labor performed, payroll tax expense for taxes paid on the salary, utility expense for electricity, and interest expense for the use of money.

In fact, expenses are expired costs—costs that have been used up, or consumed, while carrying on business. Revenues and expenses affect the equity of the business. The inflow of revenues increases equity, whereas the outflow of expenses decreases equity. In nonprofit organizations, the term is fund balance rather than equity. This is because a nonprofit organization, by its nature, is not in business to make a profit. Thus, it should not have equity. However, the principle of inflow and outflow remains the same. In the case of nonprofits, the inflow of revenues increases fund balance, and the outflow of expenses decreases fund balance.

Many managers use the terms expense and cost interchangeably. Expense in its broadest sense includes every expired (used up) cost that is deductible from revenue. A narrower interpretation groups expenses into categories such as operating expenses, administrative expenses, and so on. Cost is the amount of cash expended (or property transferred, services performed, or liability incurred) in consideration of goods or services received or to be received. As we have already said,

Progress Notes

After completing this chapter, you should be able to

1. Understand the distinction between expense and cost.
2. Understand how disbursements for services represent an expense stream (an outflow).
3. Follow how expenses are grouped in different ways for planning and control.
4. Recognize why cost reports have influenced expense formats.

costs can be either expired or unexpired. Expired costs are used up in the current period and are thus matched against current revenues. Unexpired costs are not yet used up and will be matched against future revenues.[1]

For example, an electric bill for $500 is recorded in the books of the clinic as an expense. The administrator sees the $500 as the cost of electricity for that month in the clinic. And the administrator is actually correct in seeing the $500 as a cost because it has been used up (expired) within the month.

Confusion also exists in healthcare reporting over the term cost versus the term charges. Charges are revenue, or inflow. Costs are expenses, or outflow. Charges add; costs take away. Because the two are inherently different, they should never be intermingled.

DISBURSEMENTS FOR SERVICES

There are two types of disbursements for services:

1. Payment when expense is incurred. If an expense is paid for at the point where it is incurred, it does not enter the accounts payable account. In large organizations, it is relatively rare to see payments when expenses are incurred. The only place where this usually occurs is the petty cash fund.
2. Payment after expense is incurred. In most healthcare organizations, expenses are paid at a later time and not at the point when the expense is incurred. If this is the case, the expense is recorded in the accounts payable account. It is cleared from accounts payable when payment is made. One measurement of operations is "days in accounts payable," whereby the operating expenses for the organization are reduced to a rate per day and compared with the amount in accounts payable.

GROUPING EXPENSES FOR PLANNING AND CONTROL

Cost Centers

A cost center is one form of a responsibility center. In a responsibility center, the manager is responsible, as the name implies, for a particular set of activities. In the case of a cost center, a particular unit of the organization is given responsibility for controlling costs of the operations over which it holds authority. The medical records division is an example of a cost center. The billing and collection office might be another example. A cost center might be a division, an office, or an entire department, depending on how the organization is structured.

In healthcare organizations, it is common to find departments as cost centers. This is often a logical way to designate a cost center because the lines of authority are generally organized by department. Cost centers can then be grouped into larger groups that have something in common. Within this method of grouping, the manager of a cost center may receive his or her own reports and figures, but not those of the entire group. The director or officer that is in charge of all of those particular departments receives the larger report that contains multiple cost centers. The chief executive officer receives a total report because he or she is ultimately responsible for overseeing the operations of all of the cost centers involved in that segment of the organization.

Exhibit 5–1 illustrates this concept. It contains 20 different cost centers, all of which are revenue producing. The 20 cost centers are divided into two groups: nursing services and other professional services. There are five cost centers in the nursing services group, ranging from operating room to obstetrics–nursery. There are 15 cost centers in the other professional services group. In the hospital that uses the grouping shown in Exhibit 5–1, however, not all of the 20 cost centers are departments. Some are divisions within departments. For example, EKG and EEG operate out of the same department but are two separate cost centers.

Exhibit 5–2 shows 11 different cost centers that are not directly revenue producing. (The dietary department yields some cafeteria revenue, but that revenue is not central to the major business of the organization, which is to provide healthcare services.) The 11 cost centers are divided into two groups: general services and support services. The 6 cost centers in the general services group happen to all be departments in this hospital. (Other hospitals might not have security as a separate department. The other cost centers—dietary, maintenance, laundry, housekeeping, and medical records—would be separate departments.) The 5 cost

Exhibit 5–1 Nursing Services and Other Professional Services Cost Centers

Nursing Services Cost Center	
Routine Medical-Surgical	$390,000
Operating Room	30,000
Intensive Care Units	40,000
OB–Nursery	15,000
Other	35,000
Total	$510,000

Other Professional Services Cost Center	
Laboratory	$220,000
Radiology	139,000
CT Scanner	18,000
Pharmacy	128,000
Emergency Service	89,000
Medical and Surgical Supply	168,000
Operating Rooms and Anesthesia	142,000
Respiratory Therapy	48,000
Physical Therapy	64,000
EKG	16,000
EEG	1,000
Ambulance Service	7,000
Substance Abuse	43,000
Home Health and Hospice	120,000
Other	12,000
Total	$1,215,000

centers in the support services group include a "general" cost center that contains administrative costs; the remaining 4 are related to employee salaries and wages. These 4 are insurance, Social Security taxes, employee welfare, and pension cost centers, all of which will probably be in the same department. It is the prerogative of management to set up cost centers specific to the organization's own needs and preferences. It is the responsibility of management to make the cost centers match the proper lines of authority.

Exhibit 5–2 illustrates two categories of healthcare expense: general services and support. A third related category is operations expense. An operations expense provides service directly related to patient care. Examples are radiology expense and drug expense. A general services expense provides services necessary to maintain the patient, but the service is not directly related to patient care. Examples are laundry and dietary. Support services expenses, on the other hand, provide support to both general services expenses and operations expenses. A support service expense is necessary for support, but it is neither directly related to patient care nor is

Exhibit 5–2 General Services and Support Services Cost Centers

General Services Cost Center	
Dietary	$97,000
Maintenance	92,000
Laundry	27,000
Housekeeping	43,000
Security	5,000
Medical Records	30,000
Total	$294,000

Support Services Cost Center	
General	$455,000
Insurance	24,000
Social Security Taxes	112,000
Employee Welfare	188,000
Pension	43,000
Total	$822,000

it a service necessary to maintain the patient. Examples of support services are insurance and payroll taxes.

Diagnoses and Procedures

It is common to group expenses by diagnoses and procedures for purposes of planning and control. This grouping is beneficial because it matches costs against common classifications of revenues. Much of the revenue in many healthcare organizations is designated by either diagnoses or procedures. One prevalent method groups costs into cost centers by major diagnostic categories (MDCs). The 23 MDCs serve as the basic classification system for diagnosis-related groups (DRGs). (Each DRG represents a category of patients. This category contains patients whose resource consumption, on statistical average, is equivalent. DRGs are part of the prospective payment reimbursement methodology.) **Exhibit 5–3** provides a listing of the 23 MDCs.[2] (The number of MDCs may increase when ICD-10 coding is fully implemented.)

How does the hospital use the MDC grouping? **Exhibit 5–4** shows a departmental and cost center grouping in actual use. This hospital uses 27 cost center codes: the 23 MDCs plus 4 other codes ("Special Drugs," "HIV," "Unassigned," and "Outpatient"). The special drugs and HIV cost centers represent high-cost elements that management wants to track separately. Unassigned is a default category and should have little assigned to it. Outpatient is a separate cost center at the preference of management.

Exhibit 5–5 illustrates the grouping of costs for MDC 18 (Infectious Diseases). The hospital's departmental code is 18, per Exhibit 5–4. The DRG classification, ranging from 415 to 423, appears in the next column. The description of the particular DRG appears in the third column, and the related cost appears in the fourth and final column. These costs can now be readily matched to equivalent revenues.

Outpatient services in particular are generally designated by procedure codes. Procedure codes, known as Current Procedural Terminology (CPT) codes, are commonly used to group cost centers for outpatient services. (CPT codes represent a listing of descriptive terms and identifying codes for identifying medical services and procedures performed.) However, procedures can be—and are—also used for purposes of grouping inpatient costs, generally within a certain cost center. A hospital example of reporting radiology department costs by procedure code appears in **Table 5–1**. In this example, the procedure code is in the left column, the description of the procedure is in the middle column, and the departmental cost for the particular procedure appears in the right column. These costs can now be readily matched to equivalent revenue.

Exhibit 5–3 Major Diagnostic Categories

MDC 1	Diseases and Disorders of the Nervous System
MDC 2	Eye
MDC 3	Ear, Nose, Mouth, and Throat
MDC 4	Respiratory System
MDC 5	Circulatory System
MDC 6	Digestive System
MDC 7	Hepatobiliary System and Pancreas
MDC 8	Musculoskeletal System and Connective Tissue
MDC 9	Skin, Subcutaneous Tissue, and Breast
MDC 10	Endocrine, Nutritional, and Metabolic
MDC 11	Kidney and Urinary Tract
MDC 12	Male Reproductive System
MDC 13	Female Reproductive System
MDC 14	Pregnancy, Childbirth, and the Puerperium
MDC 15	Newborns and Other Neonates with Conditions Originating in the Perinatal Period
MDC 16	Blood and Blood-Forming Organs and Immunological Disorders
MDC 17	Myeloproliferative and Poorly and Differentiated Neoplasms
MDC 18	Infections and Parasitic Diseases (Systemic or Unspecified Sites)
MDC 19	Mental Diseases and Disorders
MDC 20	Alcohol/Drug Use and Alcohol/Drug-Induced Organic Mental Disorders
MDC 21	Injuries, Poisoning, and Toxic Effect of Drugs
MDC 22	Burns
MDC 23	Factors Influencing Health Status and Other Contacts with Health Services

Exhibit 5–4 Hospital Departmental Code List Based on Major Diagnostic Categories

1	Nervous System
2	Eye
3	Ear, Nose, Mouth, and Throat
4	Respiratory System
5	Circulatory System
6	Digestive System
7	Hepatobiliary System
8	Musculoskeletal System and Connective Tissue
9	Skin, Subcutaneous Tissue, and Breast
10	Endocrine, Nutritional, and Metabolic
11	Kidney and Urinary Tract
12	Male Reproductive System
13	Female Reproductive System
14	Obstetrics
15	Newborns
16	Immunology
17	Oncology
18	Infectious Diseases
19	Mental Diseases
20	Substance Use
21	Injury, Poison, and Toxin
22	Burns
23	Other Health Services
24	Special Drugs
25	HIV
26	Unassigned
59	Outpatient

Care Settings and Service Lines

Expenses can be grouped by care setting, which recognizes the different sites at which services are delivered. "Inpatient" versus "outpatient" is a basic type of care setting grouping. Or expenses can be classified by service lines, a method that groups similar services.[3]

If revenues are grouped by care setting or by service line, as discussed in the previous chapter, then expenses should also be grouped by these categories. In that way,

Exhibit 5–5 Example of Hospital Departmental Costs Classified by Diagnoses, MDC, and DRG

Hospital Departmental Code	DRG	Description	Cost
18 INFECTIOUS DISEASES	415	O/R—INFECT/PARASITIC DIS	$4,000
18 INFECTIOUS DISEASES	416	SEPTICEMIA 17	10,000
18 INFECTIOUS DISEASES	417	SEPTICEMIA 0–17	20,000
18 INFECTIOUS DISEASES	418	POSTOP/POSTTRAUMA INFECT	2,000
18 INFECTIOUS DISEASES	419	FEVER—UKN ORIG 17W/C	3,000
18 INFECTIOUS DISEASES	420	FEVER—UKN ORIG 17W/OC	6,000
18 INFECTIOUS DISEASES	421	VIRAL ILLNESS 17	4,000
18 INFECTIOUS DISEASES	422	VIR ILL/FEVER UNK 0–17	1,000
18 INFECTIOUS DISEASES	423	OT/INFECT/PARASITIC DX	3,000

Table 5–1 Example of Radiology Department Costs Classified by Procedure Code

Procedure Code	Procedure Description	Department Cost
557210	Ribs, Unilateral	$ 60,000
557230	Spine Cervical Routine	125,000
557280	Pelvis	33,000
557320	Limb—Shoulder	55,000
557360	Limb—Wrist	69,000
557400	Limb—Hip, Unilateral	42,000
557410	Limb—Hip, Bilateral	14,000
557430	Limb—Knee Only	62,000
	Total	$460,000

matching of revenues and expenses can readily occur. A more detailed discussion of care settings and service lines, with examples, was presented in the preceding chapter.

Programs

A program can be defined as a project that has its own objectives and its own program indicators. Within management's functions of planning, controlling, and decision making, the program must stand on its own. A program is often funded separately and for finite periods of time. For example, funds from a grant might fund a specific project for—as an example—three years. Often programs—especially those funded separately from the revenue stream of the main organization—have to arrange their expenses in a special format that is specified by the entity that provides the grant funds.

Program expenses should be grouped in such a way that they are distinguishable. Also, if such programs have been specially funded, the reporting of their expenses should not be commingled. An example of a program cost center is given in **Exhibit 5–6**. This cost center example has received special funds and must be reported separately, as shown.

COST REPORTS AS INFLUENCERS OF EXPENSE FORMATS

Cost reports are required by both the Medicare program (Title XVIII) and the Medicaid program (Title XIX). Every provider participating in the program is required to file an annual cost report. A selection of providers who must file cost reports is illustrated in **Table 5–2**. The arrangement of expense headings on the cost reports has been primarily consistent since the advent of such reports in 1966. Therefore, this standard and traditional arrangement has strongly influenced the arrangement of expenses in many healthcare information systems.

Exhibit 5–6 Program Cost Center: Southside Homeless Intake Center

Program:	Southside Homeless Intake Center
Department:	Feeding Ministry
For the Month of:	January 2XXX

Raw Food	$14,050
Dietary Supplies	200
Paper Supplies	300
Minor Equipment	50
Consultant Dietitian	50
Utilities	300
Telephone	50
Program Total	$15,000

The cost report uses a method of cost finding. Its focus is what is called a cost center. The concept is not the same as the type of responsibility center "cost center" that has been discussed earlier in this chapter. Instead, the cost-finding "cost center" is, broadly speaking, a type of cost pool used in the cost-finding process. The primary purpose of the cost pool/cost center in cost finding is to assist in allocating overhead.

The central worksheets for cost finding are Worksheet A, Worksheet B, and Worksheet B-1. Worksheet A contains the basic trial balance of all expenses for the facility. (Trial balances are discussed in a preceding chapter.) The beginning trial balance is reflected in the first three columns:

[Column 1]   [Column 2]   [Column 3]
"Salaries" + "Other"   =   "Total"
(all other expenses)

The trial balance is grouped at the outset into cost center categories. The placement of these categories and their respective line items on the page stay constant throughout the flow of Worksheets A, B, and B-1. The cost centers are grouped into seven categories:

1. General service
2. Inpatient routine service
3. Ancillary service
4. Outpatient service
5. Other reimbursable
6. Special purpose
7. Nonreimbursable

Table 5–2 Selected Cost Report Forms

Type	Form
Hospital and Hospital Healthcare Complex	CMS 2552-10
Skilled Nursing Facility and Skilled Nursing Facility Complex	CMS 2540-10
Home Health Agencies	CMS 1728-94

The line items within these seven categories represent the long-lived traditional arrangement that has strongly influenced the arrangement of expenses in so many healthcare information systems.

 INFORMATION CHECKPOINT

What is needed?	A report that shows expense in your organization.
Where is it found?	With your supervisor.
How is it used?	Examine the report to find various types of expenses; look for how the expense flow is handled on the report.
What is needed?	A report that groups expenses by some type of classification.
Where is it found?	With your supervisor or in the information services division.
How is it used?	Examine the report to discover the methods that are used for grouping. You will probably find that these groupings are used for performance measures. They can also be used for control and planning.

 KEY TERMS

Cost
Diagnoses
Expenses
Expired Costs
General Services Expenses
Support Services Expenses
Operations Expenses
Procedures
Unexpired Costs

 DISCUSSION QUESTIONS

1. Have you worked with cost centers in your duties? If so, how have you been exposed to them?
2. Have you had to manage from a cost center type of report? If so, how was it categorized?
3. Do you believe that grouping expenses by diagnoses and procedures (based on type of services provided) is better to use for control and planning than grouping expenses by care setting (based on location of service provided)?
4. If so, why?
5. What grouping of expenses do you believe your organization uses (traditional cost centers, diagnoses/procedures, care settings, other)?
6. From your perspective, would there be a better grouping possible? If so, why do you think it is not used?

NOTES

1. S. A. Finkler, *Essentials of Cost Accounting for Health Care Organizations*, 2nd ed. (Gaithersburg, MD: Aspen Publishers, Inc., 1999).
2. At the time of this writing, 23 major diagnostic categories (MDCs) serve as the basic classification system for diagnosis-related groups (DRGs). When ICD-10 is fully implemented, it is probable that the number of MDCs will be increased. It is also possible that the terminology itself (MDCs) may be changed to some other designation.
3. G. F. Longshore, "Service-line Mmanagement/Bottom-line Management for Health Care," *Journal of Health Care Finance*, 24, no. 4 (1998): 72–79.

Cost Classifications

DISTINCTION BETWEEN DIRECT AND INDIRECT COSTS

Direct costs can be specifically associated with a particular unit or department or patient. The critical distinction for the manager is that the cost is directly attributable. Whatever the manager is responsible for—that is, the unit, the department, or the patient—is known as a *cost object*.

The somewhat vague definition of a cost object is any unit for which a separate cost measurement is desired. It might help the manager to think of a *cost object* as a *cost objective* instead.[1] The important thing is that direct costs can be traced. Indirect costs, on the other hand, cannot be specifically associated with a particular cost object. The controller's office is an example of indirect cost. The controller's office is essential to the overall organization itself, but its cost is not specifically or directly associated with providing healthcare services. The critical distinction for the manager is that indirect costs usually cannot be traced, but instead must be allocated or apportioned in some manner.[2] **Figure 6–1** illustrates the direct–indirect cost distinction.

To summarize, it is helpful to recognize that direct costs are incurred for the sole benefit of a particular operating unit—a department, for example. As a rule of thumb, if the answer to the following question is "yes," then the cost is a direct cost: "If the operating unit (such as a department) did not exist, would this cost not be in existence?"

Indirect costs, in contrast, are incurred for the overall operation and not for any one unit. Because they are shared, indirect costs are sometimes called joint costs or

Progress Notes

After completing this chapter, you should be able to

1. Distinguish between direct and indirect costs.
2. Understand why the difference is important to management.
3. Understand the composition and purpose of responsibility centers.
4. Distinguish between product and period costs.

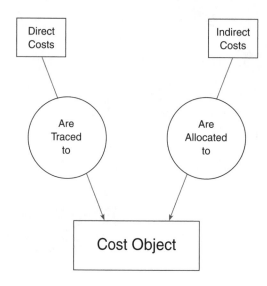

Figure 6–1 Assigning Costs to the Cost Object.

common costs. As a rule of thumb, if the answer to the following question is "yes," then the cost is an indirect cost: "Must this cost be allocated in order to be assigned to the unit (such as a department)?"

EXAMPLES OF DIRECT COST AND INDIRECT COST

It is important for managers to recognize direct and indirect costs and how they are treated on reports. Two sets of examples illustrate the reporting of direct and indirect costs. The first example concerns a rehab cost center; the second concerns an ambulance service center.

Table 6–1 represents a report of both direct cost and indirect cost for a rehab cost center. The report concerns three types of therapy—physical, occupational, and speech therapy—and a total. In this report, the manager can observe the proportionate differences between direct and indirect costs and can also see the differences among the three types of therapies.

Greater detail is provided to the manager in **Table 6–2**, which presents the method of allocating indirect costs and the result of such allocation. Managers should notice that the "Total Indirect Costs" in Table 6–2 carry forward and become the "Indirect Costs" in Table 6–1. Thus, this report showing allocation of indirect costs is considered a subsidiary report because it is supporting, or subsidiary to, the preceding main report. This use of one

Table 6–1 Examples of Rehab Cost Center Direct and Indirect Cost Totals

Rehab Cost Centers	Direct Cost	Indirect Cost	Total
Physical Therapy (PT)	$410,000	$107,500	$517,500
Occupational Therapy (OT)	190,000	44,000	234,000
Speech Therapy (ST)	120,000	33,500	153,500
Total	$720,000	$185,000	$905,000

Note: Direct Cost proportions, rounded, are as follows:

PT = 57%/OT = 26%/ST = 17%/Total = 100%

Courtesy of J.J. Baker and R.W. Baker, Dallas, Texas.

Table 6–2 Example of Indirect Costs Allocated to Rehab Cost Center

	Clerical Salaries	Administrative Salaries	Computer Services	Total Indirect Cost
Allocation Basis:	A	B	C	
Indirect Cost to Be Allocated	$60,000	$50,000	$75,000	$185,000
Allocated to:				
Physical Therapy (PT)	34,000	28,500	45,000	107,500
Occupational Therapy (OT)	16,000	13,000	15,000	44,000
Speech Therapy (ST)	10,000	8,500	15,000	33,500
Proof Total	$60,000	$50,000	$75,000	$185,000

Allocation Key:

A = # Visits (Volume): PT = 8500/OT = 4000/ST = 2500/Total = 15,000 (15,000 x $4.00 = $60,000)

B = Proportion of Direct Costs: PT = 57%/OT = 26%/ST = 17%/Total = 100% (% x $50,000)

C = # Computers in Service: PT = 9/OT = 3/ST = 3/Total = 15 (15 x $5,000 each = $75,000)

Courtesy of J.J. Baker and R.W. Baker, Dallas, Texas.

or more supporting reports to reveal details behind the main report is quite common in managerial reports. The allocation of indirect costs subsidiary report contains quite a lot of information. It shows what particular expenses (clerical salaries, administrative salaries, computer services) are contained in the $185,000 total. It also shows how each of these expenses are allocated across the three separate types of therapy. And the report also shows how each item was allocated; see the Allocation Key containing codes A, B and C. The basis for allocation is presented in the Key (A = # visits; B = proportion of direct costs, by percentage; C = number of computers in service) and the computation detail by therapy type is also noted. This set of tables is worthy of further study by the manager.

Exhibit 6–1 sets out the direct costs for an ambulance service center. These costs, as direct costs, are what the organization's managers believe can be traced to the specific operation of the freestanding center. **Exhibit 6–2** sets out the indirect costs for a freestanding ambulance service center. These costs are what the organization's managers believe are not directly attributable to the specific operation of the freestanding center. The decisions about what will and what will not be considered direct or indirect costs will almost always have been made for the manager.[3] What is important is that the manager understand two things: first, why

Exhibit 6–1 Example of Ambulance Direct Costs

Ambulance salaries & benefits	$32,500
RN salaries & benefits	9,600
Vehicle expense	21,300
Supplies	5,000
Uniforms	1,200
Employee education	3,900
Purchased services	1,900
Purchased maintenance	2,600
Utilities & telephone	5,000
Vehicle depreciation	15,000
Miscellaneous expense	2,000
Total direct costs	$100,000

Exhibit 6–2 Example of Ambulance Indirect Costs

Administrative costs	$12,000
Facility costs	8,000
Total indirect costs	$20,000

this is so, and second, how the relationship between the two works. Remember the rule of thumb discussed earlier in this chapter. If the answer to the following question is "yes," then the cost is a direct cost: "If the operating unit (such as a department) did not exist, would this cost not be in existence?"

RESPONSIBILITY CENTERS

We previously discussed revenue centers, whereby managers are responsible for generating revenue (or volume). We also previously discussed cost centers, whereby managers are responsible for managing and controlling cost. The responsibility center (R/C) makes a manager responsible for both the revenue/volume (inflow) side and the expense (outflow) side of a department, division, unit, or program. In other words, the manager is responsible for generating revenue/volume and for controlling costs. Another term for responsibility center is *profit center.*

We will examine the type of information a manager receives about his or her own responsibility center by reviewing the Westside Center operations. Westside Center offers two basic types of services: an ambulatory surgery center (ASC) and a rehabilitation center. The management of Westside is overseen by Bill, the director. Joe manages the ambulatory surgery center. Bonnie manages the rehabilitation center. Denise, a part-time radiologist, provides radiology services on an as-needed basis. Joe, Bonnie, and Denise, the managers, all report to Bill, the director. **Figure 6–2** illustrates the managerial relationships.

To restate the relationships shown in Figure 6–2, Joe manages a responsibility center for ambulatory surgery services. Bonnie manages a responsibility center for rehabilitation services. These services represent the business of Westside Center. Denise manages the

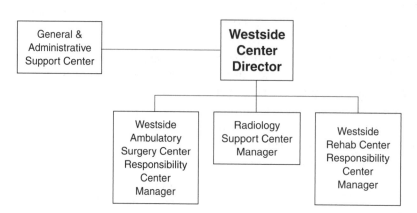

Figure 6–2 Lines of Managerial Responsibility at Westside Center.
Courtesy of Resource Group, Ltd., Dallas, Texas.

radiology services, but this is not a responsibility center in the Westside organization. Instead, it is a support center. Bill, the director, manages a bigger responsibility center that includes all of the functions just described, plus the general and administrative support center.

Bill, the director, receives a managerial report, shown in **Exhibit 6–3**. Bill's "Director's Summary" contains the data for the entire Westside operation.

Figure 6–3 illustrates the reports received by each manager at Westside. Joe's report for the ambulatory surgery center is at the top right of Figure 6–3. His report shows the controllable revenues he is responsible for ($225,000), less the controllable expenses he is responsible for ($155,000). The difference is labeled "ASC Responsibility Center Surplus" on his report. The surplus amounts to $70,000 ($225,000 minus $155,000).

Bonnie's report for the rehabilitation center is the second report on the right of Figure 6–3. Her report shows the controllable revenues she is responsible for ($300,000), less the controllable expenses she is responsible for ($215,000). The difference is labeled "Rehab Responsibility Center Surplus" on her report. The surplus amounts to $85,000 ($300,000 minus $215,000).

Denise's report for radiology services is at the bottom right of Figure 6–3. Her report shows the controllable expenses she is responsible for, which amount to $20,000. Her report shows only expenses because it is a support center, not a responsibility center. Therefore, Denise is responsible for expenses but not for revenue/volume.

Bill, the director, receives a report for the general and administrative (G&A) expenses, as shown second from the bottom on the right of Figure 6–3. This report shows the G&A controllable expenses that Bill himself is responsible for at Westside, which amount to $80,000. The G&A report shows only expenses because it also is a support center, not a responsibility center. Therefore, Bill is responsible for expenses but not for revenue/volume in the case of G&A.

However, Bill is also responsible for the entire Westside operation. That is, the overall Westside operation is his responsibility center. Therefore, Bill's director's summary, reproduced on the left side of Figure 6–3, contains the results of both responsibility centers and both support centers. The surplus figures from Joe and Bonnie's reports are positive figures of $70,000 and $85,000, respectively. The expense-only figures from Bill's G&A support center report and from Denise's radiology support center report are negative figures of $80,000 and $20,000, respectively. Therefore, to find the result of operations for Bill's entire Westside operation, the $80,000 and the $20,000 expense figures are subtracted from the surplus figures to arrive at a net surplus for Westside of $55,000.

Although the lines of managerial responsibility will vary in other organizations, the relationships between and among responsibility centers, support centers, and overall supervision will remain as shown in this example.

Exhibit 6–3 Director's Summary of Westside ASC and Rehab Responsibility Center

ASC R/C Surplus	$70,000.00
Rehab R/C Surplus	85,000.00
Less G&A Support Ctr	(80,000.00)
Less Radiology Support Ctr	(20,000.00)
Net Surplus	$55,000.00

Courtesy of Resource Group, Ltd., Dallas, Texas.

Westside ASC Responsibility Center Medical/Surgical Manager		
Controllable revenues:		
Patient fees		$225,000.00
Controllable expenses:		
Wages	100,000.00	
Payroll taxes, other fringes	25,000.00	
Billable supplies	20,000.00	
Medical supplies	10,000.00	
Total expenses		155,000.00
ASC R/C surplus		$70,000.00

Westside ASC Responsibility Center Therapy Manager		
Controllable revenues:		
Patient fees		$300,000.00
Controllable expenses:		
Wages	120,000.00	
Payroll taxes, other fringes	30,000.00	
Billable supplies	50,000.00	
Medical supplies	10,000.00	
Continuing education	3,000.00	
Licenses and permits	2,000.00	
Total expenses		215,000.00
Rehab R/C surplus		$85,000.00

Director's Summary of Westside ASC & Rehab Center	
ASC R/C Surplus	$70,000.00
Rehab R/C Surplus	85,000.00
Less G&A Support Ctr	(80,000.00)
Less Radiology Support Ctr	(20,000.00)
Net Surplus	$55,000.00

General & Administrative Support Center	
Salaries	$40,000.00
Payroll taxes, other fringes	10,000.00
Office supplies	1,200.00
Telephone	2,400.00
Rent	10,800.00
Utilities	4,800.00
Insurance	1,200.00
Depreciation	9,600.00
Total expenses	$80,000.00

Radiology Support Center Radiology Manager	
Salaries	$12,000.00
Payroll taxes, other fringes	3,000.00
Radiology supplies	5,000.00
Total expenses	$20,000.00

Figure 6–3 Westside Costs by Responsibility Center.
Courtesy of Resource Group, Ltd., Dallas, Texas.

DISTINCTION BETWEEN PRODUCT AND PERIOD COSTS

Product costs is a term that was originally associated with manufacturing rather than with services. The concept of product costs assumes that a product has been manufactured and placed into inventory while waiting to be sold. Then, whenever that product is sold, the product is matched with revenue and recognized as a cost. Thus, *cost of sales* is the common usage for manufacturing firms. (The concept of matching revenues and expenses has been discussed in a preceding chapter.)

Period costs, in the original manufacturing interpretation, are not connected with the manufacturing process. They are matched with revenue on the basis of the period during which the cost is incurred (thus *period costs*). The term comes from the span of time in which matching occurs, known as *time period*.

Service organizations have no manufacturing process as such. The business of healthcare service organizations is service delivery, not the manufacturing of products. Although the overall concept of product versus period cost is not as vital to service delivery, the distinction remains important for managers in health care to know.

In healthcare organizations, product cost can be viewed as traceable to the cost object of the department, division, or unit. A period cost is not traceable in this manner. Another way to view this distinction is to think of product costs as those costs necessary to actually deliver the service, whereas period costs are costs necessary to support the existence of the organization itself.

Finally, medical supply and pharmacy departments do have inventories on hand. In their case, a product is purchased (rather than manufactured) and placed into inventory while waiting to be dispensed. Then, whenever that product is dispensed, the product is matched with revenue and recognized as a cost of providing the service to the patient. Therefore, the product cost concept is important to managers of departments that hold a significant amount of inventory.

 INFORMATION CHECKPOINT

What is needed?	Example of a management report that uses direct/indirect cost.
Where is it found?	With your supervisor, in administration, or in information services.
How is it used?	To track operations directly associated with the unit.
What is needed?	Example of a management report that uses responsibility centers.
Where is it found?	With your supervisor, in administration, or in information services.
How is it used?	To reflect operations that a manager is specifically responsible for and to measure those operations for planning and control.

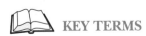 KEY TERMS

Cost Object
Direct Cost

Indirect Cost
Joint Cost
Responsibility Centers

 DISCUSSION QUESTIONS

1. In your own workplace, can you give a good example of a direct cost? An indirect cost?
2. What is the difference?
3. Does your organization use responsibility centers?
4. If not, do you think they should? Why?
5. If so, do you believe the responsibility centers operate properly? Would you make changes? Why?

NOTES

1. C. Horngren et al., *Cost Accounting: A Managerial Emphasis*, 9th ed. (Englewood Cliffs, NJ: Prentice Hall, 1998), 70.
2. J. J. Baker, *Activity-Based Costing and Activity-Based Management for Health Care* (Gaithersburg, MD: Aspen Publishers, Inc., 1998).
3. D. A. West, T. D. West, and P. J. Malone, "Managing Capital and Administrative (indirect) Costs to Achieve Strategic Objectives: The Dialysis Clinic versus the Outpatient Clinic," *Journal of Health Care Finance*, 25, no. 2 (1998): 20–24.

Tools to Analyze and Understand Financial Operations

Cost Behavior and Break-Even Analysis

DISTINCTIONS AMONG FIXED, VARIABLE, AND SEMIVARIABLE COSTS

This chapter emphasizes the distinctions among fixed, variable, and semivariable costs because this knowledge is a basic working tool in financial management. The manager needs to know the difference between fixed and variable costs to compute contribution margins and break-even points. The manager also needs to know about semivariable costs to make good decisions about how to treat these costs.

Fixed costs are costs that do not vary in total when activity levels (or volume) of operations change. This concept is illustrated in **Figure 7–1**. The horizontal axis of the graph shows number of residents in the Jones Group Home, and the vertical axis shows total monthly fixed cost in dollars. In this graph, the total monthly fixed cost for the group home is $3,000, and that amount does not change, whether the number of residents (the activity level or volume) is low or high. A good example of a fixed cost is rent expense. Rent would not vary whether the home was almost full or almost empty; thus, rent is a fixed cost.

Variable costs, on the other hand, are costs that vary in direct proportion to changes in activity levels (or volume) of operations. This concept is illustrated in **Figure 7–2**. The horizontal axis of the graph shows number of residents in the Jones Group Home, and the vertical axis shows total monthly variable cost in dollars. In this graph, the monthly variable cost for the group home changes proportionately with the number of

Progress Notes

After completing this chapter, you should be able to

1. Understand the distinctions among fixed, variable, and semivariable costs.
2. Be able to analyze mixed costs by two methods.
3. Understand the computation of a contribution margin.
4. Be able to compute the cost-volume-profit (CVP) ratio.
5. Be able to compute the profit-volume (PV) ratio.

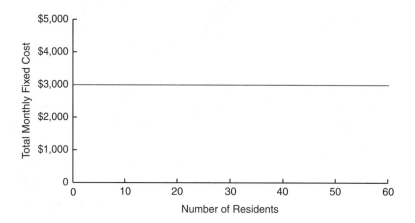

Figure 7–1 Fixed Costs—Jones Group Home.

residents (the activity level or volume) in the home. A good example of a variable cost is food for the group home residents. Food would vary directly, depending on the number of individuals in residence; thus, food is a variable cost.

Semivariable costs vary when the activity levels (or volume) of operations change, but not in direct proportion. The most frequent pattern of semivariable costs is the step pattern, where the semivariable cost rises, flattens out for a bit, and then rises again. The step pattern of semivariable costs is illustrated in **Figure 7–3**. The horizontal axis of the graph shows number of residents in the Jones Group Home, and the vertical axis shows total monthly semivariable cost. In this graph, the behavior of the cost line resembles stair steps: thus, the "step pattern" name for this configuration. The most common example

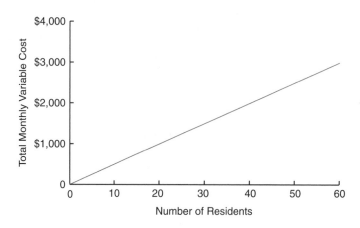

Figure 7–2 Variable Cost—Jones Group Home.

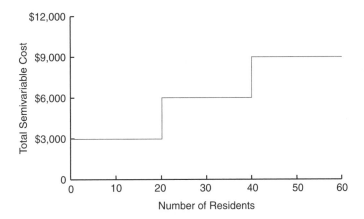

Figure 7–3 Semivariable Cost—Jones Group Home.

of a semivariable expense in health care is supervisors' salaries. A single supervisor, for example, can perform adequately over a range of rises in activity levels (or volume). When another supervisor has to be added, the rise in the step pattern occurs.

It is important to know, however, that there are two ways to think about fixed cost. The usual view is the flat line illustrated on the graph in Figure 7–1. That flat line represents total monthly cost for the group home. However, another perception is presented in **Figure 7–4**. The top view of fixed costs in Figure 7–4 is the usual flat line just discussed. The bottom view is fixed cost per resident. Think about the figure for a moment: the top view is dollars in total for the home for the month, and the bottom view is fixed-cost dollars by number of residents. The line is no longer flat but declines because this view of cost declines with each additional resident.

We can also think about variable cost in two ways. The usual view of variable cost is the diagonal line rising from the bottom of the graph to the top, as illustrated in Figure 7–2. That steep diagonal line represents monthly cost varying in direct proportion with number of residents in the home. However, another perception is presented in **Figure 7–5**. The top view of variable costs in Figure 7–5 represents total monthly variable cost and is the usual diagonal line just discussed. The bottom view is variable cost per resident. Think about this figure for a moment: the top view is dollars in total for the home for the month, and the bottom view is variable-cost dollars by number of residents. The line is no longer diagonal but is now flat because this view of variable cost stays the same proportionately for each resident. A good way to think about Figures 7–4 and 7–5 is to realize that they are close to being mirror images of each other.

Semifixed costs are sometimes used in healthcare organizations, especially in regard to staffing. Semifixed costs are the reverse of semivariable costs: that is, they stay fixed for a time as activity levels (or volume) of operations change, but then they will rise; then they will plateau; then they will rise. Thus, semifixed costs can exhibit a step pattern similar to

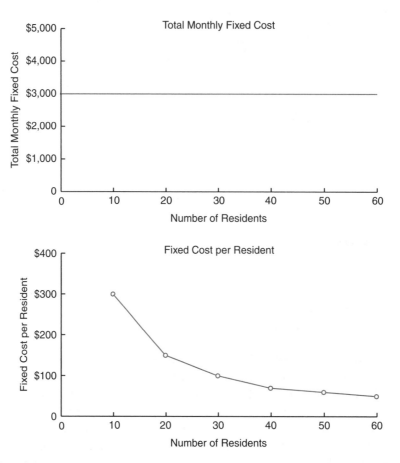

Figure 7–4 Two Views of Fixed Costs.

that of variable costs.[1] However, the semifixed cost "steps" tend to be longer between rises in cost. In summary, both semifixed and semivariable costs have mixed elements of fixed and variable costs. Thus, both semivariable and semifixed costs are called mixed costs.

EXAMPLES OF VARIABLE AND FIXED COSTS

Studying examples of expenses that are designated as variable and fixed helps to understand the differences between them. It should also be mentioned that some expenses can be variable to one organization and fixed to another because they are handled differently by the two organizations. Operating room fixed and variable costs are illustrated in **Table 7–1**. Thirty-two expense accounts are listed in Table 7–1: 11 are variable, 20 are

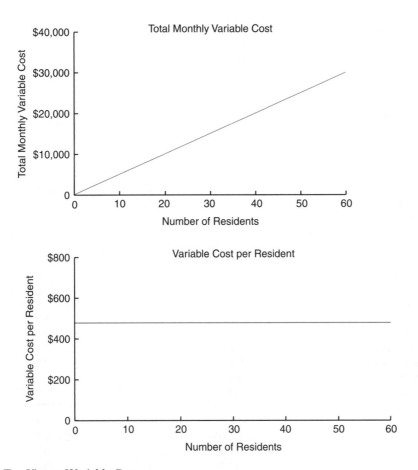

Figure 7–5 Two Views of Variable Costs.

designated as fixed by this hospital, and 1, equipment depreciation, is listed separately.[2] (The separate listing is because of the way this hospital's accounting system handles equipment depreciation.)

Another example of semivariable and fixed staffing is presented in **Table 7–2**. The costs are expressed as full-time equivalent staff (FTEs). Each line-item FTE will be multiplied times the appropriate wage or salary to obtain the semivariable and fixed costs for the operating room. (The further use of FTEs for staffing purposes is fully discussed in the chapter on staffing.) The supervisor position is fixed, which indicates that this is the minimum staffing that can be allowed. The single aide/orderly and the clerical position are also indicated as fixed. All the other positions—technicians, RNs, and LPNs—are listed as semivariable, which indicates that they are probably used in the semivariable step pattern that has been previously discussed in this chapter. This table is a good

Table 7–1 Operating Room Fixed and Variable Costs

Account	Total	Variable	Fixed	Equipment
Social Security	$ 60,517	$ 60,517	$	$
Pension	20,675	20,675		
Health Insurance	8,422	8,422		
Child Care	4,564	4,564		
Patient Accounting	155,356	155,356		
Admitting	110,254	110,254		
Medical Records	91,718	91,718		
Dietary	27,526	27,526		
Medical Waste	2,377	2,377		
Sterile Procedures	78,720	78,720		
Laundry	40,693	40,693		
Depreciation—Equipment	87,378			87,378
Depreciation—Building	41,377		41,377	
Amortization—Interest	(5,819)		(5,819)	
Insurance	4,216		4,216	
Administration	57,966		57,966	
Medical Staff	1,722		1,722	
Community Relations	49,813		49,813	
Materials Management	64,573		64,573	
Human Resources	31,066		31,066	
Nursing Administration	82,471		82,471	
Data Processing	17,815		17,815	
Fiscal	17,700		17,700	
Telephone	2,839		2,839	
Utilities	26,406		26,406	
Plant	77,597		77,597	
Environmental Services	32,874		32,874	
Safety	2,016		2,016	
Quality Management	10,016		10,016	
Medical Staff	9,444		9,444	
Continuous Quality Improvement	4,895		4,895	
EE Health	569		569	
Total Allocated	$1,217,756	$600,822	$529,556	$87,378

Adapted from J.J. Baker, *Activity-Based Costing and Activity-Based Management for Health Care*, p. 191, © 1998, Aspen Publishers, Inc.

example of how to show clearly which costs will be designated as semivariable and which costs will be designated as fixed.

Another example illustrates the behavior of a single variable cost in a doctor's office. In **Table 7–3**, we see an array of costs for the procedure code 99214 office visit type. Nine costs are listed. The first cost is variable and is discussed momentarily. The other eight costs are all shown at the same level for a 99214 office visit: supplies, for example, is the same amount in all four columns. The single figure that varies is the top line, which is "report of lab tests," meaning laboratory reports. This cost directly varies with the proportion of activity or volume, as variable cost has been defined. Here we see a variable cost at work: the first column on the left has no lab report, and the cost is zero; the second column has one lab report, and the cost is $3.82; the third column has two lab reports, and the cost is $7.64; and the fourth column has three lab reports, and the cost is $11.46. The total cost rises by the same proportionate increase as the increase in the first line.

Table 7–2 Operating Room Semivariable and Fixed Staffing

Job Positions	Total No. of FTEs	Semivariable	Fixed
Supervisor	2.2		2.2
Techs	3.0	3.0	
RNs	7.7	7.7	
LPNs	1.2	1.2	
Aides, orderlies	1.0		1.0
Clerical	1.2		1.2
Totals	16.3	11.9	4.4

ANALYZING MIXED COSTS

It is important for planning purposes for the manager to know how to deal with mixed costs because they occur so often. For example, telephone, maintenance, repairs, and utilities are all actually mixed costs. The fixed portion of the cost is that portion representing having the service (such as telephone) ready to use, and the variable portion of the cost represents a portion of the charge for actual consumption of the service. We briefly discuss

Table 7–3 Office Visit with Variable Cost of Tests

Service Code	99214 No Test	99214 1 Test	99214 2 Tests	99214 3 Tests
Report of lab tests	$0.00	$3.82	$7.64	$11.46
Fixed overhead	$31.00	$31.00	$31.00	$31.00
Physician	11.36	11.36	11.36	11.36
Medical assistant	1.43	1.43	1.43	1.43
Bill	0.45	0.45	0.45	0.45
Checkout	1.00	1.00	1.00	1.00
Receptionist	1.28	1.28	1.28	1.28
Collection	0.91	0.91	0.91	0.91
Supplies	0.31	0.31	0.31	0.31
Total visit cost	$47.74	$51.56	$55.38	$59.20

two very simple methods of analyzing mixed costs, then we examine the high–low method and the scatter graph method.

Predominant Characteristics and Step Methods

Both the predominant characteristics and the step method of analyzing mixed costs are quite simple. In the predominant characteristic method, the manager judges whether the cost is more fixed or more variable and acts on that judgment. In the step method, the manager examines the "steps" in the step pattern of mixed cost and decides whether the cost appears to be more fixed or more variable. Both methods are subjective.

High–Low Method

As the name implies, the high–low method of analyzing mixed costs requires that the cost be examined at its high level and at its low level. To compute the amount of variable cost involved, the difference in cost between high and low levels is obtained and is divided by the amount of change in the activity (or volume). Two examples are examined.

The first example is for an employee cafeteria. **Table 7–4** contains the basic data required for the high–low computation. With the formula described in the preceding paragraph, the following steps are performed:

1. Find the highest volume of 45,000 meals at a cost of $165,000 in September (see Table 7–4) and the lowest volume of 20,000 meals at a cost of $95,000 in March.
2. Compute the variable rate per meal:

	No. of Meals	Cafeteria Cost
Highest volume	45,000	$165,000
Lowest volume	20,000	95,000
Difference	25,000	70,000

3. Divide the difference in cost ($70,000) by the difference in number of meals (25,000) to arrive at the variable cost rate:

$70,000 divided by 25,000 meals = $2.80 per meal

Table 7–4 Employee Cafeteria Number of Meals and Cost by Month

Month	No. of Meals	Employee Cafeteria Cost ($)
July	40,000	164,000
August	43,000	167,000
September	45,000	165,000
October	41,000	162,000
November	37,000	164,000
December	33,000	146,000
January	28,000	123,000
February	22,000	91,800
March	20,000	95,000
April	25,000	106,800
May	30,000	130,200
June	35,000	153,000

4. Compute the fixed overhead rate as follows:
   a. At the highest level:

Total cost	$165,000
Less: variable portion	
[45,000 meals × $2.80 @]	(126,000)
Fixed portion of cost	$ 39,000

   b. At the lowest level

Total cost	$ 95,000
Less: variable portion	
[20,000 meals × $2.80 @]	(56,000)
Fixed portion of cost	$ 39,000

   c. Proof totals: $39,000 fixed portion at both levels

The manager should recognize that large or small dollar amounts can be adapted to this method. A second example concerns drug samples and their cost. In this example, a supervisor of marketing is concerned about the number of drug samples used by the various members of the marketing staff. She uses the high–low method to determine the portion of fixed cost. **Table 7–5** contains the basic data required for the high–low computation. Using the formula previously described, the following steps are performed:

1. Find the highest volume of 1,000 samples at a cost of $5,000 (see Table 7–5) and the lowest volume of 750 samples at a cost of $4,200.
2. Compute the variable rate per sample:

	No. of Samples	Cost
Highest volume	1,000	$5,000
Lowest volume	750	4,200
Difference	250	$ 800

3. Divide the difference in cost ($800) by the difference in number of samples (250) to arrive at the variable cost rate:

   $800 divided by 250 samples = $3.20 per sample

4. Compute the fixed overhead rate as follows:
   a. At the highest level:

Total cost	$5,000
Less: variable portion	
[1,000 samples × $3.20 @]	(3,200)
Fixed portion of cost	$1,800

Table 7–5 Number of Drug Samples and Cost for November

Rep.	No. of Samples	Cost ($)
J. Smith	1,000	5,000
A. Jones	900	4,300
B. Baker	850	4,600
G. Black	975	4,500
T. Potter	875	4,750
D. Conner	750	4,200

   b. At the lowest level

Total cost	$4,200
Less: variable portion	
[750 samples × $3.20 @]	(2,400)
Fixed portion of cost	$1,800

   c. Proof totals: $1,800 fixed portion at both levels

The high–low method is an approximation that is based on the relationship between the highest and the lowest levels, and the computation assumes a straight-line relationship. The advantage of this method is its convenience in the computation method.

CONTRIBUTION MARGIN, COST-VOLUME-PROFIT, AND PROFIT-VOLUME RATIOS

The manager should know how to analyze the relationship of cost, volume, and profit. This important information assists the manager in properly understanding and controlling operations. The first step in such analysis is the computation of the contribution margin.

Contribution Margin

The contribution margin is calculated in this way:

		% of Revenue
Revenues (net)	$500,000	100%
Less: variable cost	(350,000)	70%
Contribution margin	$150,000	30%
Less: fixed cost	(120,000)	
Operating income	$30,000	

The contribution margin of $150,000 or 30%, in this example, represents variable cost deducted from net revenues. The answer represents the contribution margin, so called because it contributes to fixed costs and to profits.

The importance of dividing costs into fixed and variable becomes apparent now, for a contribution margin computation demands either fixed or variable cost classifications; no mixed costs are recognized in this calculation.

Cost-Volume-Profit (CVP) Ratio or Break Even

The break-even point is the point when the contribution margin (i.e., net revenues less variable costs) equals the fixed costs. When operations exceed this break-even point, an excess of revenues over expenses (income) is realized. But if operations does not reach the break-even point, there will be an excess of expenses over revenues, and a loss will be realized.

The manager must recognize there are two ways of expressing the break-even point: either by an amount per unit or as a percentage of net revenues. If the contribution margin is expressed as a percentage of net revenues, it is often called the profit-volume (PV) ratio. A PV ratio example follows this cost-volume-profit (CVP) computation.

The CVP example is given in **Figure 7–6**. The data points for the chart come from the contribution margin as already computed:

		% of Revenue
Revenues (net)	$500,000	100%
Less: variable cost	(350,000)	70%
Contribution margin	$150,000	30%
Less: fixed cost	(120,000)	
Operating income	$30,000	

Three lines were first drawn to create the chart. They were total fixed costs of $120,000, total revenue of $500,000, and variable costs of $350,000. (All three are labeled on the chart.) The break-even point appears at the point where the total cost line intersects the revenue line. Because this point is indeed the break-even point, the organization will have no profit and no loss but will break even. The wedge shape to the left of the break-even point is potential net loss, whereas the narrower wedge to the right is potential net income (both are labeled on the chart).

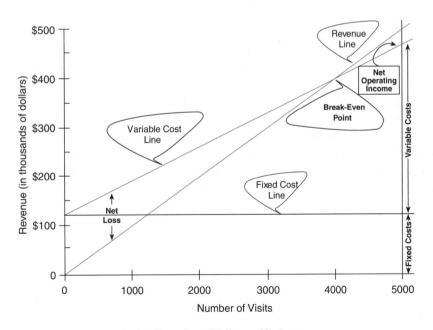

Figure 7–6 Cost-Volume-Profit (CVP) Chart for a Wellness Clinic.
Courtesy of Resource Group, Ltd., Dallas, Texas.

CVP charts allow a visual illustration of the relationships that is very effective for the manager.

Profit-Volume (PV) Ratio

Remember that the second method of expressing the break-even point is as a percentage of net revenues and that if the contribution margin is expressed as a percentage of net revenues, it is called the profit-volume (PV) ratio. **Figure 7–7** illustrates the method. The basic data points used for the chart were as follows:

Revenue per visit	$100.00	100%
Less variable cost per visit	(70.00)	70%
Contribution margin per visit	$ 30.00	30%
Fixed costs per period	$120,000	

$30.00 contribution margin per visit divided by $100 price per visit = 30% PV Ratio

On our chart, the profit pattern is illustrated by a line drawn from the beginning level of fixed costs to be recovered ($120,000 in our case). Another line has been drawn straight across the chart at the break-even point. When the diagonal line begins at $120,000, its intersection with the break-even or zero line is at $400,000 in revenue (see left-hand dotted line on chart). We can prove out the $120,000 versus $400,000 relationship as follows. Each dollar of revenue reduces the potential of loss by $0.30 (or 30% × $1.00). Fixed costs are fully recovered at a revenue level of $400,000, proved out as $120,000 divided by .30 = $400,000. This can be written as follows:

$$.30R = \$120,000$$
$$R = \$400,000 \; [120,000 \text{ divided by } .30 = 400,000]$$

The PV chart is very effective in planning meetings because only two lines are necessary to show the effect of changes in volume. Both PV and CVP are useful when working with the effects of changes in break-even points and revenue volume assumptions.

Contribution margins are also useful for showing profitability in other ways. An example appears in **Figure 7–8**, which shows the profitability of various DRGs, using contribution margins as the measure of profitability. Case volume (the number of cases of each DRG) is on the vertical axis of the matrix, and the dollar amount of contribution margin per case is on the horizontal axis of the matrix.[3]

Scatter Graph Method

In performing a mixed-cost analysis, the manager is attempting to find the mixed cost's average rate of variability. The scatter graph method is more accurate than the high–low method previously described. It uses a graph to plot all points of data, rather than the

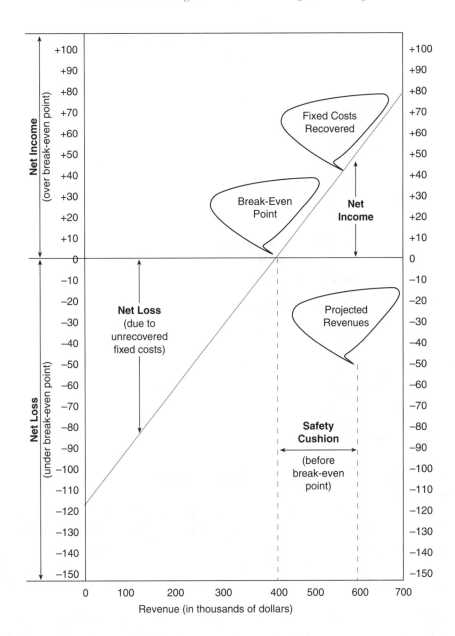

Figure 7–7 Profit-Volume (PV) Chart for a Wellness Clinic.
Courtesy of Resource Group, Ltd., Dallas, Texas.

highest and lowest figures used by the high–low method. Generally, cost will be on the vertical axis of the graph, and volume will be on the horizontal axis. All points are plotted, each point being placed where cost and volume intersect for that line item. A regression line is then fitted to the plotted points. The regression line basically represents the average—or a

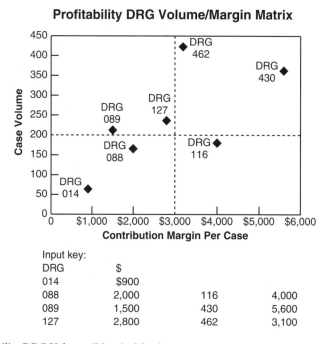

Profitability DRG Volume/Margin Matrix

Input key:

DRG	$		
014	$900		
088	2,000	116	4,000
089	1,500	430	5,600
127	2,800	462	3,100

Figure 7–8 Profitability DRG Volume/Margin Matrix.
Modified from R. Hankins and J.J. Baker, *Management Accounting for Health Care Organizations* (Sudbury, MA: Jones & Bartlett 2004), 189.

line of averages. The average total fixed cost is found at the point where the regression line intersects with the cost axis.

Two examples are examined. They match the high–low examples previously calculated. **Figure 7–9** presents the cafeteria data. The costs for cafeteria meals have been plotted on the graph, and the regression line has been fitted to the plotted data points. The regression line strikes the cost axis at a certain point; that amount represents the fixed cost portion of the mixed cost. The balance (or the total less the fixed cost portion) represents the variable portion.

The second example also matches the high–low example previously calculated. **Figure 7–10** presents the drug sample data. The costs for drug samples have been plotted on the graph, and the regression line has been fitted to the plotted data points. The regression line again strikes the cost axis at the point representing the fixed-cost portion of the mixed cost. The balance (the total less the fixed cost portion) represents the variable portion. Further discussions of this method can be found in Examples and Exercises at the back of this book.

The examples presented here have regression lines fitted visually. However, computer programs are available that will place the regression line through statistical analysis as a

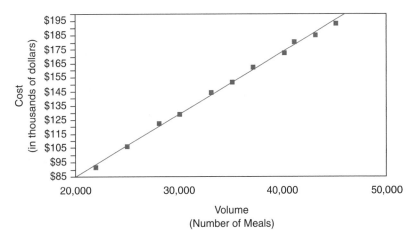

Figure 7–9 Employee Cafeteria Scatter Graph.

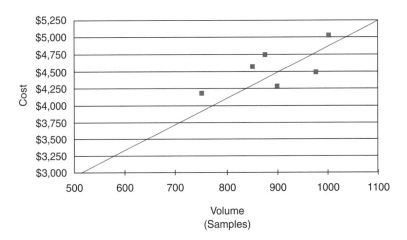

Figure 7–10 Drug Sample Scatter Graph for November.

function of the program. This method is called the least-squares method. Least squares means that the sum of the squares of the deviations from plotted points to regression line is smaller than would occur from any other way the line could be fitted to the data: in other words, it is the best fit. This method is, of course, more accurate than fitting the regression line visually.

INFORMATION CHECKPOINT

What is needed?	Revenues, variable cost, and fixed cost for a unit, division, DRG, and so on.
Where is it found?	In operating reports.
How is it used?	Use the multiple-step calculations in this chapter to compute the CPV or the PV ratio; use to plan and control operations.

KEY TERMS

Break-Even Analysis
Cost-Profit-Volume
Contribution Margin
Fixed Cost
Mixed Cost
Profit-Volume Ratio
Semifixed Cost
Semivariable Cost
Variable Cost

DISCUSSION QUESTIONS

1. Have you seen reports in your workplace that set out the contribution margin?
2. Do you believe that contribution margins can help you manage in your present work? In the future? How?
3. Have you encountered break-even analysis in your work?
4. If so, how was it used (or presented)?
5. How do you think you would use break-even analysis?
6. Do you believe your organization could use these analysis tools more often than is now happening? What do you believe the benefits would be?

NOTES

1. C. Horngren et al., *Cost Accounting: A Managerial Emphasis,* 9th ed. (Englewood Cliffs, NJ: Prentice Hall, 1998).
2. J. J. Baker, *Activity-Based Costing and Activity-Based Management for Health Care* (Gaithersburg, MD: Aspen Publishers, Inc., 1998).
3. It is possible that the term "diagnosis-related groups" (DRGs) may be changed to some new terminology as a consequence of ICD-10 implementation.

Understanding Inventory and Depreciation Concepts

OVERVIEW: THE INVENTORY CONCEPT

This overview concerns both the inventory concept and types of inventories.

Concept of Inventory in Healthcare Organizations

"Inventory" includes all the items (goods) that an organization has for sale in the normal course of its business. Inventory is an asset, owned by the company. It appears on the balance sheet as a current asset, because the individual items that compose the inventory are expected to be "used" (sold) within a 12 month period.

Types of Inventory in Healthcare Organizations

Various healthcare organizations (or departments within organizations) deal with inventory and must account for it. The hospital gift shop and the cafeteria, for example, own inventory and must account for it. All pharmacies (hospital-based, retail brick-and-mortar, or mail order pharmacies) own inventory in the normal course of their business.

In manufacturing companies, inventory typically consists of three parts: raw materials, work in progress, and the finished goods that are for sale. We might think that most inventory items for sale in a healthcare organization are not manufactured, but are finished goods instead. However, consider this example: the hospital cafeteria purchases flour, eggs, butter, and so on (raw materials), mixes the ingredients (work in progress), and produces a cake (finished goods) that is for sale. (Another example might be a pharmacy that compounds drugs.)

After completing this chapter, you should be able to

1. Understand the interrelationship between inventory and cost of goods sold.
2. Understand the difference between LIFO and FIFO inventory methods.
3. Be able to calculate inventory turnover.
4. Understand the interrelationship between depreciation expense and the reserve for depreciation.
5. Understand how to compute the net book value of a fixed asset.
6. Be able to identify the five methods of computing book depreciation.

INVENTORY AND COST OF GOODS SOLD ("GOODS" SUCH AS DRUGS)

The interrelationship between inventory and cost of goods sold is at the heart of the inventory concept.

Turning Inventory into Cost of Goods (or Drugs) Sold

The completed inventory item ("finished goods") is sold. That is how an item moves out of inventory and is recognized as cost. When the item is recognized as cost, it becomes "cost of goods sold." (Also note that different terminology may be used. In some organizations cost of goods sold is called "cost of sales.") For a business such as a retail pharmacy, the cost of inventory sold to its customers is the largest single expense of the business.

Recording Inventory and Cost of Goods (or Drugs) Sold

Recording inventory and cost of goods (or drugs) sold is a sequence of events. **Figure 8–1** illustrates the sequence as follows:

- Beginning inventory (inventory at the start of the period) is recorded.
- Purchases during the period are recorded.
- Beginning inventory plus purchases equal "cost of goods available for sale."
- Ending inventory (inventory at the end of the period) is recorded.
- Cost of goods available for sale less ending inventory equals "cost of goods sold."

Purchases added to inventory will typically include "freight in," or the shipping costs to deliver the items to you. Any discounts received on the purchases should be subtracted from the purchase cost. Thus the purchases become "net purchases"; that is, net of discounts.

Sometimes the ending inventory is estimated. An example of "Estimating the Ending Pharmacy Inventory" is shown in the chapter about estimates and benchmarking.

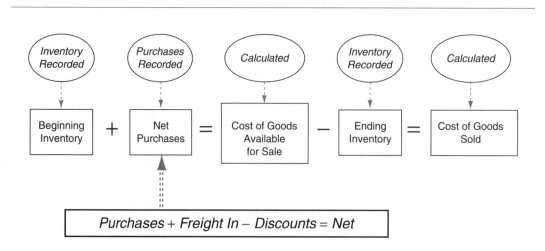

Figure 8–1 Recording Inventory in the Accounting Cycle.

Gross Margin Computation

Gross margin equals revenue from sales less the cost of goods sold. Gross margin is often expressed as a percentage. Thus, a pharmacy's gross margin might appear as follows:

Sales	100%
Cost of goods (drugs) sold	65%
Gross margin	35%

An organization's gross margin percentage can be readily compared to industry standards.

INVENTORY METHODS

How is the inventory to be valued? The two most commonly used inventory valuation methods are First-In, First-Out (FIFO) and Last-In, First-Out (LIFO). The method chosen will affect the organization's financial statements, as explained in the following sections.

First-In, First-Out (FIFO) Inventory Method

The First-In, First-Out, or FIFO inventory costing method, recognizes the first costs placed into inventory as the first costs moved out into cost of goods sold when a sale occurs. How will this method affect the organization's financial statements? Under FIFO, the ending inventory figure will be higher (because when the oldest inventory moves out first, the ending inventory will be based on the costs of the latest purchases, which we assume will have cost more). **Exhibit 8–1** illustrates this effect.

Last-In, First-Out (LIFO) Inventory Method

The Last-In, First-Out, or LIFO inventory costing method, recognizes the latest, or last, costs placed into inventory as the first costs moved out into cost of goods sold when a sale occurs. How will this method affect the organization's financial statements? Under LIFO, the ending inventory figure will be lower (because when the latest inventory moves out first, the ending inventory will be based on costs of the earliest purchases, which we assume will have cost less). **Exhibit 8–2** illustrates this effect.

Other Inventory Treatments

Two other inventory treatments deserve mention, as follows.

Weighted Average Inventory Method

This inventory costing method is based on the weighted average cost of inventory during the period. (The weighted average inventory method is also called the "average cost method.") The weighted average inventory cost is determined as follows: divide the cost of goods available for sale by the number of units available for sale.

Exhibit 8–1 FIFO Inventory Effect

	Assumptions	FIFO Inventory Effect	
Sales (Revenue)	20 units @$25 =		$500
Cost of Sales:			
Beginning Inventory	10 units @$5 =	$50	
Plus: Purchases	10 units @$10 = $100 &		
	10 units @$15 = $150	250	
Subtotal		$300	
Less: Ending Inventory	10 units @$15 =	(150)	
Cost of Sales			150
Gross Profit			$350
Operating Expenses			(50)
Earnings Before Tax			$300
Income Tax			(90)
Earnings After Tax			$210

Note: Ending inventory computed as number of units in the beginning inventory plus number of units purchased less number of units sold–count oldest units sold first.

No Method: Inventory Never Recognized

This inventory costing method is no method at all. That is, inventory is never recognized. For example, a physician's office may expense all drug purchases as supplies at the time of purchase and never count such drugs as inventory. This treatment might be justified when such supplies were only a small part of the practice expenses. However, if the physician is purchasing very expensive drugs and administering them in the office (infusing expensive drugs is a good example), then not recognizing any such drugs being held as inventory on the financial statements is misleading.

INVENTORY TRACKING

The two most typical inventory tracking systems are described as follows.

Exhibit 8–2 LIFO Inventory Effect

	Assumptions	LIFO Inventory Effect
Sales (Revenue)	20 units @$25 =	$500
Cost of Sales:		
Beginning Inventory	10 units @$5 =	$50
Plus: Purchases	10 units @$10 = $100 &	
	10 units @$15 = $150	250
Subtotal		$300
Less: Ending Inventory	10 units @$5 =	(50)
Cost of Sales		250
Gross Profit		$250
Operating Expenses		(50)
Earnings Before Tax		$200
Income Tax		(60)
Earnings After Tax		$140

Note: Ending inventory computed as number of units purchased plus number of units in the beginning inventory less number of units sold–count newest units sold first.

Perpetual Inventory System

With a perpetual inventory system, the healthcare organization keeps a continuous, or perpetual, record for every individual inventory item. Thus the amount of inventory on hand can be determined at any time. (A real-time system is a variation of the perpetual inventory system, whereby transactions are entered simultaneously.)

A perpetual inventory system requires, of course, a specific identification method for each inventory item. Bar coding is often used for this purpose. You are most likely to find a perpetual inventory system in the pharmacy department of a hospital.

Periodic Inventory System

With a periodic inventory system, the healthcare organization does not keep a continuous record that identifies every individual inventory item on hand. Instead, at the end of the period the organization physically counts the inventory items on hand. Then costs per item are attached to the inventory counts in order to arrive at the cost of the inventory at the end of the period (the ending inventory).

Necessary Adjustments

Certain inventory adjustments will commonly become necessary, as discussed here.

Shortages

When the periodic inventory results are compared to the inventory balance on the financial statements, it is not uncommon to find that the actual physical inventory amount is less than the amount recorded on the books. This difference, or shortage, is commonly termed "shrinkage." The inventory amount on the books must be reduced to the actual amount per the periodic inventory, and the resulting shrinkage cost must be recorded as an expense.

Obsolete Items

Most inventories will inevitably come to contain certain obsolete items. For example, the pharmacy inventory will contain drugs that have "sell by" or "use by" expiration dates. Obsolete inventory items should be discarded. Their cost must be removed from the cost of inventory on hand, and the resulting obsolescence cost must be recorded as an expense.

CALCULATING INVENTORY TURNOVER

Inventory turnover is a ratio that shows how fast inventory is sold, or "turns over." The computation is in two steps as follows. **Figure 8–2** illustrates the sequence.

Step 1. First compute "Average Inventory":
Beginning Inventory plus Ending Inventory divided by two equals Average Inventory

Step 2. Next compute "Inventory Turnover":
Cost of Goods Sold (or Cost of Sales) divided by Average Inventory equals Inventory Turnover

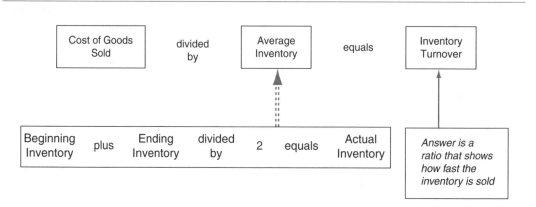

Figure 8–2 Calculating Inventory Turnover.

For example,

Step 1. $100,000 (beginning inventory) plus $150,000 (ending inventory) divided by 2 equals $125,000 (average inventory).

Step 2. $500,000 (cost of goods sold, or cost of sales) divided by $125,000 (average inventory) equals 4.0 (inventory turnover).

An organization's inventory turnover ratio can be readily compared to industry standards.

OVERVIEW: THE DEPRECIATION CONCEPT

Depreciation expense spreads, or allocates, the cost of a fixed asset over the useful life of that asset, as discussed here.

Fixed Assets and Depreciation Expense

Fixed assets, also known as long-term assets, are classified as long-term and placed on the balance sheet as such because they will not be converted into cash in the coming 12 months. The purchase of a fixed asset is a capital expenditure. (Capital expenditures involve the acquisition of assets that are long lasting, such as buildings and equipment.) "Capitalizing" means recording these assets as long-term assets on the balance sheet.

We recognize the cost of owning buildings and equipment through depreciation expense. When the cost is spread, or allocated, over a period of years, each year's financial statements (for that period of years) recognize some portion of the cost, expressed as depreciation expense.

Useful Life of the Asset

The useful life determines the period over which the fixed asset's cost will be spread. For example, a piece of laboratory equipment is purchased for $20,000. It has a useful life of five years. So depreciation expense is recognized in each of the five years until the $20,000 is used up.

Salvage Value

Before depreciation expense can be calculated, we need to know whether the fixed asset will have salvage value at the end of the depreciated period. Salvage value, also known as residual value or scrap value, represents any expected cash value of the asset at the end of its useful life. If the laboratory equipment is expected to have a salvage value of $1,000 at the end of its five-year useful life, then $19,000 will be spread over the five-year life as depreciation expense, and the $1,000 will remain undepreciated at the end of that time.

BOOK VALUE OF A FIXED ASSET AND THE RESERVE FOR DEPRECIATION

This section describes important interrelationships between and among depreciation expense, the reserve for depreciation, and net book value of an asset.

The Reserve for Depreciation

Depreciation expense over the years is accumulated into the reserve for depreciation. In other words, the reserve for depreciation holds the cumulative amount of depreciation expense that has been recognized over time, beginning with the date that the fixed asset was acquired. Another way to think about this is to view the reserve for depreciation as holding all the depreciation expense that has been recognized and recorded over the useful life of the asset.

Interrelationship of Depreciation Expense and the Reserve for Depreciation

Depreciation expense for the year is recorded in the income statement. At the same time, an equivalent amount is added to the cumulative amount that has been accumulating within the reserve for depreciation on the balance sheet. These amounts should balance each other; that is, if $25,000 is recognized as depreciation expense in the income statement, then $25,000 should be added to the reserve for depreciation on the balance sheet. This interrelationship is illustrated in **Figure 8–3**.

Net Book Value of a Fixed Asset

The net book value (also known as book value) of a fixed asset is a balance sheet figure that represents the remaining undepreciated portion of the fixed asset cost. The term derives from value recorded on the books—thus "book value."

The net book value of a fixed asset is computed as follows:

- Determine the original cost of the fixed asset on the balance sheet.
- Subtract the reserve for depreciation, which has accumulated depreciation expense as it has been recognized.
- The result equals net book value at that point in time (**Figure 8–4**).

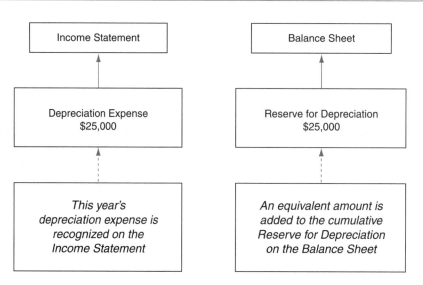

Figure 8–3 Interrelationship of Depreciation Expense and Reserve for Depreciation in the Accounting Cycle.

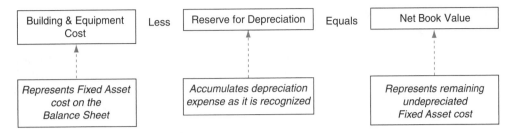

Figure 8–4 Net Book Value Computation.

Also note that fully depreciated fixed assets may still remain on the books if they are still in use. A fully depreciated fixed asset, of course, means that the depreciable cost has been exhausted because all the depreciation expense over the asset's useful life has already been recognized. Thus, the net book value would either be zero or would amount to the remaining salvage value of the asset.

FIVE METHODS OF COMPUTING BOOK DEPRECIATION

Just as "book value" means value that is recorded on the organization's books, "book depreciation" means depreciation that is recorded on the books. Book depreciation is the depreciation expense recorded in the financial accounting records and reflected on the financial statements. "Tax depreciation," on the other hand, is depreciation that is computed for tax purposes and is reflected on the applicable tax returns of the organization. Tax depreciation methods are discussed in the final section of this chapter.

You as a manager will most likely be using book depreciation in your planning, control, and decision making. Five methods of computing book depreciation are described below.

Straight-Line Depreciation Method

The straight-line depreciation method assigns an equal or even amount of depreciation expense over each year (or period) of the asset's useful life. The expense is thus spread evenly—or in a straight line—over the life of the asset. **Table 8–1** illustrates the straight-line depreciation method applied to a fixed asset costing $10,000 with a 5-year useful life and no salvage value. The depreciation expense would thus equal $2,000 for each of the 5 years ($10,000 divided by 5 equals $2,000 per year).

Table 8–2 illustrates the straight-line depreciation method applied to a fixed asset costing $10,000 with a 5-year useful life and a $1,000 salvage value. The depreciation expense would thus equal $1,800 for each year in this example, because we must leave $1,000 at the end of the asset's 5-year life ($10,000 less $1,000 equals $9,000 divided by 5 equals $1,800 per year.)

If the asset was acquired in the second half of the year, in some cases only a half-year of depreciation will be recognized in Year 1. If this is the case, the remaining half-year of depreciation will be recognized in Year 6, in order to fully depreciate the asset.

Table 8–1 Straight-Line Depreciation: 5-Year Life with No Salvage Value

	Cost (to Be Depreciated)	Depreciation Expense per Year*	Accumulated Depreciation (Reserve for Depreciation)	Net Remaining Undepreciated Cost (Net Book Value)
	$10,000			
Year 1		$2,000	$2,000	$8,000
Year 2		2,000	4,000	6,000
Year 3		2,000	6,000	4,000
Year 4		2,000	8,000	2,000
Year 5		2,000	10,000	-0-

*$10,000 divided by 5 years = $2,000 per year.

Table 8–2 Straight-Line Depreciation: 5-Year Life with Salvage Value

	Cost (to Be Depreciated)	Depreciation Expense per Year*	Accumulated Depreciation (Reserve for Depreciation)	Net Remaining Undepreciated Cost (Net Book Value)
	$10,000			$10,000
Year 1		$1,800	$1,800	8,200
Year 2		1,800	3,600	6,400
Year 3		1,800	5,400	4,600
Year 4		1,800	7,200	2,800
Year 5		1,800	9,000	1,000**

*$9,000 divided by 5 years = $1,800 per year.
**Remaining salvage value.

Accelerated Book Depreciation Methods

As the name would imply, accelerated book depreciation methods write off more depreciation in the first part of the asset's useful life. Thus, they "accelerate" recognizing depreciation expense. Three accelerated depreciation methods are briefly described here. Further details about the computations for each method appear in Appendix 8-A at the end of this chapter.

Sum-of-the-Year's Digits (SYD) Method

The Sum-of-the-Year's Digits (SYD) accelerated depreciation method computes depreciation by multiplying the depreciable cost of the asset by a fraction.

Double-Declining Balance (DDB) Method

The Double-Declining Balance (DDB) accelerated depreciation method computes depreciation by multiplying the asset's net book value at the beginning of each year by a constant percentage, or factor. In the case of DDB, the constant factor is twice the straight-line rate (thus "double-declining").

150% Declining Balance (150% DB) Method

The 150% Declining Balance (150% DB) accelerated depreciation method also computes depreciation by multiplying the asset's net book value at the beginning of each year by a constant percentage, or factor. In the case of 150% DB, however, the constant factor is half again or 150% of the straight-line rate.

Units of Service or Units of Production (UOP) Depreciation Method

The Units of Service or Units of Production (UOP) method computes depreciation by assigning a fixed amount of depreciation to each unit of service or output that is produced by equipment. "Units of Production" is a manufacturer's term for manufacturing, or producing, a product. "Units of Service" more properly describes the medical equipment providing services in healthcare organizations.

Instead of a useful life in years, equipment depreciated by the UOP method is assigned a fixed total amount of units of service. This fixed amount is the overall total for the life of the equipment. Then the number of units of service actually provided each year is depreciated.

COMPUTING TAX DEPRECIATION

The following discussion about tax depreciation is general in nature and is not to be utilized as tax advice. Any additional details about tax depreciation are beyond the scope of this text.

Overview

"Tax Depreciation," as previously defined, means depreciation that is computed for tax purposes and is reflected on the applicable tax returns of the organization. The methods of tax depreciation in effect at the time of this writing fall under the Modified Accelerated Cost Recovery System as described here.

Modified Accelerated Cost Recovery System (MACRS)

The Modified Accelerated Cost Recovery System (MACRS) is currently used to depreciate most business and investment property for tax purposes. MACRS presently consists of two depreciation systems, both of which are briefly described here.

General Depreciation System (GDS)

The General Depreciation System (GDS) is the method generally used under the U.S. Internal Revenue Service rules and regulations, although there are certain exceptions. GDS provides nine property classifications for useful life, including 3-, 5-, 7-, and 10-year property, and 15-, 20-, and 25-year property, along with residential rental property and nonresidential real property. For example, computers, calculators, and copiers fall into the 5-year property classification while office furniture and fixtures such as desks, files, and safes fall into the 7-year property classification.[1]

The GDS method allows double-declining balance, 150% declining balance, and the straight-line method of depreciation, depending upon what type of property is being depreciated. For example, nonfarm 3-, 5-, 7-, and 10-year property can use any of the three methods in most (but not all) circumstances.[2]

Alternative Depreciation System (ADS)

The Alternative Depreciation System (ADS) is required for particular properties including, for example, any tax-exempt use property.[3] ADS uses fixed ADS recovery periods, along with straight-line depreciation. ADS can also be used for certain eligible property, even though the property in question could come under GDS (certain restrictions apply).[4]

The tax law changes rapidly; thus, modifications to the tax depreciation methods described in this section may have been placed into effect at any point in time. More information can be obtained from the recent Internal Revenue Service Publication 946 "How to Depreciate Property."

 INFORMATION CHECKPOINT

What is needed?	A depreciation schedule that includes depreciation expense, reserve for depreciation, and net book value.
Where is it found?	With your supervisor or in the accounting and/or administration offices.
How is it used?	To reflect depreciation expense in order to complete the income statement.

 KEY TERMS

Book Value
Depreciation
FIFO
Inventory
Inventory Turnover
LIFO
Salvage Value
Useful Life (of an asset)

 DISCUSSION QUESTIONS

1. Do you or your supervisor have to deal with inventory? If so, please describe.
2. Have you ever had to count physical inventory? If so, please describe the process.
3. Do you or your supervisor have to deal with depreciation expense? If so, please describe.
4. Have you ever had to compute depreciation expense? If so, please describe the circumstances.

NOTES

1. Department of the Treasury, Internal Revenue Service. How to Depreciate Property. Publication 946 (Washington, DC: U.S. Government, 2011).
2. Ibid., Table 4-1.
3. Ibid., "Required Use of ADS."
4. Ibid., "Election of ADS."

A Further Discussion of Accelerated and Units of Service Depreciation Computations

ACCELERATED BOOK DEPRECIATION METHODS

As the name would imply, accelerated book depreciation methods write off more depreciation in the first part of the asset's useful life. Thus they "accelerate" recognizing depreciation expense. The computations of three accelerated depreciation methods are described in this appendix as follows.

Sum-of-the-Year's Digits (SYD) Method

The Sum-of-the-Year's Digits (SYD) accelerated depreciation method computes depreciation by multiplying the depreciable cost of the asset by a fraction. The fraction is the mechanism by which the acceleration is computed. It is calculated as follows:

- The numerator of the SYD fraction starts with the asset's useful life expressed in years and decreases by one each year thereafter. (Thus, for a 5-year useful life, the numerators are 5; 4; 3; 2; 1 respectively.)
- The denominator of the SYD fraction is the sum of the years' digits of the asset's life. (Thus, for a 5-year useful life, the sum of $5 + 4 + 3 + 2 + 1$ equals 15, which is the denominator.)

Table 8-A–1 illustrates the computation for each year. The depreciable cost of $10,000 is divided by 15 to arrive at $666.66. Thus, one-fifteenth or $666.66 is multiplied by 5 for the first year ($3,333 depreciation expense); by 4 for the second year ($2,667 depreciation expense), and so on.

Double-Declining Balance (DDB) Method

The Double-Declining Balance (DDB) accelerated depreciation method computes depreciation by multiplying the asset's net book value at the beginning of each year by a constant percentage, or factor. In the case of DDB, the constant factor is twice the straight-line rate (thus "double-declining").

Table 8-A–2 illustrates the computation for each year of a 5-year useful life with no salvage value. The double-declining factor is computed as follows:

- $10,000 cost of the fixed asset divided by the asset's useful life of 5 years equals 20% or a factor of 0.20.
- Multiply the 0.20 by 2 (or double) to arrive at the 0.40 double-declining factor.

Table 8-A–1 Sum-of-the-Years' Digits Depreciation: 5-Year Life with No Salvage Value

	Cost (to Be Depreciated)	Depreciation Computation				Accumulated Depreciation (Reserve for Depreciation)	Net Remaining Undepreciated Cost (Net Book Value)
		Depreciable Cost (for Computation)	×	Sum-of-the-Years' Digits* Fraction**	= Annual Depreciation Expense		
	$10,000						
Year 1		$10,000		5/15	$3,333	$3,333	$6,667
Year 2		10,000		4/15	2,667	6,000	4,000
Year 3		10,000		3/15	2,000	8,000	2,000
Year 4		10,000		2/15	1,333	9,333	667
Year 5		10,000		1/15	667	10,000	-0-

*Sum-of-the-Years' Digits = 15 = (1 + 2 + 3 + 4 + 5).
**One-fifteenth of $10,000 = $666.66.

Table 8-A-2 Double-Declining Balance Depreciation: 5-Year Life with No Salvage Value

Cost (to Be Depreciated)	Depreciation Computation			Accumulated Depreciation (Reserve for Depreciation)	Net Remaining Undepreciated Cost (Net Book Value)
	Carry-forward Book Value (for Computation)	Double Declining Balance Factor	Annual Depreciation Expense		
$10,000		x	=		
Year 1	$10,000	0.40*	$4,000	$4,000	$6,000
Year 2	6,000	0.40	2,400	6,400	3,600
Year 3	3,600	0.40	1,440	7,840	2,160
Year 4	2,160	S/L**	1,080	8,920	1,080
Year 5	1,296	S/L	1,080	10,000	-0-

*$10,000 divided by 5 years equals 0.20 times 2 (double) equals 0.40 factor.
**Double-Declining Balance changes to straight-line method when straight-line yields a higher depreciation. (See Table 8-A-3.)

The computation continues as follows:

- For Year 1, $10,000 times 0.40 equals $4,000 Year 1 depreciation expense. Accumulated depreciation for Year 1 also equals $4,000. The accumulated depreciation of $4,000 is subtracted from the $10,000 cost to arrive at the net remaining undepreciated cost, or net book value, of $6,000 at the end of Year 1.
- For Year 2, the factor of 0.40 is multiplied times the $6,000 net book value to equal $2,400 Year 2 depreciation expense. The Year 2 depreciation of $2,400 is added to the accumulated depreciation for a total of $6,400 ($4,000 plus $2,400 equals $6,400). The $6,400 is subtracted from the $10,000 cost to arrive at the net remaining undepreciated cost, or net book value, of $3,600 at the end of Year 2.
- For Year 3, the factor of 0.40 is multiplied times the $3,600 net book value to equal $1,440 Year 3 depreciation expense. The Year 3 depreciation of $1,440 is added to the accumulated depreciation for a total of $7,840 ($6,400 plus $1,440 equals $7,840). The $7,840 is subtracted from the $10,000 cost to arrive at the net remaining undepreciated cost, or net book value, of $2,160 at the end of Year 3.

The declining-balance method has a peculiarity in that it switches back to the straight-line method at the point where the straight-line computation yields a higher annual depreciation than does the declining-balance computation. Thus, as we arrive at Year 4 in this example, we must test the double-declining computation against the straight-line computation.

- To compute Year 4 double-declining, the factor of 0.40 is multiplied times the net book value of $2,160 to arrive at a DDB of $864.
- To compute a comparative Year 4 by the straight-line method, the remaining net book value of $2,160 is divided by the remaining years of useful life, which in this case would be 2 years. Thus $2,160 divided by 2 years equals straight-line depreciation per year for Year 4 and for Year 5 of $1,080 per year.
- The Year 4 straight-line method is greater ($1,080) than the Year 4 DDB ($864). Thus the switch to straight line is made for the remaining Year 4 and Year 5, as illustrated in Table 8-A–2.

The point at which the straight-line method overtakes the declining-balance method varies, of course, with the method and with the number of years of useful life. **Table 8-A–3** illustrates the first year for which the straight-line depreciation method gives an equal or greater deduction. (Note that the 5-year Property Class [or Useful Life Class] for 200% declining balance [or double-declining balance] shows the fourth year as the point at which the switch to straight line would be made. This is consistent with our example in Table 8-A–2.)

150% Declining Balance Method

The 150% Declining Balance (150% DB) accelerated depreciation method also computes depreciation by multiplying the asset's net book value at the beginning of each year by a constant percentage, or factor. In the case of 150% DB, however, the constant factor is half again or 150% of the straight-line rate.

Table 8-A–3 Declining Balance Rates by Property Class

Property Class	Method	Declining Balance Rate	Year*
3-year	200% DB	66.667%	3rd
5-year	200% DB	40.000%	4th
7-year	200% DB	28.571%	5th
10-year	200% DB	20.00%	7th
15-year	150% DB	10.0	7th
20-year	150% DB	7.5	9th

*Indicates the first year for which the straight-line depreciation method gives an equal or greater deduction.
Reproduced from Internal Revenue Service, Publication 946, "How to Depreciate Property," p. 43.

Table 8-A–4 illustrates the computation for each year of a 5-year useful life with no salvage value. The 150% DB factor is computed as follows:

- $10,000 cost of the fixed asset divided by the asset's useful life of 5 years equals 20% or a factor of 0.20.
- Multiply the 0.20 by 150% (or half again) to arrive at the 0.30 150% DB factor.

The 150% DB computation follows the same pattern as the double-declining example just described, with two exceptions:

- The factor applied is 0.30 per year, as just explained.
- The 150% DB switches to straight line in Year 3 instead of Year 4 as in the previous example.

Units of Service or Units of Production (UOP) Depreciation Method

The Units of Service or Units of Production (UOP) method computes depreciation by assigning a fixed amount of depreciation to each unit of service or output that is produced by equipment. The "Units of Production" is a manufacturer's term for manufacturing, or producing, a product. "Units of Service" more properly describes the medical equipment providing services in healthcare organizations.

Instead of a useful life in years, equipment depreciated by the UOP method is assigned a fixed total amount of units of service. This fixed amount is the overall total for the life of the equipment. Then the number of units of service actually provided each year is depreciated.

Table 8-A–5 illustrates the UOP method. The depreciation per unit of service is computed as follows:

- The total depreciable units of service over 5 years are determined to be 5,000 units. The equipment cost to be depreciated of $10,000 is divided by 5,000 units to arrive at depreciation of $2.00 per unit.
- Units of Service in Year 1 total 1,000. Thus 1,000 units times $2.00 per unit equals $2,000 Year 1 depreciation.

Table 8-A-4 150% Declining Balance Depreciation: 5-Year Life with No Salvage Value

		Depreciation Computation				
Cost (to Be Depreciated)	Carry-Forward Book Value (for Computation)	×	150% Declining Balance Factor	= Annual Depreciation Expense	Accumulated Depreciation (Reserve for Depreciation)	Net Remaining Undepreciated Cost (Net Book Value)
$10,000						
Year 1	$10,000		0.30*	$3,000	$3,000	$7,000
Year 2	7,000		0.30	2,100	5,100	4,900
Year 3	4,900		S/L**	1,663	6,733	3,267
Year 4	3,267		S/L	1,633	8,366	1,634
Year 5	1,634		S/L	1,634	10,000	-0-

*$10,000 divided by 5 years equals 0.20 times half again (150%) equals 0.30 factor.

**150% Declining Balance changes to straight-line method when straight-line method yields a higher depreciation.

Table 8-A–5 Units of Service (Units of Production) Depreciation: 5-Years of Service with No Salvage Value

Depreciation Computation

Cost (to Be Depreciated)	Units of Service per Year	×	Depreciation per Unit	=	Annual Depreciation Expense	Accumulated Depreciation (Reserve for Depreciation)	Net Remaining Undepreciated Cost (Net Book Value)
$10,000							
Year 1	$1,000		$2.00*		$2,000	$2,000	$8,000
Year 2	900		2.00		1,800	3,800	6,200
Year 3	800		2.00		1,600	5,400	4,600
Year 4	1,100		2.00		2,200	7,600	2,400
Year 5	1,200		2.00		2,400	10,000	-0-
Total Units	5,000						

*$10,000 divided by total units (5,000) equals depreciation per unit of $2.00.

- Units of Service in Year 2 total 900. Thus 900 units times $2.00 per unit equals $1,800 Year 2 depreciation.

The computation continues in this manner until the total 5,000 units of service are exhausted. The equipment is then fully depreciated.

Staffing: The Manager's Responsibility

STAFFING REQUIREMENTS

In most businesses, a position is filled if the employee works five days a week, generally Monday through Friday. But in health care, many positions must be filled, or covered, all seven days of the week. Furthermore, in most businesses, a position is filled for that day if the employee works an eight-hour day—from 9:00 to 5:00, for example. But in health care, many positions must also be filled, or covered, 24 hours a day. The patients need care on Saturday and Sunday, as well as Monday through Friday, and patients need care around the clock, 24 hours a day.

Thus, healthcare employees work in shifts. The shifts are often eight-hour shifts, because three such shifts times eight hours apiece equals 24-hour coverage. Some facilities have gone to 12-hour shifts. In their case, two 12-hour shifts equal 24-hour coverage. The manager is responsible for seeing that an employee is present and working for each position and for every shift required for that position. Therefore, it is necessary to understand and use the staffing measurement known as the full-time equivalent (FTE). Two different approaches are used to compute FTEs: the annualizing method and the scheduled-position method. Full-time equivalent is a measure to express the equivalent of an employee (annualized) or a position (staffed) for the full time required. We examine both methods in this chapter.

FTEs FOR ANNUALIZING POSITIONS

Why Annualize?

Annualizing is necessary because each employee that is eligible for benefits (such as vacation days) will not be on duty for the full number of hours paid for by the

Progress Notes

After completing this chapter, you should be able to

1. Understand the difference between productive time and nonproductive time.
2. Understand computing full-time equivalents to annualize staff positions.
3. Understand computing full-time equivalents to fill a scheduled position.
4. Tie cost to staffing.

organization. Annualizing thus allows the full cost of the position to be computed through a burden approach. In the burden approach, the net hours desired are inflated, or burdened, in order to arrive at the gross number of paid hours that will be needed to obtain the desired number of net hours on duty from the employee.

Productive Versus Nonproductive Time

Productive time actually equates to the employee's net hours on duty when performing the functions in his or her job description. Nonproductive time is paid-for time when the employee is not on duty: that is, not producing and therefore "nonproductive." Paid-for vacation days, holidays, personal leave days, and/or sick days are all nonproductive time.[1]

Exhibit 9–1 illustrates productive time (net days when on duty) versus nonproductive time (additional days paid for but not worked). In Exhibit 9–1, Bob, the security guard, is

Exhibit 9–1 Metropolis Clinic Security Guard Staffing

The Metropolis laboratory area has its own security guard from 8:30 AM to 4:30 PM seven days per week. Bob, the security guard for the clinic area, is a full-time Metropolis employee.

He works as follows:

1. The area assigned to Bob is covered seven days per week for every week of the year. Therefore,

Total days in business year	364	
2. Bob doesn't work on weekends	(104)	
(2 days per week × 52 weeks = 104 days)		
Bob's paid days total per year amount to	260	
(5 days per week × 52 weeks = 260 days)		

3. During the year Bob gets paid for:

Holidays	9
Sick days	7
Vacation days	7
Education days	2
	(25)

4. Net paid days Bob actually works   235

Jim, a police officer, works part time as a security guard for the Metropolis laboratory area. Jim works on the days when Bob is off, as follows:

Weekends	104	
Bob's holidays	9	
Bob's sick days	7	
Bob's vacation days	7	
Bob's education days	2	
	129	
5. Paid days Jim works		129
6. Total days lab area security guard position is covered		364

paid for 260 days per year (total paid days) but works for only 235 days per year. The 235 days are productive time, and the remaining 25 days of holidays, sick days, vacation days, and education days are nonproductive time.

FTE for Annualizing Positions Defined

For purposes of annualizing positions, the definition of FTE is as follows: the equivalent of one full-time employee paid for one year, including both productive and nonproductive (vacation, sick, holiday, education, etc.) time. Two employees each working half-time for one year would be the same as one FTE.

Staffing Calculations to Annualize Positions

Exhibit 9–2 contains a two-step process to perform the staffing calculation by the annualizing method. The first step computes the net paid days worked. In this step, the number of paid days per year is first arrived at; then paid days not worked are deducted to arrive at net paid days worked. The second step of the staffing calculation converts

---

Exhibit 9–2 Basic Calculation for Annualizing Master Staffing Plan

Step 1: How Many Net Paid Days Are Worked?
  (a) A *business year* has 364 days.
  (b) In this example the employee works five days per week. The other two days off are not paid for. Thus two days off per week times 52 weeks equals 104 *non-paid days.*
  (c) Therefore the number of *paid days per year* equals 364 less 104, or 260 days.
  (d) But not all paid days per year are worked. In this example each employee (RN, LPN, & Nurse Assistant [NA]) receives 35 *personal leave days.* (The personal leave days are intended to include holidays, sick leave, and vacation days.)
  (e) In addition these employees are entitled to *continuing professional education (CPE) days.* These are also paid days not worked, as follows: RNs = 5 days; LPNs = 3 days; NAs = 2 days.
  (f) Therefore the *net paid days worked* are as follows:

$$RN = 260 \text{ days } (35) \ (5) = 220$$
$$LPN = 260 \text{ days } (35) \ (3) = 222$$
$$NA = 260 \text{ days } (35) \ (3) = 223$$

Step 2: How Are Net Paid Days Worked Converted to a Factor?
The factor is calculated by dividing total days in the business year (364) by the net paid days worked, as follows:

$$RN = 364/220 = 1.6545$$
$$LPN = 364/222 = 1.6396$$
$$NA = 364/223 = 1.6323$$

Courtesy of J.J. Baker and R.W. Baker, Dallas, Texas.

Exhibit 9–3 Master Staffing Plan for Nursing Unit

8-Hour Shifts	RNs	LPNs	NAs
Day Shift	3	1	6
Evening Shift	2	2	5
Night Shift	1	2	2
24-Hour Total	6	5	13

Courtesy of J.J. Baker and R.W. Baker, Dallas, Texas.

the net paid days worked to a factor. In the example in Exhibit 9–2, the factor averages out to about 1.6.

This calculation is for a 24-hour around-the-clock staffing schedule. Thus, the 364 in the step 2 formula equates to a 24-hour staffing expectation. **Exhibit 9–3** illustrates such a master staffing plan.

NUMBER OF EMPLOYEES REQUIRED TO FILL A POSITION: ANOTHER WAY TO CALCULATE FTEs

Why Calculate by Position?

The calculation of number of FTEs by the scheduled-position method—in other words, to fill a position—is used in controlling, planning, and decision making. **Exhibit 9–4** sets out the schedule and the FTE computation. A summarized explanation of the calculation in Exhibit 9–4 is as follows. One full-time employee (as shown) works 40 hours per week. One 8-hour shift per day times 7 days per week equals 56 hours on duty. Therefore, to cover 7 days per week, or 56 hours, requires 1.4 times a 40-hour employee (56 hours divided by 40 hours equals 1.4), or 1.4 FTEs.

Exhibit 9–4 Staffing Requirements Example

Emergency Department Scheduling for 8-Hour Shifts:

Position:	Shift 1 Day	Shift 2 Evening	Shift 3 Night	=	24-Hour Scheduling Total
Emergency Room Intake	1	1	1	=	3 8-hour shifts
To Cover Position 7 Days per Week Equals FTEs of:	1.4	1.4	1.4	=	4.2 FTEs

One full-time employee works 40 hours per week. One 8-hour shift per day times 7 days per week equals 56 hours on duty. Therefore, to cover 7 days per week or 56 hours requires 1.4 times a 40-hour employee (56 hours divided by 40 hours equals 1.4), or 1.4 FTEs.

Staffing Calculations to Fill Scheduled Positions

The term "staffing," as used here, means the assigning of staff to fill scheduled positions. The staffing measure used to compute coverage is also called the FTE. It measures what proportion of one single full-time employee is required to equate the hours required (i.e., full-time equivalent) for a particular position. For example, the cast room has to be staffed 24 hours a day, 7 days a week because it supports the emergency room and therefore has to provide service at any time. In this example, the employees are paid for an 8-hour shift. The three shifts required to fill the position for 24 hours are called the day shift (7:00 AM to 3:00 PM), the evening shift (3:00 PM to 11:00 PM), and the night shift (11:00 PM to 7:00 AM).

One 8-hour shift times 5 days per week equals a 40-hour work week. One 40-hour work week times 52 weeks equals a person-year of 2,080 hours. Therefore, one person-year of 2,080 hours equals a full-time position filled for one full year. This measure is our baseline.

It takes seven days to fill the day shift cast room position from Monday through Sunday, as required. Seven days is 140% of five days (seven divided by five equals 140%), or, expressed another way, is 1.4. The FTE for the day shift cast room position is 1.4. If a seven-day schedule is required, the FTE will be 1.4.

This method of computing FTEs uses a basic 40-hour work week (or a 37-hour work week, or whatever is the case in the particular institution). The method computes a figure that will be necessary to fill the position for the desired length of time, measuring this figure against the standard basic work week. For example, if the standard work week is 40 hours and a receptionist position is to be filled for just 20 hours per week, then the FTE for that position would be 0.5 FTE (20 hours to fill the position divided by a 40-hour standard work week). **Table 9–1** illustrates the difference between a standard work year at 40 hours per week and a standard work year at 37.5 hours per week.

Table 9–1 Calculations to Staff the Operating Room

Job Position	No. of FTEs	No. of Annual Hours Paid at 2,080 Hours*	No. of Annual Hours Paid at 1,950 Hours**
Supervisor	2.2	4,576	4,290
Techs	3.0	6,240	5,850
RNs	7.7	16,016	15,015
LPNs	1.2	2,496	2,340
Aides, orderlies	1.0	2,080	1,950
Clerical	1.2	2,496	2,340
Totals	16.3	33,904	31,785

*40 hours per week × 52 weeks = 2,080.

**37.5 hours per week × 52 weeks = 1,950.

TYING COST TO STAFFING

In the case of the annualizing method, the factor of 1.6 already has this organization's vacation, holiday, sick pay, and other nonproductive days accounted for in the formula (review Exhibit 9–2 to check out this fact). Therefore, this factor is multiplied times the base hourly rate (the net rate) paid to compute cost.

In the case of the scheduled-position method, however, the FTE figure of 1.4 will be multiplied times a burdened hourly rate. The burden on the hourly rate reflects the vacation, holiday, sick pay, and other nonproductive days accounted for in the formula (review Exhibit 9–4 to see the difference). The scheduled-position method is often used in the forecasting of new programs and services.

Actual cost is attached to staffing in the books and records through a subsidiary journal and a basic transaction record (both discussed in a preceding chapter). **Exhibit 9–5** illustrates a subsidiary journal in which employee hours worked for a one-week period are recorded. Both regular and overtime hours are noted. The hourly rate, base pay, and overtime premiums are noted, and gross earnings are computed. Deductions are noted and deducted from gross earnings to compute the net pay for each employee in the final column.

Exhibit 9–6 illustrates a time card for one employee for a week-long period. This type of record, whether it is generated by a time clock or an electronic entry, is the original record upon which the payroll process is based. Thus, it is considered a basic transaction record. In this example, time in and time out are recorded daily. The resulting regular and overtime hours are recorded separately for each day worked. Although the appearance of the time card may vary, and it may be recorded within a computer instead of on a hard copy, the essential transaction is the same: this recording of daily time is where the payroll process begins.

Exhibit 9–7 represents an emergency department staffing report. Actual productive time is shown in columns 1 and 2, with regular time in column 1 and overtime in column 2. Nonproductive time is shown in column 3, and columns 1, 2, and 3 are totaled to arrive at column 4, labeled "Total [actual] Hours." The final actual figure is the FTE figure in column 5.

The report is biweekly and thus is for a 2-week period. The standard work week amounts to 40 hours, so the biweekly standard work period amounts to 80 hours. Note the first line item, which is for the manager of the emergency department nursing service. The actual hours worked in column 4 amount to 80, and the actual FTE figure in column 5 is 1.0. We can tell from this line item that the second method of computing FTEs—the FTE computation to fill scheduled positions—has been used in this case. Columns 7 through 9 report budgeted time and FTEs, and columns 10 through 12 report the variance in actual from budget. The budget and variance portions of this report structure will be more thoroughly discussed in the chapter about operating budgets.

In summary, hours worked and pay rates are essential ingredients of staffing plans, budgets, and forecasts. Appropriate staffing is the responsibility of the manager.

Exhibit 9–5 Example of a Payroll Register

Metropolis Health System
Payroll Register

Week Ended   June 10, ____

Employee No.	Name	Hours Worked			Rate	Base Pay	Overtime Premiums	Gross Earnings	Deductions			Net Pay
		Regular	Overtime	Total					Federal Income Tax	Social Security	Medicare Tax	
1071	J.F. Green	40	2	42	14.00	588.00	14.00	602.00	90.30	37.32	8.73	465.65
1084	C.B. Brown	40		40	14.00	560.00		560.00	84.00	34.72	8.62	432.66
1090	K.D. Grey	40		40	10.00	400.00		400.00	60.00	24.80	6.16	309.04
1092	R.N. Black	40	5	45	10.00	450.00	25.00	475.00	71.25	29.45	6.89	367.41

Courtesy of Resource Group, Ltd., Dallas, Texas.

Exhibit 9–6 Example of a Time Record

Metropolis Health System
Time Card

Employee ___J.F. Green___   No. ___1071___

Department ___3___   Week ending ___June 10___

Day	Regular In	Regular Out	Regular In	Regular Out	Overtime In	Overtime Out	Hours Regular	Hours Overtime
Monday	8:00	12:01	1:02	5:04			8	
Tuesday	7:56	12:00	12:59	5:03	6:00	8:00	8	2
Wednesday	7:57	12:02	12:58	5:00			8	
Thursday	8:00	12:00	1:00	5:01			8	
Friday	7:59	12:01	1:01	5:02			8	
Saturday								
Sunday								
Total regular hours							40	
Total overtime								2

Courtesy of Resource Group, Ltd., Dallas, Texas.

Exhibit 9–7 Comparative Hours Staffing Report

PR 2301

Biweekly Comparative Hours Report
for the Payroll Period Ending Sept. 20, ____

Dept. No. 3421
Emergency Room

	Job Code	Actual Productive Regular Time (1)	Overtime (2)	Non-Productive (3)	Total Hours (4)	FTEs (5)	Budget Productive (6)	Non-Productive (7)	Total Hours (8)	FTEs (9)	Variance Number Hours (10)	Number FTEs (11)	Percent (12)
Mgr Nursing Service	11075	80	0	0	80	1.0	69.8	10.2	80	1	0	0	0
Supv Charge Nurse	11403	383.2	0.1	79	462.3	5.8	456	64	520	6.5	57.7	0.7	11.1%
Medical Assistant	12007	6.2	0	0	6.2	0.1	0	0	0	0	-6.2	-0.1	100.0%
Staff RN	13401	2010.5	32.8	285.8	2329.1	29.1	2012.8	240.8	2253.6	28.2	-75.5	-0.9	-3.4%
Relief Charge Nurse	13403	81.9	4.3	0	86.2	1.1	0	0	0	0	-86.2	-1.1	100.0%
Orderly/Transporter	15483	203.8	38	20	261.8	3.3	279.8	35.3	315.1	3.9	53.3	0.6	16.9%
ER Tech	22483	244.6	27.5	67.9	340	4.3	336.2	34.5	370.7	4.6	30.7	0.3	8.3%
Secretary	22730	58.1	0	0	58.1	0.7	50.5	5.9	56.4	0.7	-1.7	0.0	-3.0%
Unit Coordinator	22780	555.1	35.6	74.9	665.6	8.3	505.4	53.8	559.2	7	-106.4	-1.3	-19.0%
Preadmission Testing Clerk	22818		6.5	0	6.5	0.1	0	0	0	0	-6.5	-0.1	100.0%
Patient Registrar	22873	617.5	78.6	105.7	801.8	10.0	718.2	57.8	776	9.7	-25.8	-0.3	-3.3%
Lead Patient Registrar	22874	0	0	0	0	0.0	73.8	6.2	80	1	80.0	1.0	100.0%
Patient Registrar (weekend)	22876	36.7	0	0	36.7	0.5	0	0	0	0	-36.7	-0.5	100.0%
Overtime	29998	0	0	0	0	0.0	38.5	0	38.5	0.5	38.5	0.5	100.0%
Department Totals		4277.6	223.4	633.3	5134.3	64.3	4541	508.5	5049.5	63.1	-84.8	-1.2	0.0

Courtesy of Resource Group, Ltd., Dallas, Texas.

INFORMATION CHECKPOINT

What is needed?	The original record of time and the subsidiary journal summary.
Where is it found?	The original record can be found at any check-in point; the subsidiary journal summary can be found with a supervisor in charge of staffing for a unit, division, and so on.
How is it used?	It is reviewed as historical evidence of results achieved. It is also reviewed by managers seeking to perform future staffing in an efficient manner.

KEY TERMS

Full-Time Equivalents (FTEs)
Nonproductive Time
Productive Time
Staffing

DISCUSSION QUESTIONS

1. Are you or your immediate supervisor responsible for staffing?
2. If so, do you use a computerized program?
3. Do you believe a computerized program is better? If so, why?
4. Does your organization report time as "productive" and "nonproductive"?
5. If not, do you believe it should? What do you believe the benefits would be?

NOTE

1. J. J. Baker, *Prospective Payment for Long-Term Care: An Annual Guide* (Gaithersburg, MD: Aspen Publishers, Inc., 1999).

Report
and Measure
Financial Results

Reporting as a Tool

UNDERSTANDING THE MAJOR REPORTS

It is not our intention to convert you into an accountant. Therefore, our discussion of the major financial reports will center on the concept of each report and not on the precise accounting entries that are necessary to make the statement balance. The first concept we will discuss is that of cash versus accrual accounting. In cash basis accounting, a transaction does not enter the books until cash is either received or paid out. In accrual accounting, revenue is recorded when it is earned—not when payment is received—and expenses are recorded when they are incurred—not when they are paid.[1] Most healthcare organizations operate on the accrual basis.

There are four basic financial statements. You can think of them as a set. They include the balance sheet, the statement of revenue and expense, the statement of fund balance or net worth, and the statement of cash flows. The four major reports we are about to examine—the financial statements—have been prepared using the accrual method.

BALANCE SHEET

The balance sheet records what an organization owns, what it owes, and basically, what it is worth (although the terminology uses *fund balance* rather than *worth* or *equity* for nonprofit organizations). The balance sheet balances. That is, the total of what the organization owns—its assets—equals the combined total of what the organization owes and what it is worth—its liabilities and

Progress Notes

After completing this chapter, you should be able to

1. Review a balance sheet and understand its components.
2. Review a statement of revenue and expense and understand its components.
3. Understand the basic concept of cash flows.
4. Know what a subsidiary report is.

its net worth, or its fund balance. This balancing of the elements in the balance sheet can be visualized as

$$\text{Assets} = \text{Liabilities} + \text{Net Worth/Fund Balance}$$

Another characteristic of the balance sheet is that it is stated at a particular point in time. A common analogy is that a balance sheet is like a snapshot: it freezes the figures and reports them as of a certain date.

Exhibit 10–1 illustrates these concepts. A single date (not a period of time) is at the top of the statement (this is the snapshot). The clinic balance sheet reflects two years in two columns, with the most current date on the left and the prior period on the right. Total assets for the current left-hand column amount to $963,000. Total liabilities and fund balance also amount to $963,000; the balance sheet balances. The total liabilities amount to $545,000 and the total fund balances amount to $418,000. The total of the two, of course, makes up the $963,000 shown at the bottom of the statement.

Three types of assets are shown: current assets; property, plant, and equipment; and other assets. Current assets are supposed to be convertible into cash within one year—thus "current" assets. Property, plant, and equipment, however, represent long-term assets. Other assets represent noncurrent items.

Two types of liabilities are shown: current liabilities and long-term debt. Current liabilities are those expected to be paid within the next year—thus "current" liabilities. Long-term debt is not due within a year. (In fact, most long-term debt is due over a period of many years.) The amount of long-term debt that will be due within the next year ($52,000) has been subtracted from the long-term debt amount and has been moved up into the current liabilities section. This treatment is consistent with the concept of "current."

Once again, because our intent is not to make an accountant of you, we will not be discussing generally accepted accounting principles (GAAP) either. Financial accounting and the resulting reports intended for third-party use must be prepared in accordance with GAAP. However, managerial accounting for internal purposes in the organization does not necessarily have to adhere to GAAP. One of the requirements of GAAP is that unrestricted fund balances be separated from restricted fund balances on the statements, so you see two appropriate line items (restricted and unrestricted) in the fund balance section.

We should also mention that the standards underlying generally accepted accounting principles within the United States are produced by the Financial Accounting Standards Board (FASB). Sometime in the (probable) near future U.S. publicly held companies may be required to adopt certain international accounting standards as produced by the International Accounting Standards Board (IASB). Benefits would include global comparability and consistency in accounting standards and financial reports while barriers to such adoption include funding, maintenance, application, and governance.[2] Any further discussion of these accounting issues is beyond the scope of this text.

STATEMENT OF REVENUE AND EXPENSE

The formula for a very condensed statement of revenue and expense would look like this:

$$\text{Operating Revenue} - \text{Operating Expenses} = \text{Operating Income}$$

Exhibit 10–1 Westside Clinic Balance Sheet

Assets		December 31, 20×4		December 31, 20×3
Current Assets				
Cash and cash equivalents		$190,000		$145,000
Accounts receivable (net)		250,000		300,000
Inventories		25,000		20,000
Prepaid Insurance		5,000		3,000
Total Current Assets		$470,000		$468,000
Property, Plant, and Equipment				
Land	$100,000		$100,000	
Buildings (net)	0		0	
Equipment (net)	260,000		300,000	
Net Property, Plant, and Equipment		360,000		400,000
Other Assets				
Investments	$133,000		$32,000	
Total Other Assets		133,000		32,000
Total Assets		$963,000		$900,000
Liabilities and Fund Balance				
Current Liabilities				
Current maturities of long-term debt	$52,000		$48,000	
Accounts payable and accrued expenses	293,000		302,000	
Total Current Liabilities		$345,000		$350,000
Long-Term Debt	$252,000		$300,000	
Less Current Maturities of Long-Term Debt	−52,000		−48,000	
Net Long-Term Debt		200,000		252,000
Total Liabilities		$545,000		$602,000
Fund Balances				
Unrestricted fund balance	$418,000		$298,000	
Restricted fund balance	0		0	
Total Fund Balances		418,000		298,000
Total Liabilities and Fund Balance		$963,000		$900,000

A statement of revenue and expense covers a period of time (rather than one single date or point in time). The concept is that revenue, or inflow, less expenses, or outflow, results in an excess of revenue over expenses if the year has been good, or perhaps an excess of expenses over revenue (resulting in a loss) if the year has been bad.

Exhibit 10–2 sets out the result of operations for two years, with the most current period in the left column. If the balance sheet is a snapshot, then the statement of revenue and expenses is a diary, because it is a record of transactions over the period of a year. Operating revenues and operating expenses are set out first, with the result being income from operations of $115,000 ($2,000,000 less $1,885,000). Then other transactions are reported; in this case, interest income of $5,000 under the heading "Nonoperating Gains (Losses)." The total of $120,000 ($115,000 plus $5,000) is reported as an increase in fund balance. This figure carries forward to the next major report, known as the statement of changes in fund balance.

Exhibit 10–2 Westside Clinic Statement of Revenue and Expenses

	For the Year Ending	
Revenue	December 31, 20X4	December 31, 20X3
Net Patient Service Revenue	$2,000,000	$1,850,000
Total Operating Revenue	$2,000,000	$1,850,000
Operating Expenses		
Medical/surgical services	$600,000	$575,000
Therapy services	860,000	806,000
Other professional services	80,000	75,000
Support services	220,000	220,000
General services	65,000	60,000
Depreciation	40,000	40,000
Interest	20,000	24,000
Total Operating Expenses	1,885,000	1,800,000
Income from Operations	$115,000	$50,000
Nonoperating Gains (Losses)		
Interest Income	$5,000	$2,000
Net Nonoperating Gains	5,000	2,000
Revenue and Gains in Excess of Expenses and Losses	$120,000	$52,000
Increase in Unrestricted Fund Balance	$120,000	$52,000

STATEMENT OF CHANGES IN FUND BALANCE/NET WORTH

Remember that our formula for a basic statement of revenue and expense looked like this:

$$\text{Operating Revenue} - \text{Operating Expenses} = \text{Operating Income}$$

The excess of revenue over expenses flows back into equity or fund balance through the mechanism of the statement of fund balance/net worth. **Exhibit 10–3** shows a balance at the first of the year, then it adds the excess of revenue over expenses (in the amount of $115,000) plus some interest income (in the amount of $5,000) to arrive at the balance at the end of the year.

If you refer back to the balance sheet, you will see the $418,000 balance at the end of the year appearing on it. So we can think of the balance sheet, the statement of revenue and expenses, and the statement of changes in fund balance/net worth as locked together, with the statement of changes in fund balance being the mechanism that links the other two statements.

But there is one more major report—the statement of cash flows—and we will examine it next.

STATEMENT OF CASH FLOWS

To perceive why a statement of cash flows is necessary, we must first revisit the concept of accrual basis accounting. If cash is not paid or received when revenues and expenses are entered on the books—the usual situation in accrual accounting—what happens? The other side of the entry for revenues is accounts receivable, and the other side of the entry for expenses is accounts payable. These accounts rest on the balance sheet and have not yet been turned into cash. Another characteristic of accrual accounting is the recognition of depreciation. A capital asset—a piece of equipment, for example—is purchased for $20,000. It has a usable life of five years. So depreciation expense is recognized in each of the five years until the $20,000 is used up, or depreciated. (Land is an exception to this rule: it is never depreciated.) Depreciation is recognized within each year as an expense, but it does not represent a cash expense. This is a concept that now enters into the statement of cash flows.

Exhibit 10–3 Westside Clinic Statement of Changes in Fund Balance

	For the Year Ending	
Statement of Changes in Fund Balance	December 31, 20×4	December 31, 20×3
Balance First of Year	$298,000	$246,000
Revenue in Excess of Expenses	115,000	50,000
Interest Income	5,000	2,000
Balance End of Year	$418,000	$298,000

Exhibit 10–4 Westside Clinic Statement of Cash Flows

Statement of Cash Flows	For the Year Ending	
	December 31, 20×4	December 31, 20×3
Operating Activities		
Income from Operations	$115,000	$50,000
Adjustments to reconcile income from operations to net cash flows from operating activities		
Depreciation and amortization	40,000	40,000
Interest expense	20,000	24,000
Changes in asset and liability accounts		
Patient accounts receivable	50,000	−250,000
Inventories	−5,000	−5,000
Prepaid expenses and other assets	−2,000	−1,000
Accounts payable and accrued expenses	−9,000	185,000
Net Cash Flow from Operating Activities	$209,000	$43,000
Cash Flows from Noncapital Financing Activities	0	0
Cash Flows from Capital and Related Financing Activities		
Acquisition of equipment	$ 0	$ (300,000)
Proceeds from loan for equipment	0	300,000
Interest paid on long-term obligations	−20,000	0
Repayment of long-term obligations	−48,000	0
Net Cash Flows from Capital and Related Financing Activities	−68,000	0
Cash Flows from Investing Activities		
Interest income received	$5,000	$2,000
Investments purchased (net)	−101,000	0
Net Cash Flows from Investing Activities	−96,000	2,000
Net Increase (Decrease) in Cash and Cash Equivalents	$45,000	$45,000
Cash and Cash Equivalents, Beginning of Year	145,000	100,000
Cash and Cash Equivalents, End of Year	$190,000	$145,000

Exhibit 10–4 presents the current period cash flow. In effect, this statement takes the accrual basis statements and converts them to a cash flow for the period through a series of reconciling adjustments that account for the noncash amounts.

Understanding the cash/noncash concept makes sense of this statement. The starting point is the income from operations, the subtotal from the statement of revenue and expense. Depreciation and interest are added back, and changes in asset and liability accounts, both positive and negative, are recognized. These adjustments account for operating activities. Next, capital and related financing activities are addressed, then investing activities are adjusted. The result is a net increase in cash and cash equivalents of $45,000 in our example. This figure is added to the cash balance at the beginning of the year ($145,000) to arrive at the cash balance at the end of the year ($190,000). Now refer back to the balance sheet, and you will find the cash balance is indeed $190,000. So the fourth major report—the statement of cash flows—interlocks with the other three major reports.

SUBSIDIARY REPORTS

The subsidiary reports are just that; subsidiary to the major reports. These reports support the major reports by providing more detail. For example, patient service revenue totals on the statement of revenue and expenses are often expanded in more detail on a subsidiary report. The same thing is true of operating expense. These reports are called "schedules" instead of "statements"—a sure sign that they are subsidiary reports.

SUMMARY

The four major reports fit together; each makes its own contribution to the whole. A checklist for balance sheet review (**Exhibit 10–5**) and a checklist for review of the statement of revenue and expense (**Exhibit 10–6**) are provided.

Exhibit 10–5 Checklist for the Balance Sheet Review

1. What is the date on the balance sheet?
2. Are there large discrepancies in balances between the prior year and the current year?
3. Did total assets increase over the prior year?
4. Did current assets increase, decrease, or stay about the same?
5. Did current liabilities increase, decrease, or stay about the same?
6. Did land, plant, and equipment increase or decrease significantly over the prior year?
7. Did long-term debt increase or decrease significantly over the prior year?

Exhibit 10–6 Checklist for Review of the Statement of Revenue and Expense

1. What is the period reported on the statement of revenue and expense?
2. Is it one year or a shorter period? If it is a shorter period, why is that?
3. Are there large discrepancies in balances between the prior year operations and the current year operations?
4. Did total operating revenue increase over the prior year?
5. Did total operating expenses increase, decrease, or stay about the same? Is any particular line item unusually large or small?
6. Did income from operations increase, decrease, or stay about the same?
7. Are there unusual nonoperating gains or losses?
8. Did the current year result in an excess of revenue over expense? Is it as much as the prior year?
9. Did long-term debt increase or decrease significantly over the prior year?

INFORMATION CHECKPOINT

What is needed?	A set of financial statements, ideally containing the four major reports plus subsidiary reports for additional detail.
Where is it found?	Possibly in the files of your supervisor or in the finance office or in the office of the administrator.
How is it used?	Study the financial statement to see how they fit together; use the checklists included in this chapter to assist in your review. Understanding how the statements work will give you another valuable managerial tool.

 KEY TERMS

Accrual Basis Accounting
Balance Sheet
Cash Basis Accounting
Statement of Cash Flows
Statement of Fund Balance/Net Worth
Statement of Revenue and Expense
Subsidiary Reports

 DISCUSSION QUESTIONS

1. Can you give an example of an asset? A liability?
2. Does the concept of revenue less expense equaling an increase in equity or fund balance make sense to you? If not, why not?
3. Are you familiar with the current maturity of long-term debt? What example of it can you give in your own life (either at work or at home)?
4. Do you get a chance to review financial statements at your place of work? Would you like to? Why?

NOTES

1. S. A. Finkler, et al., *Essentials of Cost Accounting for Health Care Organizations*, 3rd ed. (Sudbury MA: Jones & Bartlett Publishers, 2007).
2. K. Tysiac, "Still in Flux: Future of IFRS in U.S. Remains Unclear After SEC report" *Journal of Accountancy* (September 2012). *Source:* www.journalofaccountancy.com/Issues /2012/Sep/20126059.htm

Financial and Operating Ratios as Performance Measures

THE IMPORTANCE OF RATIOS

Ratios are convenient and uniform measures that are widely adopted in healthcare financial management. They are important because they are so widely used, especially because they are used for credit analysis. But a ratio is only a number. It has to be considered within the context of the operation. There is another caveat: ratio analysis should be conducted as a comparative analysis. In other words, one ratio standing alone with nothing to compare it with does not mean very much. When interpreting ratios, the differences between periods must be considered, and the reasons for such differences should be sought. It is a good practice to compare results with equivalent computations from outside the organization—regional figures from similar institutions would be a good example of such outside sources. Caution and good managerial judgment must always be exercised when working with ratios.

Financial ratios basically pull together two elements of the financial statements: one expressed as the numerator and one as the denominator. To calculate a ratio, divide the bottom number (the denominator) into the top number (the numerator). The Mini-Case Study that is entitled "Comparative Analysis (Financial Ratios and Benchmarking) Helps Turn Around a Hospital" uses financial ratios as indicators of financial position. We highly recommend that you spend time with this Case Study, as it will add depth and background to the contents of this chapter.

In this chapter we examine liquidity, solvency, and profitability ratios. **Exhibit 11–1** sets out eight basic ratios

Progress Notes

After completing this chapter, you should be able to

1. Understand four types of liquidity ratios.
2. Understand two types of solvency ratios.
3. Understand two types of profitability ratios.
4. Successfully compute ratios.

Exhibit 11–1 Eight Basic Ratios Used in Health Care

Liquidity Ratios

1. Current Ratio

$$\frac{\text{Current Assets}}{\text{Current Liabilities}}$$

2. Quick Ratio

$$\frac{\text{Cash and Cash Equivalents + Net Receivables}}{\text{Current Liabilities}}$$

3. Days Cash on Hand (DCOH)

$$\frac{\text{Unrestricted Cash and Cash Equivalents}}{\text{Cash Operation Expenses} \div \text{No. of Days in Period (365)}}$$

4. Days Receivables

$$\frac{\text{Net Receivables}}{\text{Net Credit Revenues} \div \text{No. of Days in Period (365)}}$$

Solvency Ratios

5. Debt Service Coverage Ratio (DSCR)

$$\frac{\text{Change in Unrestricted Net Assets (net income)} + \text{Interest, Depreciation, Amortization}}{\text{Maximum Annual Debt Service}}$$

6. Liabilities to Fund Balance

$$\frac{\text{Total Liabilities}}{\text{Unrestricted Fund Balances}}$$

Profitability Ratios

7. Operating Margin (%)

$$\frac{\text{Operating Income (Loss)}}{\text{Total Operating Revenues}}$$

8. Return on Total Assets (%)

$$\frac{\text{EBIT (Earnings Before Interest and Taxes)}}{\text{Total Assets}}$$

Courtesy of Resource Group, Ltd., Dallas, Texas.

that are widely used in healthcare organizations: four liquidity types, two solvency types, and two profitability types. All are discussed in this chapter.

LIQUIDITY RATIOS

Liquidity ratios reflect the ability of the organization to meet its current obligations. Liquidity ratios measure short-term sufficiency. As the name implies, they measure the ability of the organization to "be liquid": in other words, to have sufficient cash—or assets that can be converted to cash—on hand.

Current Ratio

The current ratio equals current assets divided by current liabilities. For instance, consider this example:

$$\frac{\text{Current Assets}}{\text{Current Liabilities}} = \frac{\$120,000}{\$60,000} = 2 \text{ to } 1$$

This ratio is considered to be a measure of short-term debt-paying ability. However, it must be carefully interpreted. The standard by which the current ratio is measured is 2 to 1, as computed.

Quick Ratio

The quick ratio equals cash plus short-term investments plus net receivables divided by current liabilities:

$$\frac{\text{Cash and Cash Eqivalents} + \text{Net Receivables}}{\text{Current Liabilities}} = \frac{\$65,000}{\$60,000} = 1.08 \text{ to } 1$$

The standard by which the quick ratio is measured is generally 1 to 1. This computation, at 1.08 to 1, is a little better than the standard.

This ratio is considered to be an even more severe test of short-term debt-paying ability (even more than the current ratio). The quick ratio is also known as the acid-test ratio, for obvious reasons.

Days Cash on Hand

The days cash on hand (DCOH) equals unrestricted cash and investments divided by cash operating expenses divided by 365:

$$\frac{\text{Unrestricted Cash and Cash Equivalents}}{\substack{\text{Cash Operating Expenses} \\ \div \text{ No. of Days in Period}}} = \frac{\$330,000}{\$11,000} = 30 \text{ days}$$

There is no concrete standard for this computation.

This ratio indicates cash on hand in relation to the amount of daily operating expense. This example indicates the organization has 30 days worth of operating expenses represented in the amount of (unrestricted) cash on hand.

Days Receivables

The days receivables computation is represented as net receivables divided by net credit revenues divided by 365:

$$\frac{\text{Net Receivables}}{\text{Net Credit Revenue/No. of Days in Period}} = \frac{\$720,000}{\$12,000} = 60 \text{ days}$$

This computation represents the number of days in receivables. The older a receivable is, the more difficult it becomes to collect. Therefore, this computation is a measure of worth as well as performance.

There is no hard and fast rule for this computation because much depends on the mix of payers in your organization. This example indicates that the organization has 60 days worth of credit revenue tied up in net receivables. This computation is a common measure of billing and collection performance. There are many "days receivables" regional and national figures to compare with your own organization's computation.

Figure 11–1 shows how the information for the numerator and the denominator of each calculation is obtained. It takes the Westside Clinic balance sheet and the statement of revenue and expense that were discussed in the preceding chapter and illustrates the source of each figure in the four ratios just discussed. The multiple computations for days cash on hand and for days receivables are further broken down into a three-step process. If you study Figure 11–1 and work with the Mini-Case Study entitled "Comparative Analysis (Financial Ratios and Benchmarking) Helps Turn Around a Hospital", you will soon master this process.

SOLVENCY RATIOS

Solvency ratios reflect the ability of the organization to pay the annual interest and principal obligations on its long-term debt. As the name implies, they measure the ability of the organization to "be solvent": in other words, to have sufficient resources to meet its long-term obligations.

Debt Service Coverage Ratio

The debt service coverage ratio (DSCR) is represented as change in unrestricted net assets (net income) plus interest, depreciation, and amortization divided by maximum annual debt service:

$$\frac{\begin{array}{c}\text{Change in Unrestricted Net Assets (Net Income)}\\ + \text{ Interest, Depreciation, and Amortization}\end{array}}{\text{Maximum Annual Debt Service}} = \frac{\$250,000}{\$100,000} = 2.5$$

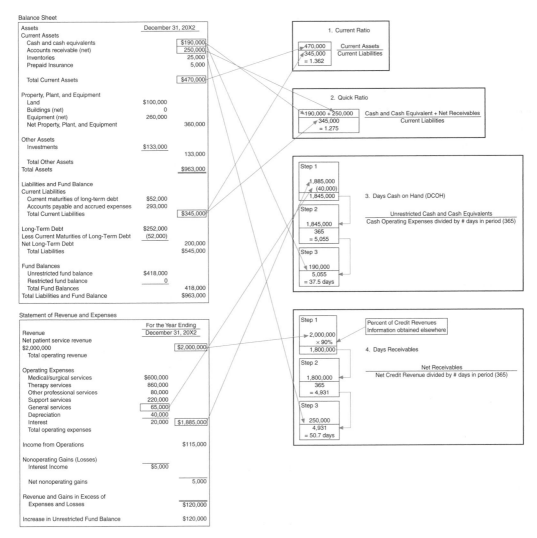

Figure 11–1 Examples of Liquidity Ratio Calculations.
Courtesy of Resource Group, Ltd, Dallas, Texas.

This ratio is universally used in credit analysis and figures prominently in the Mini-Case Study.

Each lending institution has its particular criteria for the DSCR. Lending agreements often have a provision that requires the DSCR to be maintained at or above a certain figure.

Liabilities to Fund Balance (or Debt to Net Worth)

The liabilities to fund balance or net worth computation is represented as total liabilities divided by unrestricted net assets (i.e., fund balances or net worth) or total debt divided by tangible net worth:

$$\frac{\text{Total Liabilities}}{\text{Unrestricted Fund Balances}} = \frac{\$2,000,000}{\$2,250,000} = 0.80$$

This figure is a quick indicator of debt load.

Another indicator that is more severe is long-term debt to net worth (fund balance), which is computed as long-term debt divided by fund balance. This computation is somewhat equivalent to the quick ratio discussed previously in its restrictiveness to net worth computation.

A mirror image of total liabilities to fund balance is total assets to fund balance, which is computed as total assets divided by fund balance.

Figure 11–2 shows how the information for the numerator and the denominator of each calculation is obtained. This figure again takes the Westside Clinic balance sheet and statement of revenue and expense that were discussed in the preceding chapter and illustrates the source of each figure in the two solvency ratios just discussed, along with each figure in the two profitability ratios still to be discussed. When multiple computations are necessary, they are further broken down into a two-step process.

PROFITABILITY RATIOS

Profitability ratios reflect the ability of the organization to operate with an excess of operating revenue over operating expense. Nonprofit organizations may not call this result a profit, but the measurement ratios are still generally called profitability ratios, whether they are applied to for-profit or nonprofit organizations.

Operating Margin

The operating margin, which is generally expressed as a percentage, is represented as operating income (loss) divided by total operating revenues:

$$\frac{\text{Operating Income (Loss)}}{\text{Total Operating Revenues}} = \frac{\$250,000}{\$5,000,000} = 5.0\%$$

This ratio is used for a number of managerial purposes and also sometimes enters into credit analysis. It is therefore a multipurpose measure. It is so universal that many outside sources are available for comparative purposes. The result of the computation must still be carefully considered because of variables in each period being compared.

Return on Total Assets

The return on total assets is represented as earnings before interest and taxes (EBIT) divided by total assets:

$$\frac{\text{EBIT}}{\text{Total Assets}} = \frac{\$400,000}{\$4,000,000} = 10\%$$

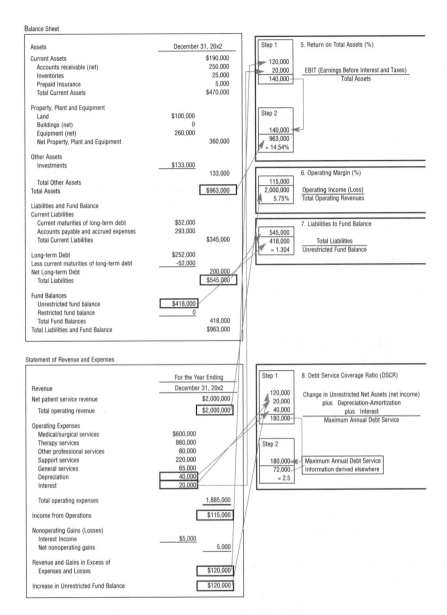

Figure 11–2 Examples of Solvency and Profitability Ratio Calculations.
Courtesy of Resource Group, Ltd, Dallas, Texas.

This is a broad measure in common use. Note the acronym EBIT, as its use is widespread in credit analysis circles. (Some analysts use an alternative computation for Return on Total Assets. They compute this ratio as Net Income divided by Total Assets.)

This concludes the description of solvency and profitability ratios. Again, if you study Figure 11–2 and work with the Mini-Case Study entitled "Comparative Analysis (Financial Ratios and Benchmarking) Helps Turn Around a Hospital", you will master this process too.

INFORMATION CHECKPOINT

What is needed?	Reports that use ratios as measures.
Where is it found?	Possibly in your supervisor's file; in the administrator's office; in the chief executive officer's office.
How is it used?	Use as a measure against outside benchmarks (as discussed in this chapter); also use as internal benchmarks for departments/divisions/units; also use as benchmarks at various points over time.

 KEY TERMS

Current Ratio
Days Cash on Hand (DCOH)
Days Receivables
Debt Service Coverage Ratio (DSCR)
Liabilities to Fund Balance
Liquidity Ratios
Operating Margin
Profitability Ratios
Quick Ratio
Return on Total Assets
Solvency Ratios

 DISCUSSION QUESTIONS

1. Are there ratios in the reports you receive at your workplace?
2. If so, do you use them? How?
3. If not, do you believe ratios should be on the reports? Which reports?
4. Can you think of good outside sources that could be used to obtain ratios for comparative purposes? If the outside information was available, what ratios would you choose to use? Why?

The Time Value of Money

PURPOSE

The purpose of these computations is to evaluate the use of money. The manager has many options as to where resources of the organization should be spent.[1] These calculations provide guides to assist in evaluating the alternatives.

UNADJUSTED RATE OF RETURN

The unadjusted rate of return is a relatively unsophisticated return-on-investment method, and the answer is only an estimate, containing no precision. The computation of the unadjusted rate of return is as follows:

$$\frac{\text{Average Annual Net Income}}{\text{Original Investment Amount}} = \text{Rate of Return}$$

OR

$$\frac{\text{Average Annual Net Income}}{\text{Average Investment Amount}} = \text{Rate of Return}$$

The original investment amount is a matter of record. The average investment amount is arrived at by taking the total unrecovered asset cost at the beginning of estimated useful life plus the unrecovered asset cost at the end of estimated useful life and dividing by two. This method has the advantage of accommodating whatever depreciation method has been chosen by the organization. This method is sometimes called the accountant's method because information necessary for the computation is obtained from the financial statements.

After completing this chapter, you should be able to

1. Compute an unadjusted rate of return.
2. Understand how to use a present-value table.
3. Compute an internal rate of return.
4. Understand the payback period theory.

PRESENT-VALUE ANALYSIS

The concept of present-value analysis is based on the time value of money. Inherent in this concept is the fact that the value of a dollar today is more than the value of a dollar in the future: thus the "present value" terminology. Furthermore, the further in the future the receipt of your dollar occurs, the less it is worth. Think of a dollar bill dwindling in size more and more as its receipt stretches further and further into the future. This is the concept of present-value analysis.

We learned about compound interest in math class. We learned that

$500 invested at the beginning of year 1
.05   earns interest (assumed) at a rate of 5% for one year,
$525 and we have a compound amount at the end of year 1 amounting to $525,
.05   which earns interest (assumed) at the rate of 5% for another year,
$551 and we have a compound amount at the end of year 2 amounting to $551 (rounded), and so on.

Using this concept, it is possible to restate the present values of $1 to be paid out or received at the end of each of these years. It is possible to use equations, but that is not necessary because we have present-value tables (also called "look-up tables," because one can "look-up" the answer). A present-value table is included at the end of this chapter in Appendix 12-A. All of the figures on the present-value table represent the value of a dollar. The interest rate available on this version of the table is on the horizontal columns and ranges from 1% to 20%. The number of years in the period is on the vertical; in this version of the table, the number of years ranges from 1 to 30. To look up a present value, find the column for the proper interest. Then find the line for the proper number of years. Then trace down the interest column and across the number-of-years line item. The point where the two lines meet is the number (or factor) that represents the value of $1 according to your assumptions. For example, find the year 10 by reading down the left-hand column labeled "Year." Then read across that line until you find the column labeled "10%." The point where the two lines meet is found to be 0.3855. The present value of $1 under these assumptions (10 year/10%) is about 38.5 cents (shown as 0.3855 on the table).

Besides using the look-up table, you can also compute this factor on a business analyst calculator. A reference to business analyst calculators is contained in the Appendix entitled "Web-Based and Software Learning Tools." This can be found at the end of this text. Besides using either the look-up table or the business calculator, you can use a function on your computer spreadsheet to produce the factor. The important point is this: no matter which method you use, you should get the same answer.

Now that you have the present value of $1, by whichever method, it is simple to find the present value of any other number. You merely multiply the other number by the factor you found on the table—or in the calculator or the computer. Say, for example, you want to find the present value of $8,000 under the assumption used above (10 years/10%). You simply multiply $8,000 by the factor of 0.3855 you found in the table. The present value of $8,000 is $3,084 (or $8,000 times 0.3855).

A compound interest table is also included at the end of this chapter in Appendix 12-B, along with a table showing the present value of an annuity of $1.00 in Appendix 12-C, so that you have the tools for computation at your disposal.

INTERNAL RATE OF RETURN

The internal rate of return (IRR) is another return on investment method. It uses a discounted cash flow technique. The internal rate of return is the rate of interest that discounts future net inflows (from the proposed investment) down to the amount invested. The return for a particular investment can therefore be known. The IRR recognizes the elements contained in the previous two methods discussed, but it goes further. It also recognizes the time pattern in which the earnings occur. This means more precision in the computation because IRR calculates from period to period, whereas the other two methods rely on an average investment.

The IRR computation is not very complicated. The computation requires two assumptions and three steps to compute. Assumption 1: Find the initial cost of the investment. Assumption 2: Find the estimated annual net cash inflow the investment will generate. Assumption 3: Find the useful life of the asset (generally expressed in number of years, known as periods for this computation). Step 1: Divide the initial cost of the investment (Assumption 1) by the estimated annual net cash inflow it will generate (Assumption 2). The answer is a ratio. Step 2: Now use the look-up table. Find the number of periods (Assumption 3). Step 3: Look across the line for the number of periods and find the column that approximates the ratio computed in Step 1. That column contains the interest rate representing the rate of return.

How is IRR used? It can take the rate of return obtained and restate it. The restated figure represents the maximum rate of interest that can be paid for capital over the entire span of the investment without incurring a loss. (You can think of that restated figure as a kind of break-even point for investment purposes.) The fact that a rate of return can be computed is the benefit of using an IRR method.

PAYBACK PERIOD

The payback period is the length of time required for the cash coming in from an investment to equal the amount of cash originally spent when the investment was acquired. In other words, if we invested $1,000, under a particular set of assumptions, how long would it take to get our $1,000 back? The payback period concept is used extensively in evaluating whether to invest in a plant and/or equipment. In that case, the question can be restated as follows: If we invested $1,200,000 in a magnetic resonance imaging machine, under a particular set of assumptions, how long would it take to get the hospital's $1,200,000 back?

The assumptions are key to the computation of the payback period. In the case of equipment, volume of usage is a critical assumption and is sometimes very difficult to predict. Therefore, it is prudent to run more than one payback period computation based on different circumstances. Generally a "best case" and a "worst case" run are made.

The computation itself is simple, although it has multiple steps. The trick is to break it into segments.

For example, Doctor Green is considering the purchase of a machine for his office laboratory. It will cost $300,000. He wants to find the payback period for this piece of equipment. To begin, Dr. Green needs to make the following assumptions. Assumption 1: Purchase price of the equipment. Assumption 2: Useful life of the equipment. Assumption 3:

Revenue the machine will generate per year. Assumption 4: Direct operating costs associated with earning the revenue. Assumption 5: Depreciation expense per year (computed as purchase price per Assumption 1 divided by useful life per Assumption 2).

Dr. Green's five assumptions are as follows:

1. Purchase price of equipment = $300,000
2. Useful life of the equipment = 10 years
3. Revenue the machine will generate per year = $10,000 after taxes
4. Direct operating costs associated with earning the revenue = $150,000
5. Depreciation expense per year = $30,000

Now that the assumptions are in place, the payback period computation can be made. It is in three steps, as follows:

Step 1: Find the machine's expected net income after taxes.

Revenue (Assumption #3)		$200,000
Less		
Direct operating costs		
(Assumption 4)	$150,000	
Depreciation		
(Assumption 5)	30,000	
		180,000
Net income before taxes		$20,000
Less income taxes of 50%		10,000
Net income after taxes		$10,000

Step 2: Find the net annual cash inflow after taxes the machine is expected to generate (in other words, convert the net income to a cash basis).

Net income after taxes	$10,000
Add back depreciation (a noncash expenditure)	30,000
Annual net cash inflow after taxes	$40,000

Step 3: Compute the payback period.

$$\frac{\$300{,}000 \text{ Machine Cost*}}{\$40{,}000**} = 7.5 \text{ year Payback Period}$$

Investment
Net Annual
Cash Flow
after Taxes

*Assumption 1 above
**per Step 2 above

The machine will pay back its investment under these assumptions in 7.5 years.

Payback period computations are very common when equipment purchases are being evaluated. The evaluation process itself is the final subject we consider in this chapter.

EVALUATIONS

Evaluating the use of resources in healthcare organizations is an important task. There are never enough resources to go around, and it is important to use an objective process to evaluate which investments will be made by the organization. A uniform use of a chosen method of evaluating return on investment and/or payback period makes the evaluation process more manageable.

It is important to choose a method that is understood by the managers who will be using it. It is equally important to choose a method that can be readily calculated. If a multiple-page worksheet has to be constructed to set up the assumptions for a modestly priced piece of equipment, the evaluation method is probably too complex. This comment actually touches on the cost-benefit of performing the evaluation.

Sometimes a computer program is chosen that performs a uniform computation of investment returns and payback periods. Such a program is a suitable choice if the managers who use it understand the printouts it produces. Understanding both input and output is key for the managers. In summary, evaluations should be objective, the process should not be too cumbersome, and the responsible managers should understand how the computation was achieved.

RESOURCES

Three look-up tables are presented as appendices to this chapter. They include the following:

A. Present-Value Table (the present value of $1.00)
B. Compound Interest Table (the future value of $1.00)
C. Present Value of an Annuity of $1.00

These tables provide an ongoing resource for you.

 INFORMATION CHECKPOINT

What is needed?	Information sufficient to perform these calculations.
Where is it found?	In the files of your supervisor; also in the office of the financial analyst; probably also in the strategic planning office.
How is it used?	To measure the time value of money.

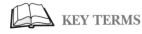 KEY TERMS

Internal Rate of Return
Payback Period

Present-Value Analysis
Time Value of Money
Unadjusted Rate of Return

 DISCUSSION QUESTIONS

1. Can you compute an unadjusted rate of return now? Would you use it? Why?
2. Are you able to use the present-value look-up table now? Would you prefer a computer to compute it?
3. Have you seen the payback period concept used in your workplace? If not, do you think it ought to be used? What are your reasons?
4. Have you had a chance to participate in an evaluation of an equipment purchase at your workplace? If so, would you have done it differently if you had supervised the evaluation? Why?

NOTE

1. S. Williamson et al., *Fundamentals of Strategic Planning for Healthcare Organizations* (New York: The Haworth Press, 1997).

APPENDIX

Present-Value Table
(The Present Value of $1.00)

12-A

Year	1%	2%	3%	4%	5%	6%	7%	8%	9%	10%
1	0.9901	0.9804	0.9709	0.9615	0.9524	0.9434	0.9346	0.9259	0.9174	0.9091
2	0.9803	0.9612	0.9426	0.9246	0.9070	0.8900	0.8734	0.8573	0.8417	0.8264
3	0.9706	0.9423	0.9151	0.8890	0.8638	0.8396	0.8163	0.7938	0.7722	0.7513
4	0.9610	0.9238	0.8885	0.8548	0.8227	0.7921	0.7629	0.7350	0.7084	0.6830
5	0.9515	0.9057	0.8626	0.8219	0.7835	0.7473	0.7130	0.6806	0.6499	0.6209
6	0.9420	0.8880	0.8375	0.7903	0.7462	0.7050	0.6663	0.6302	0.5963	0.5645
7	0.9327	0.8706	0.8131	0.7599	0.7107	0.6651	0.6227	0.5835	0.5470	0.5132
8	0.9235	0.8535	0.7894	0.7307	0.6768	0.6274	0.5820	0.5403	0.5019	0.4665
9	0.9143	0.8368	0.7664	0.7026	0.6446	0.5919	0.5439	0.5002	0.4604	0.4241
10	0.9053	0.8203	0.7441	0.6756	0.6139	0.5584	0.5083	0.4632	0.4224	0.3855
11	0.8963	0.8043	0.7224	0.6496	0.5847	0.5268	0.4751	0.4289	0.3875	0.3505
12	0.8874	0.7885	0.7014	0.6246	0.5568	0.4970	0.4440	0.3971	0.3555	0.3186
13	0.8787	0.7730	0.6810	0.6006	0.5303	0.4688	0.4150	0.3677	0.3262	0.2987
14	0.8700	0.7579	0.6611	0.5775	0.5051	0.4423	0.3878	0.3405	0.2992	0.2633
15	0.8613	0.7430	0.6419	0.5553	0.4810	0.4173	0.3624	0.3152	0.2745	0.2394
16	0.8528	0.7284	0.6232	0.5339	0.4581	0.3936	0.3387	0.2919	0.2519	0.2176
17	0.8444	0.7142	0.6050	0.5134	0.4363	0.3714	0.3166	0.2703	0.2311	0.1978
18	0.8360	0.7002	0.5874	0.4936	0.4155	0.3503	0.2959	0.2502	0.2120	0.1799
19	0.8277	0.6864	0.5703	0.4746	0.3957	0.3305	0.2765	0.2317	0.1945	0.1635
20	0.8195	0.6730	0.5537	0.4564	0.3769	0.3118	0.2584	0.2145	0.1784	0.1486
21	0.8114	0.6598	0.5375	0.4388	0.3589	0.2942	0.2415	0.1987	0.1637	0.1351
22	0.8034	0.6468	0.5219	0.4220	0.3418	0.2775	0.2257	0.1839	0.1502	0.1228
23	0.7954	0.6342	0.5067	0.4057	0.3256	0.2618	0.2109	0.1703	0.1378	0.1117
24	0.7876	0.6217	0.4919	0.3901	0.3101	0.2470	0.1971	0.1577	0.1264	0.1015
25	0.7798	0.6095	0.4776	0.3751	0.2953	0.2330	0.1842	0.1460	0.1160	0.0923
26	0.7720	0.5976	0.4637	0.3607	0.2812	0.2198	0.1722	0.1352	0.1064	0.0839
27	0.7644	0.5859	0.4502	0.3468	0.2678	0.2074	0.1609	0.1252	0.0976	0.0763
28	0.7568	0.5744	0.4371	0.3335	0.2552	0.1956	0.1504	0.1159	0.0895	0.0693
29	0.7493	0.5631	0.4243	0.3207	0.2429	0.1846	0.1406	0.1073	0.0822	0.0630
30	0.7419	0.5521	0.4120	0.3083	0.2314	0.1741	0.1314	0.0994	0.0754	0.0573

Year	11%	12%	13%	14%	15%	16%	17%	18%	19%	20%
1	0.9009	0.8929	0.8850	0.8772	0.8696	0.8621	0.8547	0.8475	0.8403	0.8333
2	0.8116	0.7972	0.7831	0.7695	0.7561	0.7432	0.7305	0.7182	0.7062	0.6944
3	0.7312	0.7118	0.6913	0.6750	0.6575	0.6407	0.6244	0.6086	0.5934	0.5787
4	0.6587	0.6355	0.6133	0.5921	0.5718	0.5523	0.5337	0.5158	0.4987	0.4823
5	0.5935	0.5674	0.5428	0.5194	0.4972	0.4761	0.4561	0.4371	0.4190	0.4019
6	0.5346	0.5066	0.4803	0.4556	0.4323	0.4104	0.3898	0.3704	0.3521	0.3349
7	0.4817	0.4523	0.4251	0.3996	0.3759	0.3538	0.3332	0.3139	0.2959	0.2791
8	0.4339	0.4039	0.3762	0.3506	0.3269	0.3050	0.2848	0.2660	0.2487	0.2326
9	0.3909	0.3606	0.3329	0.3075	0.2843	0.2630	0.2434	0.2255	0.2090	0.1938
10	0.3522	0.3220	0.2946	0.2697	0.2472	0.2267	0.2080	0.1911	0.1756	0.1615
11	0.3173	0.2875	0.2607	0.2366	0.2149	0.1954	0.1778	0.1619	0.1476	0.1346
12	0.2858	0.2567	0.2307	0.2076	0.1869	0.1685	0.1520	0.1372	0.1240	0.1122
13	0.2575	0.2292	0.2042	0.1821	0.1625	0.1452	0.1299	0.1163	0.1042	0.0935
14	0.2320	0.2046	0.1807	0.1597	0.1413	0.1252	0.1110	0.0985	0.0876	0.0779
15	0.2090	0.1827	0.1599	0.1401	0.1229	0.1079	0.0949	0.0835	0.0736	0.0649
16	0.1883	0.1631	0.1415	0.1229	0.1069	0.0930	0.0811	0.0708	0.0618	0.0541
17	0.1696	0.1456	0.1252	0.1078	0.0929	0.0802	0.0693	0.0600	0.0520	0.0451
18	0.1528	0.1300	0.1108	0.0946	0.0808	0.0691	0.0592	0.0508	0.0437	0.0376
19	0.1377	0.1161	0.0981	0.0829	0.0703	0.0596	0.0506	0.0431	0.0367	0.0313
20	0.1240	0.1037	0.0868	0.0728	0.0611	0.0514	0.0433	0.0365	0.0308	0.0261
21	0.1117	0.0926	0.0768	0.0638	0.0531	0.0443	0.0370	0.0309	0.0259	0.0217
22	0.1007	0.0826	0.0680	0.0560	0.0462	0.0382	0.0316	0.0262	0.0218	0.0181
23	0.0907	0.0738	0.0601	0.0491	0.0402	0.0329	0.0270	0.0222	0.0183	0.0151
24	0.0817	0.0659	0.0532	0.0431	0.0349	0.0284	0.0231	0.0188	0.0154	0.0126
25	0.0736	0.0588	0.0471	0.0378	0.0304	0.0245	0.0197	0.0160	0.0129	0.0105
26	0.0663	0.0525	0.0417	0.0331	0.0264	0.0211	0.0169	0.0135	0.0109	0.0087
27	0.0597	0.0469	0.0369	0.0291	0.0230	0.0182	0.0144	0.0115	0.0091	0.0073
28	0.0538	0.0419	0.0326	0.0255	0.0200	0.0157	0.0123	0.0097	0.0077	0.0061
29	0.0485	0.0374	0.0289	0.0224	0.0174	0.0135	0.0105	0.0082	0.0064	0.0051
30	0.0437	0.0334	0.0256	0.0196	0.0151	0.0116	0.0090	0.0070	0.0054	0.0042

Compound Interest Table 12-B

Compound Interest of $1.00
(The Future Amount of $1.00)

Year	1%	2%	3%	4%	5%	6%	7%	8%	9%	10%
1	1.010	1.020	1.030	1.040	1.050	1.060	1.070	1.080	1.090	1.100
2	1.020	1.040	1.061	1.082	1.102	1.124	1.145	1.166	1.188	1.210
3	1.030	1.061	1.093	1.125	1.156	1.191	1.225	1.260	1.295	1.331
4	1.041	1.082	1.126	1.170	1.216	1.262	1.311	1.360	1.412	1.464
5	1.051	1.104	1.159	1.217	1.276	1.338	1.403	1.469	1.539	1.611
6	1.062	1.120	1.194	1.265	1.340	1.419	1.501	1.587	1.677	1.772
7	1.072	1.149	1.230	1.316	1.407	1.504	1.606	1.714	1.828	1.949
8	1.083	1.172	1.267	1.369	1.477	1.594	1.718	1.851	1.993	2.144
9	1.094	1.195	1.305	1.423	1.551	1.689	1.838	1.999	2.172	2.358
10	1.105	1.219	1.344	1.480	1.629	1.791	1.967	2.159	2.367	2.594
11	1.116	1.243	1.384	1.539	1.710	1.898	2.105	2.332	2.580	2.853
12	1.127	1.268	1.426	1.601	1.796	2.012	2.252	2.518	2.813	3.138
13	1.138	1.294	1.469	1.665	1.886	2.133	2.410	2.720	3.066	3.452
14	1.149	1.319	1.513	1.732	1.980	2.261	2.579	2.937	3.342	3.797
15	1.161	1.346	1.558	1.801	2.079	2.397	2.759	3.172	3.642	4.177
16	1.173	1.373	1.605	1.873	2.183	2.540	2.952	3.426	3.970	4.595
17	1.184	1.400	1.653	1.948	2.292	2.693	3.159	3.700	4.328	5.054
18	1.196	1.428	1.702	2.026	2.407	2.854	3.380	3.996	4.717	5.560
19	1.208	1.457	1.754	2.107	2.527	3.026	3.617	4.316	5.142	6.116
20	1.220	1.486	1.806	2.191	2.653	3.207	3.870	4.661	5.604	6.728
25	1.282	1.641	2.094	2.666	3.386	4.292	5.427	6.848	8.632	10.835
30	1.348	1.811	2.427	3.243	4.322	5.743	7.612	10.063	13.268	17.449

Year	12%	14%	16%	18%	20%	24%	28%	32%	40%	50%
1	1.120	1.140	1.160	1.180	1.200	1.240	1.280	1.320	1.400	1.500
2	1.254	1.300	1.346	1.392	1.440	1.538	1.638	1.742	1.960	2.250
3	1.405	1.482	1.561	1.643	1.728	1.907	2.067	2.300	2.744	3.375
4	1.574	1.689	1.811	1.939	2.074	2.364	2.684	3.036	3.842	5.062
5	1.762	1.925	2.100	2.288	2.488	2.932	3.436	4.007	5.378	7.594
6	1.974	2.195	2.436	2.700	2.986	3.635	4.398	5.290	7.530	11.391
7	2.211	2.502	2.826	3.185	3.583	4.508	5.629	6.983	10.541	17.086
8	2.476	2.853	3.278	3.759	4.300	5.590	7.206	9.217	14.758	25.629
9	2.773	3.252	3.803	4.435	5.160	6.931	9.223	12.166	20.661	38.443
10	3.106	3.707	4.411	5.234	6.192	8.594	11.806	16.060	28.925	57.665
11	3.479	4.226	5.117	6.176	7.430	10.657	15.112	21.199	40.496	86.498
12	3.896	4.818	5.936	7.288	8.916	13.215	19.343	27.983	56.694	129.746
13	4.363	5.492	6.886	8.599	10.699	16.386	24.759	36.937	79.372	194.619
14	4.887	6.261	7.988	10.147	12.839	20.319	31.691	48.757	111.120	291.929
15	5.474	7.138	9.266	11.074	15.407	25.196	40.565	64.350	155.568	437.894
16	6.130	8.137	10.748	14.129	18.488	31.243	51.923	84.954	217.795	656.840
17	6.866	9.276	12.468	16.672	22.186	38.741	66.461	112.140	304.914	985.260
18	7.690	10.575	14.463	19.673	26.623	48.039	85.071	148.020	426.879	1477.900
19	8.613	12.056	16.777	23.214	31.948	59.568	108.890	195.390	597.630	2216.800
20	9.646	13.743	19.461	27.393	38.338	73.864	139.380	257.920	836.683	3325.300
25	17.000	26.462	40.874	62.669	95.396	216.542	478.900	1033.600	4499.880	25251.000
30	29.960	50.950	85.850	143.371	237.376	634.820	1645.500	4142.100	24201.432	191750.000

Present Value of an Annuity of $1.00

12-C

Periods	2%	4%	6%	8%	10%	12%	14%	16%	18%	20%	Periods
1	0.980	0.962	0.943	0.926	0.909	0.893	0.877	0.862	0.848	0.833	1
2	1.942	1.886	1.833	1.783	1.736	1.690	1.647	1.605	1.566	1.528	2
3	2.884	2.775	2.673	2.577	2.487	2.402	2.322	2.246	2.174	2.107	3
4	3.808	3.630	3.465	3.312	3.170	3.037	2.914	2.798	2.690	2.589	4
5	4.713	4.452	4.212	3.993	3.791	3.605	3.433	3.274	3.127	2.991	5
6	5.601	5.242	4.917	4.623	4.355	4.111	3.889	3.685	3.498	3.326	6
7	6.472	6.002	5.582	5.206	4.868	4.564	4.288	4.039	3.812	3.605	7
8	7.325	6.733	6.210	5.747	5.335	4.968	4.639	4.344	4.078	3.837	8
9	8.162	7.435	6.802	6.247	5.759	5.328	4.946	4.607	4.303	4.031	9
10	8.983	8.111	7.360	6.710	6.145	5.650	5.216	4.833	4.494	4.193	10
15	12.849	11.118	9.712	8.560	7.606	6.811	6.142	5.576	5.092	4.676	15
20	16.351	13.590	11.470	9.818	8.514	7.469	6.623	5.929	5.353	4.870	20
25	19.523	15.622	12.783	10.675	9.077	7.843	6.873	6.097	5.467	4.948	25

Tools to Review and Manage Comparative Data

Trend Analysis, Common Sizing, and Forecasted Data

COMMON SIZING

The process of common sizing puts information on the same relative basis. Generally, common sizing involves converting dollar amounts to percentages. If, for example, total revenue of $200,000 equals 100%, then radiology revenue of $20,000 will equal 10% of that total. Converting dollars to percentages allows comparative analysis. In other words, comparing the percentages allows a common basis of comparison. Common sizing is sometimes called "vertical analysis" (because the computation of the percentages is vertical).

Although such comparisons on the basis of percentages can, and should, be performed on your own organization's data, comparisons can also be made between or among various organizations. For example, **Table 13–1** shows how common sizing allows a comparison of liabilities for three different hospitals. In each case, the total liabilities equal 100%. Then the current liabilities of hospital 1, for example, are divided by total liabilities to find the proportionate percentage attributable to that line item (100,000 divided by 500,000 equals 20%; 400,000 divided by 500,000 equals 80%). When all the percentages have been computed, add them to make sure they add to 100%. If you use a computer, computation of these percentages is available as a spreadsheet function.

Another example of comparative analysis is contained in **Table 13-2**. In this case, general services expenses for three hospitals are compared. Once again, the total expense for each hospital becomes 100%, and the relative percentage for each of the four line items is computed ($320,000 divided by $800,000 equals 40%

Table 13–1 Common Sizing Liability Information

	Same Year for All Three Hospitals					
	Hospital 1		Hospital 2		Hospital 3	
Current liabilities	$100,000	20%	$500,000	25%	$400,000	80%
Long-term debt	400,000	80%	1,500,000	75%	100,000	20%
Total liabilities	$500,000	100%	$2,000,000	100%	$500,000	100%

and so on). The advantage of comparative analysis is illustrated by the "laundry" line item, where the dollar amounts are $80,000, $300,000, and $90,000 respectively. Yet each of these amounts is 10% of the total expense for the particular hospital.

TREND ANALYSIS

The process of trend analysis compares figures over several time periods. Once again, dollar amounts are converted to percentages to obtain a relative basis for purposes of comparison, but now the comparison is across time. If, for example, radiology revenue was $20,000 this period but was only $15,000 for the previous period, the difference between the two is $5,000. The difference of $5,000 equates to a 33.3% difference because trend analysis is computed on the earlier of the two years: that is, the base year (thus, 5,000 divided by 15,000 equals 33.3%). Trend analysis is sometimes called "horizontal analysis" (because the computation of the percentage of difference is horizontal).

An example of horizontal analysis is contained in **Table 13–3**. In this case, the liabilities of hospital 1 for year 1 are compared with the liabilities of hospital 1's year 2. Current liabilities, for example, were $100,000 in year 1 and are $150,000 in year 2, a difference of $50,000. To arrive at a percentage of difference for comparative purposes, the $50,000 difference is divided by the year 1 base figure of $100,000 to compute the relative differential (thus, 50,000 divided by 100,000 is 50%).

Table 13–2 Common Sizing Expense Information

	Same Year for All Three Hospitals					
	Hospital 1		Hospital 2		Hospital 3	
General services expense						
Dietary	$320,000	40%	$1,260,000	42%	$450,000	50%
Maintenance	280,000	35%	990,000	33%	135,000	15%
Laundry	80,000	10%	300,000	10%	90,000	10%
Housekeeping	120,000	15%	450,000	15%	225,000	25%
Total GS expense	$800,000	100%	$3,000,000	100%	$900,000	100%

Table 13–3 Trend Analysis for Liabilities

	Hospital 1					
	Year 1		Year 2		Difference	
Current liabilities	$100,000	20%	$150,000	25%	$50,000	50%
Long-term debt	400,000	80%	450,000	75%	50,000	12.5%
Total liabilities	$500,000	100%	$600,000	100%	$100,000	–

Another example of comparative analysis is contained in **Table 13–4**. In this case, general services expenses for two years in hospital 1 are compared. The difference between year 1 and year 2 for each line item is computed in dollars; then the dollar difference figure is divided by the year 1 base figure to obtain a percentage difference for purposes of comparison. Thus, housekeeping expense in year 1 was $120,000, and in year 2 was $180,000, resulting in a difference of $60,000. The difference amounts to 50% ($60,000 difference divided by $120,000 year 1 equals 50%). In Table 13–4, two of the four line items have negative differences: that is, year 2 was less than year 1, resulting in a negative figure. Also, the dollar figure difference is $100,000 when added down (subtract the negative figures from the positive figures; thus, $85,000 plus $60,000 minus $10,000 minus $35,000 equals $100,000). The dollar figure difference is also $100,000 when added across ($900,000 minus $800,000 equals $100,000).

ANALYZING OPERATING DATA

Comparative analysis is an important tool for managers, and it is worth investing the time to become familiar with both horizontal and vertical analysis. Managers will generally analyze their own organization's data most of the time (rather than performing comparisons against other organizations). With that fact in mind, we examine operating room operating data (no pun intended) that incorporate both common sizing and trend analysis.

Table 13–4 Trend Analysis for Expenses

	Hospital 1					
	Year 1		Year 2		Difference	
General services expense						
Dietary	$320,000	40%	$405,000	45%	$85,000	26.5%
Maintenance	280,000	35%	270,000	30%	(10,000)	(3.5)%
Laundry	80,000	10%	45,000	5%	(35,000)	(43.5)%
Housekeeping	120,000	15%	180,000	20%	60,000	50.0%
Total GS expense	$800,000	100%	$900,000	100%	$100,000	–

Table 13–5 Vertical and Horizontal Analysis for the Operating Room

Comparative Expenses

Account	12-Month Current Year	%	12-Month Prior Year	%	Annual Increase (Decrease)	% of Change
Social Security	60,517	4.97	68,177	5.70	(7,660)	−12.66
Pension	20,675	1.70	23,473	1.96	(2,798)	−13.53
Health Insurance	8,422	0.69	18,507	1.55	(10,085)	−119.75
Child Care	4,564	0.37	4,334	0.36	230	5.04
Patient Accounting	155,356	12.76	123,254	10.30	32,102	20.66
Admitting	110,254	9.05	101,040	8.45	9,214	8.36
Medical Records	91,718	7.53	94,304	7.88	(2,586)	−2.82
Dietary	27,526	2.26	35,646	2.98	(8,120)	−29.50
Medical Waste	2,377	0.20	3,187	0.27	(810)	−34.08
Sterile Procedures	78,720	6.46	70,725	5.91	7,995	10.16
Laundry	40,693	3.34	40,463	3.38	230	0.57
Depreciation—Equipment	87,378	7.18	61,144	5.11	26,234	30.02
Depreciation—Building	41,377	3.40	45,450	3.80	(4,073)	−9.84
Amortization—Interest	(5,819)	−0.48	1,767	0.15	(7,586)	130.37
Insurance	4,216	0.35	7,836	0.65	(3,620)	−85.86
Administration	57,966	4.76	56,309	4.71	1,657	2.86
Medical Staff	1,722	0.14	5,130	0.43	(3,408)	−197.91
Community Relations	49,813	4.09	40,618	3.39	9,195	18.46
Materials Management	64,573	5.30	72,305	6.04	(7,732)	−11.97
Human Resources	31,066	2.55	13,276	1.11	17,790	57.27
Nursing Administration	82,471	6.77	92,666	7.75	(10,195)	−12.36
Data Processing	17,815	1.46	16,119	1.35	1,696	9.52
Fiscal	17,700	1.45	16,748	1.40	952	5.38
Telephone	2,839	0.23	2,569	0.21	270	9.51
Utilities	26,406	2.17	38,689	3.23	(12,283)	−46.52
Plant	77,597	6.37	84,128	7.03	(6,531)	−8.42
Environmental Services	32,874	2.70	37,354	3.12	(4,480)	−13.63
Safety	2,016	0.17	2,179	0.18	(163)	−8.09
Quality Management	10,016	0.82	8,146	0.68	1,870	18.67
Medical Staff	9,444	0.78	9,391	0.78	53	0.56
Continuous Quality Improvement	4,895	0.40	0	0.00	4,895	100.00
EE Health	569	0.05	1,513	0.13	(944)	−165.91
Total Allocated	1,217,756	100.00	1,196,447	100.00	21,309	1.75
All Other Expenses	1,211,608	—	—	—	—	—
Total Expense	2,429,364	—	—	—	—	—

Table 13–5 sets out 32 expense items. The expense amount in dollars for each line item is set out for the current year in the left column (beginning with $60,517). The expense amount in dollars for each line item is set out for the prior year in the third column of the analysis (beginning with $68,177). The difference in dollars, labeled "Annual Increase (Decrease)," appears in the sixth column of the analysis (beginning with [$7,660]).

Vertical analysis has been performed for the current year, and the percentage results appear in the second column (beginning with 4.97%). Vertical analysis has also been performed for the prior year, and those percentage results appear in the fourth column (beginning with 5.70%). Horizontal analysis has been performed on each line item, and those percentage items appear in the far right column (beginning with 12.66%). This table is a good example of the type of operating data reports that managers receive for planning and control purposes.

Comparative analysis is especially important to managers because it creates a common ground to make judgments for planning, control, and decision-making purposes. Using comparative data is the subject of the following chapter.

IMPORTANCE OF FORECASTS

The dictionary defines "to forecast" as "to calculate or predict some future event or condition, usually as a result of study and analysis of available pertinent data."[1]

From the manager's viewpoint, forecasted data are information used for purposes of planning for the future. Forecasting, to some degree or another, is often required when producing budgets. (Budgets are the subject of two of the following chapters.) It is pretty simple today to create "what if" scenarios on the computer. But the important thing for managers to remember is that assumptions directly affect the results of forecasts.

Forecasts Versus Projections

Forecasts are different than projections, although both are considered to be "prospective" and thus "future" financial statements. Forecasts are based on assumptions that are expected to exist, and that reflect actions that are expected to occur. Projections, on the other hand, are views further into the future. Because they are further into the future, we "project" future events, projects, or operations using a set of presumed, or hypothetical, assumptions.

We are discussing forecasts in this chapter rather than projections. Therefore these forecasts are relatively short term and can be based on realistic assumptions that we expect to exist, along with actions that we can reasonably expect to occur.

Forecasting Approaches

The approach to producing a forecast usually involves three different sources of information and forecast assumptions:

- The first level derives from the personnel who are directly involved in the department or unit. They know the operation and can provide important ground-level detail.
- The second level comes from electronic and statistical information, including trend analysis. Electronic reports can provide a thicket of information, and there is a skill to selecting relevant information for forecasting purposes.
- The third level represents executive-level judgment that is typically applied to a preliminary rough draft of the forecast. For example, adjusting volume upward or downward due to the anticipated future impact of local competition would most likely be an executive-level judgment.

The amount and type of electronic information that is readily available greatly affects the forecast difficulty. Electronic templates and standardized worksheets may also greatly influence the final forecast results.

Common Types of Forecasts in Healthcare Organizations

The three most common types of forecasts found in most healthcare organizations include revenue forecasts, staffing forecasts, and operating expense forecasts. (The operating expense forecast, which is not as common, would generally cover those operating expenses other than labor.) This section will discuss revenue and staffing forecasts, as they are what most managers will need to deal with.

OPERATING REVENUE FORECASTS

Operating revenue forecasts are inputs into the operating budget. Forecast types and their assumptions are discussed in this section.

Types of Revenue Forecasts

Forecasts of revenue will cover varying time periods. Longer-range multi-year forecasts are useful for executive decision making regarding the future of the organization. **Figure 13–1** illustrates a multi-year forecast.

A single-year forecast is generally for the coming year and is thus a short-range forecast. Reliable forecasts of revenue are a vital part of the organization's planning process and are

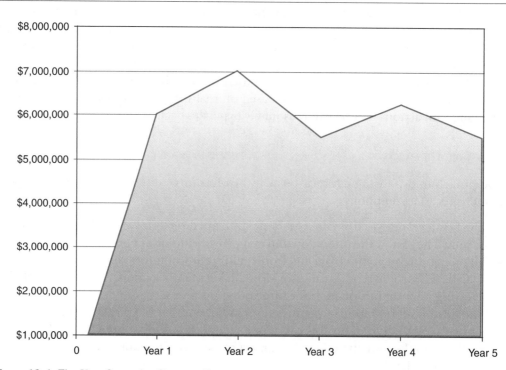

Figure 13–1 Five-Year Operating Revenue Forecast.

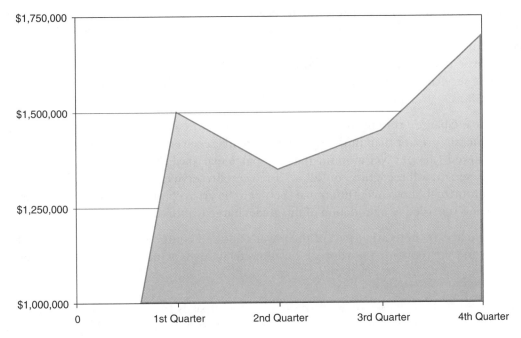

Figure 13–2 One-Year Operating Revenue Forecast.

an input into the operating budget. **Figure 13–2** illustrates a short-range forecast. Note that the graph in Figure 13–2 could be by month instead of by quarter as shown.

Building Revenue Forecast Assumptions

Five important issues regarding revenue forecast assumptions are discussed here.

Utilization Assumptions

In health care, significant changes in utilization patterns can be occurring that need to be taken into account in the manager's forecast assumptions. The inexorable shift to shorter lengths of stay for hospital inpatients over the last decade is an example of a basic shift in utilization patterns.

Patient Mix Assumptions

It is important to specify anticipated patient mix as well as his or her anticipated utilization or volume. By "patient mix" we mean whether the individual is a Medicare patient, a Medicaid patient, a patient covered by private insurance, or a private pay patient. When payers are thus identified, this information allows the appropriate payments to be associated with the service utilization assumptions.

Contractual Allowance Assumptions

The forecasted utilization of a service (or its volume) assumption is multiplied by the appropriate rate, or charges, in order to arrive at forecasted revenue stated in dollars.

A word of warning, however: revenue forecasted at "gross charges" is not a valid figure. Instead, revenue stated at "allowed charges" is the proper figure to use. Virtually all payers, including Medicare, Medicaid, and private insurers, will pay a stipulated amount for a particular service. But the amounts these different payers have agreed to pay for the same service will vary. How to handle the issue? Through a contractual allowance, as defined here:

- Gross Charge: Amount for a service as shown on the claim form; a uniform charge generally greater than most expected payments received for the service.
- Allowed Charge: Net amount that the particular payer's contract or participation agreement will recognize, or "allow," for a certain service.
- Contractual Allowance: Difference (between the gross charge and the allowed charge) that is recorded as a reduction of the gross charge within the accounting cycle.

(It should also be noted that part of the payer's allowed charge is generally due from the patient, and the remaining portion of the allowed charge is actually due from the payer.)

Trend Analysis Assumptions

One of the basic purposes of performing trend analysis is to compare data between or among years and to see the trends. If such trends are found, then it makes sense to take them into account in your forecast. A word of warning, however: the manager must determine whether the data used for comparison in the trend analysis are comparable data.

Payer Change Assumptions

Trend analysis is retrospective; that is, it is using historical data from a past period. Forecasting is prospective; that is, it is projecting into the future. If changes, say, in regulatory requirements for payment are made this year, then that fact has to be taken into account.

STAFFING FORECASTS

Staffing forecasts are also inputs into the operating budget. We have addressed staffing computations, costs, and reports in a previous chapter. This section builds upon that information in order to produce a staffing forecast. Thus forecast considerations, components, and assumptions are addressed in this section.

Staffing Forecast Considerations

Staffing forecasts are a very common type of forecast required of managers. Three important considerations when preparing staffing forecasts are discussed here.

Controllable Versus Noncontrollable Expenses

The concept of responsibility centers and controllable versus noncontrollable expenses has been discussed earlier in this book. Essentially, controllable costs are subject to a manager's own decision making, whereas noncontrollable costs are outside that manager's power. It is extremely difficult to make staffing forecasts with any degree of accuracy if noncontrollable expenses are included in the manager's forecast. The organization's structure must be recognized and taken into account when setting up assumptions for staffing forecasts. Shared services across lines of authority are workable in theory, but often do not work in actuality. **Figure 13–3** gives an example of the essential "business units" under the supervision of a director of nurses. Note the responsibility centers and the support centers on this organization chart.

Required Minimum Staff Levels

Regulatory healthcare standards may set minimum staff levels for providing service in a particular unit. These minimum levels cannot be ignored in the forecast process.

Labor Market Issues in Staffing Forecasts

We most often hear about a chronic lack of adequate staff, and certain parts of the country do have a continual shortage of certain qualified professional healthcare staff. Yet other parts of the country can have an overabundance during that same period. The status of the local labor market has a direct impact on staffing forecasts. The impact is in dollars: when there are plenty of staff available, the hourly rate to attract staff may go down, but when there is a shortage of available qualified staff, the hourly rate has to go up. As strange as it may seem, this elemental economic fact is sometimes not taken into account in forecasting assumptions.

Staffing Forecast Components

In many cases a staffing plan is first created, and the staffing forecast follows after the plan is reviewed and refined. Four components are typically required, as follows. **Figure 13–4** illustrates the sequence.

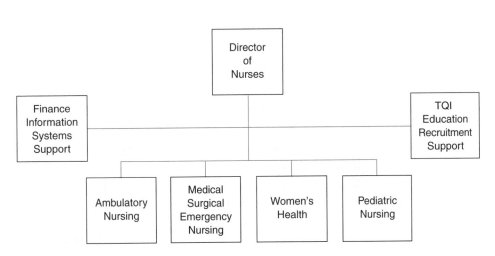

Figure 13–3 Primary Nursing Staff Classification by Line of Authority.
Courtesy of Resource Group, Ltd., Dallas, Texas.

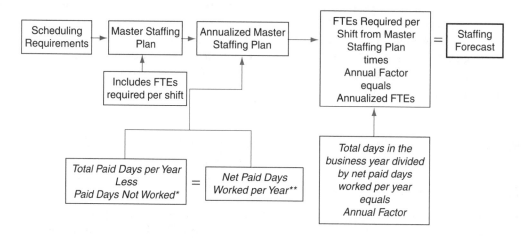

*Paid Days Not Worked = Nonproductive Days
**Net Paid Days Worked = Productive Days

Figure 13–4 Components of the Staffing Forecast.

Scheduling Requirements

Scheduling requirements should encompass all hours and days required to cover each position. For example, see the exhibit in the discussion about staffing (Chapter 9) that illustrates a single security guard position and the number of units required.

Master Staffing Plan

The master staffing plan should include all units and all hours and days required to cover all positions within the units. For example, see the exhibit in the discussion about staffing that illustrates entire units by shift, covering 24 hours per day times 7 days a week.

Computation Sequence to Annualize the Master Staffing Plan

The annualizing sequence is as follows. (This sequence is illustrated visually in Figure 13–4. An example in worksheet form appears in the chapter about staffing.)

- Compute Productive and Nonproductive Days and Net Paid Days
  The proportion of productive days (net paid days) versus nonproductive days (paid days not worked) will be based on the organization's policy as to paying for days not worked. For example, see Step 1 in the Staffing chapter's exhibit for such a computation, including "Net Paid Days." (Holidays, sick days, vacation days, and education days composed the "Paid Days Not Worked" in the worksheet example within the Staffing chapter's exhibit.)

- Convert Net Paid Days Worked to an Annual Factor
  The total days in the business year divided by net paid days worked equals a factor. Step 2 in the Staffing chapter's exhibit illustrates this computation.
- Calculate the Annual FTEs Using the Factors
  Finally, use the factor to calculate the FTEs required to fully cover the position's shifts all year long. For example, in the Staffing chapter's exhibit, the RN FTE would be 1.6 (1.6106195).

The resulting staffing forecast reflects 24 hour per day 7 days per week annual FTEs to cover all shifts.

CAPACITY LEVEL ISSUES IN FORECASTING

In the manufacturing industry, capacity levels relate to the production of, say, widgets. In the world of health care, capacity relates to services; that is, the ability to produce or provide specific healthcare services.

Space and Equipment Availability

The ability to provide services is automatically limited by the availability of both space and the proper equipment to provide certain specific services. Forecasts need to take a realistic view of these capacity levels.

Staffing Availability

Capacity is a tricky assumption to make in staffing forecasts. In some programs, particularly those in a startup phase, overcapacity (too much staff available for the amount of work required) is a problem. In some other organizations, under capacity (a chronic lack of adequate staff) is the problem. Forecasting assumptions, in the best of all worlds, take these difficulties into account. See the Mini-Case Study that demonstrates this problem of staffing in the context of the Women, Infants, and Children (WIC) federal program.[2]

Example of Forecasting Maximum Service Capacity

Exhibit 13–1 illustrates the array of elements that should be taken into account when computing maximum capacity levels. This computation is important because your forecast should take maximum capacity into account. (Alternative assumptions can also be made, of course. See the sensitivity analysis discussion in a following chapter.)

SUMMARY

In summary, the ultimate accuracy of a forecast rests on the strength of its assumptions.

Exhibit 13–1 Capacity Level Checkpoints for an Outpatient Infusion Center

---

Outpatient Infusion Center Capacity Level Checkpoints

\# infusion chairs .... 3 chairs

\# staff .... 1 RN

\# weekly operating hours .... 40 hours

\# of hours per patient infusion............. average 2 hours (for purposes of this example)

Work Flow Description

For each infusion the nurse must perform the following steps (generalized for this purpose; actual protocol is more specific):

1. Obtain and review the patient's chart
2. Obtain and prepare the appropriate drug for infusion
3. Interview the patient
4. Prepare the patient and commence the infusion
5. Monitor and record progress throughout the ongoing infusion
6. Observe the patient upon completion of the infusion
7. Complete charting

Work Flow Comments

It is impossible for one nurse to start patients' infusions in all three chairs simultaneously. Thus the theoretical treatment sequence might be as follows:

- Assume one half-hour for patient number one's Steps 1 through 4.
- Once patient number one is at Step 5, the nurse can begin the protocol for patient number two.
- Assume another one half-hour for patient number two's Steps 1 through 4.
- Once patient number two is at Step 5, theoretically the nurse can begin the protocol for patient number three.

This sequence should work, assuming all factors work smoothly; that is, the appropriate drugs in the proper amounts are at hand, the patients show up on time, and no one patient demands an unusual amount of the nurse's attention. (For example, a new patient will require more attention.)

Daily Infusion Center Capacity Level Assumption

Patient scheduling is never entirely smooth, and patient reactions during infusions are never predictable. Therefore, we realistically assume the following: Chair #1 = 3 patients per day, Chair #2 = 2 patients per day, and Chair #3 = 2 patients per day, for a daily total of 7 patients infused.

INFORMATION CHECKPOINT

What is needed?	An example of a staffing forecast created in your organization.
Where is it found?	In the files of the supervisor who is responsible for staffing.
How is it used?	Use the example to learn the nature of the assumptions that were used and the setup of the forecast itself.

KEY TERMS

Common Sizing
Controllable Expenses
Forecasts
Noncontrollable Expenses
Patient Mix
Trend Analysis
Vertical Analysis

DISCUSSION QUESTIONS

1. Do any of the reports you receive in the course of your work use trend analysis? Why do you think so?
2. Do any of the reports you receive in the course of your work use common sizing? Why do you think so?
3. Are you or your immediate supervisor involved with staffing decisions? If so, are you aware of how staffing forecasts are prepared in your organization? Describe an example.
4. Have you, in the course of your work, become involved in problems with capacity level issues such as space and equipment availability? If so, would forecasting have assisted in solving such problems? Describe why.

NOTES

1. *Merriam Webster's Collegiate Dictionary*, 10th ed., s.v. "Forecast."
2. B. A. Brotman, M. Bumgarner, and P. Prime, "Client Flow through the Women, Infants, and Children Public Health Program," *Journal of Health Care Finance*, 25, no. 1 (1998): 72–77.

Using Comparative Data

OVERVIEW

Comparative data can become an important tool for the manager. It is important, however, to fully understand the requirements and the uses of such data.

COMPARABILITY REQUIREMENTS

True comparability needs to meet three criteria: consistency, verification, and unit measurement. Each is discussed in this section.

Consistency

Three equally important elements of consistency should be considered as follows.

Time Periods

Time periods should be consistent. For example, a 10-month period should not be compared to a 12-month period. Instead, the 10-month period should be annualized, as described within this chapter.

Consistent Methodology

The same methods should be used across time periods. For example, the chapter about inventory discusses the use of two inventory methods: first-in, first-out (FIFO) versus last-in, first-out (LIFO). The same inventory method—one or the other—should always be used consistently for both the beginning of the year and the end of the year.

Progress Notes

After completing this chapter, you should be able to

1. Understand the three criteria for true comparability.
2. Understand the four uses of comparative data.
3. Annualize partial-year expenses.
4. Apply inflation factors.
5. Understand basic currency measures.

Inflation Factors

Finally, if multiple years are being compared, should inflation be taken into account? The proper application of an inflation factor is also described within this chapter.

Verification

Basically, can these data be verified? Is it reasonable? If an objective, qualified person reviewed the data, would he or she arrive at the same conclusion and/or results? You may have to do a few tests to determine if the data can in fact be verified. If so, you should retain your back-up data, because it is the evidence that supports your conclusions about verification.

Monetary Unit Measurement

With regard to comparative data, we should ask: "Is all the information being prepared or under review measured by the same monetary unit?" In the United States, we would expect all the data to be expressed in dollars and not in some other currency such as euros (used in much of Europe) or pounds (used in Britain and the United Kingdom). Most of the manager's data will automatically meet this requirement. However, currency conversions are an important part of reporting financial results for companies that have global operations, and consistency in applying such conversions can be a significant factor in expressing financial results.

A MANAGER'S VIEW OF COMPARATIVE DATA

It is important for the manager to always be aware of whether the data he or she is receiving (or preparing) are appropriate for comparison. It is equally important for the manager to perform a comprehensive review, as described here.

The Manager's Responsibility

Whether you as a manager must either review or prepare required data, your responsibility is to recall and apply the elements of consistency. Why? Because such data will typically be used for decision making. If such data are not comparable, then relying upon them can result in poor decisions, with financial consequences in the future. The actual mechanics of making a comparative review are equally important. The deconstruction of a comparative budget review follows.

Comparative Budget Review

The manager needs to know how to effectively review comparative data. To do so, the manager needs to understand, for example, how a budget report format is constructed. In general, the usual operating expense budget that is under review will have a column for actual expenditures, a column for budgeted expenditures, and a column for the difference between the two. Usually, the actual expense column and the budget column will both have a vertical analysis of percentages (as discussed in the preceding chapter). Each different line item will have a horizontal analysis (also discussed in the preceding chapter) that measures the amount of the difference against the budget.

Table 14–1 illustrates the operating expense budget configuration just described. Notice that the "Difference" column has both positive and negative numbers in it (the negative numbers being set off with parentheses). Thus, the positive numbers indicate budget overage, such as the dietary line, which had an actual expense of $405,000 against a budget figure of $400,000, resulting in a $5,000 difference. The next line is maintenance. This department did not exceed its budget, so the difference is in parentheses; the maintenance budget amounted to $290,000, and actual expenses were only $270,000, so the $20,000 difference is in parentheses. In this case, parentheses are good (under budget) and no parentheses is bad (over budget).

USES OF COMPARATIVE DATA

Four common uses of comparisons that the manager will find helpful are discussed in this section.

Compare Current Expenses to Current Budget

Managers are most likely to be responsible for comparing the current expenses of their department, division, unit, or program to their current budget. Of the four types of comparisons discussed in this section, this is the one most commonly in use.

Table 14–1 illustrates a comparison of actual expenses versus budgeted expenses. This format reflects both dollars and percentages, as is most common. Table 14–1 shows the grand totals for each department (Dietary, Maintenance, etc.) contained in General

Table 14–1 Comparative Analysis of Budget Versus Actual

	Hospital 1					
	Year 2 Actual		Year 2 Budget		Difference	
	$$	%	$$	%	$$	%
General Services Expense						
Dietary	$405,000	45	$400,000	46	$5,000	12.5
Maintenance	270,000	30	290,000	33	(20,000)	(6.9)
Laundry	45,000	5	50,000	6	(5,000)	(10.0)
Housekeeping	180,000	20	130,000	15	50,000	38.5
Total GS Expense	$900,000	100	$870,000	100	$30,000	3.5

Services expense for this hospital. There is, of course, a detailed budget for each of these departments that adds up to the totals shown on Table 14–1. Thus, for example, all the detailed expenses of the Laundry department (labor, supplies, etc.) are contained in a supporting detailed budget whose total actual expenses amount to $45,000 and whose total budgeted expenses amount to $50,000.

The department manager will be responsible for analyzing and managing the detailed budgets of his or her own department. A manager at a higher level in the organization—the chief financial officer (CFO), perhaps—will be responsible for making a comparative analysis of the overall operations of the organization. This comparative analysis at a higher level will condense each department's details into a departmental grand total, as shown in Table 14–1, for convenience and clarity in review.

The CFO may also convert this comparative data into charts or graphs in order to "tell the story" in a more visual manner. For example, the total General Service expense in Table 14–1 can be readily converted into a graph. **Figure 14–1** illustrates such a graph.

Compare Current Actual Expenses to Prior Periods in Own Organization

Trend analysis, as explained in the preceding chapter, allows comparison of current actual expenses to expenses incurred in prior periods of the same organization. For example, consider total general services expenses of $800,000 for year 1 and $900,000 for year 2. The CFO could easily convert this information into a graph, as shown in **Figure 14–2**. This

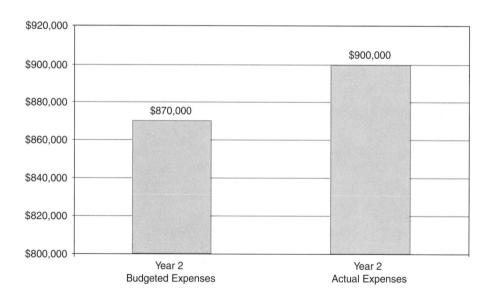

Figure 14–1 A Comparison of Hospital One's Budgeted and Actual Expenses.

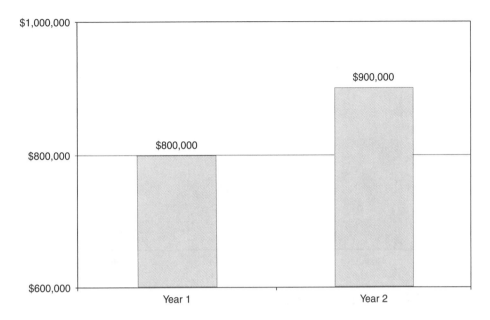

Figure 14–2 A Comparison of Hospital One's Expenses Over Time.

information might be even more valuable for decision-making input if the CFO used five years instead of the two years that are shown here.

Compare to Other Organizations

Common sizing, as explained in the preceding chapter, allows comparison of your organization to other similar organizations. To illustrate, refer to the table in a preceding chapter (Table 13–1) entitled "Common Sizing Liability Information." Here we see the liabilities of three hospitals that are the same size expressed in both dollars and in percentages. Therefore, our CFO can convert the percentages into an informative graph, as shown in **Figure 14–3**.

Be warned that the basis for some comparisons will be neither useful nor valid. For example, see **Figure 14–4**. Here we have a graph of the grand totals from the table in a preceding chapter (Table 13–2) entitled "Common Sizing Expense Information." The percentages shown are for the General Services departments of each hospital and have been common sized to percentages, as is perfectly correct. However, Figure 14–4 attempts to compare the total General Services expense (the total of all four general services departments) in dollars. As we can see here, hospital 1 and hospital 3 are both 100 beds, while hospital 2 is 400 beds. Obviously a 400-bed hospital will incur much more expense than a 100-bed hospital, so this graph cannot possibly show a valid comparison among the three organizations.

Instead, the CFO should find a standard measure that can be used as a valid basis for comparison. In this case, he or she can choose size (number of beds) for this purpose. The

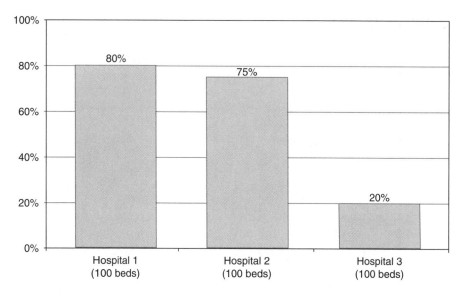

Figure 14–3 A Comparison of Three 100-Bed Hospitals' Long-Term Debt.

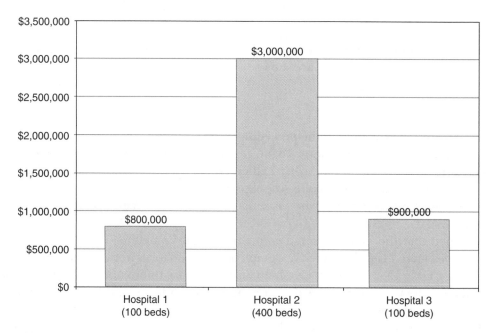

Figure 14–4 A Comparison of Three Hospitals' Total Expenses.

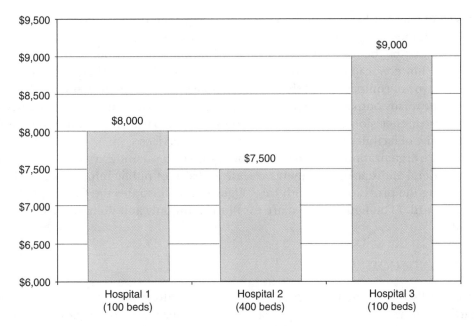

Figure 14–5 A Comparison of Three Hospitals' Expenses per Bed.

resulting graph is shown in **Figure 14–5**. As you can see, hospital 1's cost per bed is $8,000, computed as follows. The total expense of $800,000 for hospital 1 is divided by 100 beds (its size) to arrive at the $8,000 expense per bed shown on the graph in Figure 14–5. Hospital 2 ($3,000,000 total expense divided by 400 beds to equal $7,500 per bed) and hospital 3 ($900,000 total expense divided by 100 beds to equal $9,000 per bed) have the same computations performed on their equivalent figures.

In actual fact, another step in this computation should be performed in order to make the comparisons completely valid. A per-bed computation implies inpatient expenses incurred, because beds are occupied by admitted inpatients. (Outpatients, on the other hand, use a different mix of services.) Therefore, a more accurate comparison would adjust the overall total expense using one subtotal for inpatients and another subtotal for outpatients. Let us assume, for purposes of illustration, that the CFO of hospital 1 has determined that 70% of General Services expense can be attributed to inpatients and that the remaining 30% can be attributed to outpatients. Let us further assume that hospital 1's General Services expense of $800,000 as shown, is indeed a hospital-wide expense. The CFO would then multiply $800,000 by 70% to arrive at $420,000, representing the inpatient portion of General Services expense.

Compare to Industry Standards

In the example just given in the paragraph above, the CFO has computed his or her own hospital's percentage of inpatient versus outpatient utilization of General Services expense.

But this CFO may not have any way to know these equivalent percentages for hospitals 2 and 3. If this is the case, computing the per-bed expense using overall expense, as shown in Figure 14–5, may be the only way to show a three-hospital comparison.

The CFO, however, can use the 70% inpatient and 30% outpatient expense breakdown for another type of comparison. It should be possible to find industry standards that break out inpatient versus outpatient expense percentages. The use of industry standards is of particular use for decision making because it positions the particular organization within a large grouping of facilities that provide a similar set of services.

Healthcare organizations are particularly well suited to use industry standards because both the federal and state governments release a wealth of public information and statistics regarding the provision of health care. **Figure 14–6** illustrates the CFO's graph using such a standard. (The figures shown are for illustration only and do not reflect an actual standard.)

MAKING DATA COMPARABLE

This section discusses annualizing partial-year expenses, along with using inflation factors, standardized measures, and currency measures. The manager needs to know how to make data comparable as a basis for properly preparing and/or reviewing budgets and reports.

Annualizing

Because comparability requires consistency, the manager needs to know how to annualize partial-year expenses. **Table 14–2** sets out the actual 10-month expenses for the operating

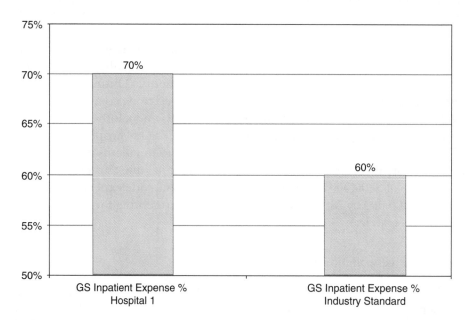

Figure 14–6 A Comparison of Hospital One's GS Inpatient Expenses with Industry Standards.

Table 14–2 Annualizing Operating Room Partial-Year Expenses

	Expenses	
Account	Actual 10 Month	Annualized 12 Month
Social Security	50,431	60,517
Pension	17,229	20,675
Health Insurance	7,018	8,422
Child Care	3,803	4,564
Patient Accounting	129,463	155,356
Admitting	91,878	110,254
Medical Records	76,432	91,718
Dietary	22,938	27,526
Medical Waste	1,981	2,377
Sterile Procedures	65,600	78,720
Laundry	33,911	40,693
Depreciation—Equipment	72,815	87,378
Depreciation—Building	34,481	41,377
Amortization—Interest	(4,849)	(5,819)
Insurance	3,513	4,216
Administration	48,305	57,966
Medical Staff	1,435	1,722
Community Relations	41,511	49,813
Materials Management	53,811	64,573
Human Resources	25,888	31,066
Nursing Administration	68,726	82,471
Data Processing	14,846	17,815
Fiscal	14,750	17,700
Telephone	2,366	2,839
Utilities	22,005	26,406
Plant	64,664	77,597
Environmental Services	27,395	32,874
Safety	1,680	2,016
Quality Management	8,347	10,016
Medical Staff	7,870	9,444
Continuous Quality Improvement	4,079	4,895
EE Health	474	569
Total Allocated	1,014,796	1,217,756
All Other Expenses	1,009,673	1,211,608
Total Expense	2,024,469	2,429,364

room. But these expenses are going to be compared against a 12-month budget. What to do? The actual 10-month expenses are converted, or annualized, to a 12-month basis, as shown in the second column of Table 14–2.

These computations were performed on a computer spreadsheet; however, the calculation is as follows. Using the first line as an example, $50,431 is 10-months worth of expenses; therefore, 1 month's expense is one-tenth of $50,431, or $5,043. To annualize for 12-months worth of expenses, the 10-month total of $50,431 is increased by 2 more months at $5,043 apiece ($50,431 plus $5,043 for month 11, plus another $5,043 for month 12, equals $60,517, the annualized 12-month figure for the year).

Inflation Factors

Inflation means "an increase in the volume of money and credit relative to available goods and services resulting in a continuing rise in the general price level."[1] An inflation factor is used to compute the effect of inflation.

Let's assume that hospital 1's General Services expenses for Year 1 were $800,000, versus $900,000 for Year 2. We can assume that these amounts reflect actual dollars expended in each year. But let us also now assume that inflation caused these expenses to rise by 5% in Year 2. If the Chief Financial Officer (CFO) decides to take such inflation into account, a government source will be available to provide the appropriate inflation rate. (The 5% in our example is for illustration only and does not reflect an actual rate.)

The inflation factor for this example is expressed as a factor of 1.05 (1.00 plus 5% [expressed as .05] equals 1.05). The CFO might apply the inflation factor to year 1 in order to give it a spending power basis equivalent to that of year 2. (Applying an inflation factor for a two-year comparison is not usually the case, but let us assume the CFO has a good reason for doing so in this case.) The computation would thus be $800,000 year 1 expense times the 1.05 inflation factor equals an inflation-adjusted year 1 expense figure of $840,000.

However, if the CFO wants to apply an inflation factor to a whole series of years, he or she must account for the cumulative effect over time. An example appears in **Table 14–3**. We assume a base of $500,000 and an annual inflation rate of 10%. The inflation factor for the first year is 10%, converted to 1.10, just as in the previous example, and $500,000 multiplied by 1.10 equals $550,000 in nominal dollars.

Beyond the first year, however, we must determine the cumulative inflation factor. For this purpose we turn to the Compound Interest Table. It shows "The Future Amount of $1.00," and appears in Appendix B of the chapter about time value of money. "The Future Amount of $1.00" table has years down the left side (vertical) and percentages across the top (horizontal). We find the 10% column and read down it for years one, two, three, and so on.

As shown in **Table 14–3.2**, the factor for year 2 is 1.210; for year 3 is 1.331, and so on. We carry those factors to column C of **Table 14–3.1**. Now we multiply the $500,000 in column B

Table 14–3 Applying a Cumulative Inflation Factor

Table 14–3.1

SOURCE OF FACTOR IN COLUMN C ABOVE:
From the Compound Interest Look-Up Table
"The Future Amount of $1.00" (Appendix 12-B)

Year	Factors as shown at 10%
1	1.100
2	1.210
3	1.331
4	1.464

Table 14–3.2

	(A)	(B)	(C)	(D)
	Year	Real Dollars	Cumulative Inflation Factor*	Nominal Dollars**
	1	$500,000	$(1.10)^1 = 1.100$	$550,000
	2	500,000	$(1.10)^2 = 1.210$	605,000
	3	500,000	$(1.10)^3 = 1.331$	665,500
	4	500,000	$(1.10)^4 = 1.464$	732,050

*Assume an annual inflation rate of 10%. Thus 1.00 + 0.10 = the 1.10 factor in Column C.
**Column D "Nominal Dollars" equals Column B times Column C.

times the factor for each year to arrive at the cumulative inflated amount in column D. Thus $500,000 times the year 2 factor of 1.210 equals $605,000, and so on.

Currency Measures

Monetary unit measurement, and the related currency measures and currency conversions, are typically beyond most manager's responsibilities. Nevertheless, it is important for the manager to understand that consistency in applying such measures and conversions will be a significant factor in expressing financial results of companies that have global operations.

Therefore, for comparative purposes we must determine if all the information being prepared or under review is measured by the same monetary unit. A few foreign currency examples are illustrated in **Exhibit 14–1**. Currencies are typically converted for financial reporting purposes using the U.S.-dollar foreign exchange rates as of a certain date.

Exchange rates may be expressed in two ways: "in U.S. dollars" or "per U.S. dollars." For example, assume the euro is trading at 1.3333 in U.S. dollars and at 0.7500 per U.S. dollars. That means if you were spending your U.S. dollar in, say, France (part of the "euro area"), it would take a third as much (1.33) in your dollars to buy products priced in euros. If your French friend, on the other hand, was spending euros for products priced in U.S. dollars, he or she could buy one-quarter more for his or her money (because the U.S. dollar would be worth only three quarters [0.7500] of the euro at that particular exchange rate).

Standardized Measures

A final word about standardized measures. Standardized measures aid comparability. They especially assist in performance measurement. Types of standardized measures include the typical hospital per-bed measure along with work load measures.

There is, of course, a whole array of uses for standardized measures. Managed care plans, for example, may use a standard set of measures that are applied to every physician who contracts with the plan. Each physician then receives a report from the plan that illustrates his or her performance.

Exhibit 14–1 Foreign Currency Examples

Country (or Area)	*Currency*
Canada	Canadian dollar
China	Yuan
Euro Area	Euro
Japan	Yen
Mexico	Peso
United Kingdom	Pound

Finally, electronic medical records (as further discussed in following chapters) depend upon standardized input. The input into various fields is standardized (and thus made comparable) by the very nature of the electronic system design.

CONSTRUCTING CHARTS TO SHOW THE DATA

Managers use charts to explain their projects and to report their results. Thus constructing accurate and effective charts is a valuable skill.

Types of Charts

There are four basic chart styles as follows:

- Column chart
- Pie chart
- Bar chart
- Line chart

The column chart's data is presented in vertical columns. The pie chart is typically circular (like a pie, thus its name). The bar chart presents data in horizontal bars. The line chart generally uses multiple lines that track along a grid.

Chart Content and Format

Constructing the chart means answering a series of questions about content and format, as follows:

- What is the subject of the chart?
- What are the specific elements to be included?
- What type of chart will best serve my purpose?
- Is the information accurate and consistent?
- If applicable, is the information comparable?
- What are the dimensions of the chart?
- If applicable, what is the span between high and low?

Chart Templates

A variety of chart templates are now available online. They are generally found within office suite programs. Each template typically offers a drop-down menu for specifics of the format and a second drop-down menu for the chart's data input. Electronic templates also provide quick and easy color choices for your chart presentation. You can experiment with various colors to reach the best combination for your project.

To summarize, the chart you construct can be simple or elaborate. It can be black and white or it can be multi-colored. But whatever its style, your chart must contain accurate and comparable data.

INFORMATION CHECKPOINT

What is needed?	Example of a detailed comparative budget review (comparing budget to actual).
Where is it found?	With the supervisor responsible for the budget.
How is it used?	To find whether data are stated in comparable terms between actual amounts and budget amounts.

KEY TERMS

Annualize
Inflation Factor
Monetary Unit

DISCUSSION QUESTIONS

1. Do you believe your organization uses a flexible or static budget? Why do you think so?
2. If you reviewed a budget at your workplace, do you think the major increases and decreases could be explained? If so, why? If not, why not?
3. Have you ever in the course of your work reviewed a report that had been annualized? If so, did you agree with how it appeared to be annualized?
4. Were you also able to see the assumptions used to annualize? If so, were you able to recalculate the results using the same assumptions?
5. Have you ever in the course of your work reviewed a financial report that applied inflation factors? If so, were you able to see the assumptions used to apply the factors? If not, why not? Please describe.

NOTE

1. *Merriam Webster's Collegiate Dictionary*, 10th ed., s.v. "Inflation."

Construct and Evaluate Budgets

Operating Budgets

OVERVIEW

A budget is an organization-wide instrument. The organization's objectives define the specific activities to be performed, how they will be assembled, and the particular levels of operation, whereas the organization's performance standards or norms set out the anticipated levels of individual performance. The budget is the instrument through which activities are quantified in financial terms.

Objectives for the Budgeting Process

A healthcare standard view of budgeting is illustrated by the American Hospital Association's (AHA's) objectives for the budgeting process:

1. To provide a written expression, in quantitative terms, of a hospital's policies and plans.
2. To provide a basis for the evaluation of financial performance in accordance with a hospital's policies and plans.
3. To provide a useful tool for the control of costs.
4. To create cost awareness throughout the organization.[1]

Operating Budgets Versus Capital Expenditure Budgets

Operating budgets generally deal with actual short-term revenues and expenses necessary to operate the facility. The usual period covered is the next year (a 12-month period). Capital expenditure budgets, on the other hand,

After completing this chapter, you should be able to

1. Understand the difference between operating budgets and capital expenditure budgets.
2. Understand what budget expenses will most likely be identifiable versus allocated expenses.
3. Understand how to build an operating budget.
4. Understand the difference between static and flexible budgets.

may cover the next year as well, but are linked into a more futuristic view. Thus, capital expenditure budgets may cover a 5- or even a 10-year period.

BUDGET VIEWPOINTS

Responsibility Centers

In a responsibility center the manager is responsible for a particular set of activities. (We have discussed responsibility centers in a previous chapter.) In the context of operating budgets there are two common types of responsibility centers: cost centers and profit centers. As shown in **Figure 15–1**, in cost centers the manager is responsible for controlling costs. In profit centers the manager is responsible for both costs and revenues. Thus, we expect that a cost center operating budget will show costs only, while a profit center budget should show both revenues and costs.

Transactions Outside the Operating Budget

Certain transactions are outside the operating budget, as shown in **Figure 15–2**. For example, many grants received by healthcare organizations are restricted funds. The monies in a restricted fund are not to be commingled with general operations monies. Also, a restricted fund generally requires altogether separate accounting and reporting.

Foundation transactions are also outside the operating budget. Foundations are legally separate organizations that require separate accounting and reporting of their funds. Therefore, we would not expect any of their costs to be included in operations.

BUDGET BASICS: A REVIEW

A brief review of budget basics is advisable as we move into constructing an operating budget.

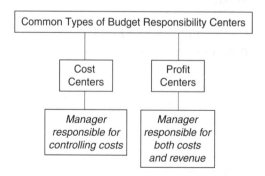

Figure 15–1 Two Common Budget Responsibility Centers.

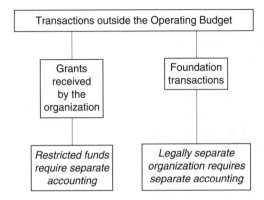

Figure 15–2 Transactions Outside the Operating Budget.

Identifiable Versus Allocated Budget Costs

Within a departmental budget, certain costs will be specifically identifiable while others will be allocated instead, as shown in **Figure 15–3**:

- Direct patient care and supporting patient care should be mostly identifiable.
- General and administrative expense and patient-related expense will probably be mostly allocated costs.
- Financial-related expense, such as interest expense, may not be included at all in the manager's budget.

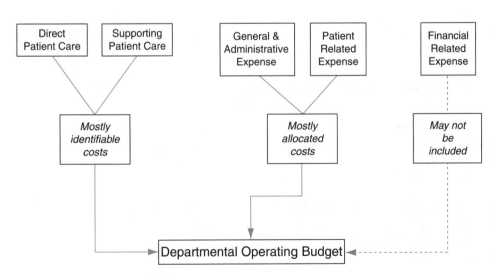

Figure 15–3 Identified Versus Allocated Costs.

Fixed Versus Variable Costs

You will recall that fixed costs do not change in total, even though volume rises or falls (within a wide range). Variable costs, however, rise or fall in proportion to a change (a rise or fall) in volume. You will further recall that volume, in the case of healthcare organizations, generally means number of procedures (outpatient services) or number of patient days (inpatient services) or perhaps, prescriptions filled (pharmacy services). **Figure 15–4** illustrates this principle, while **Exhibit 15–1** provides examples of fixed and variable cost categories that would typically be found within an operating budget.

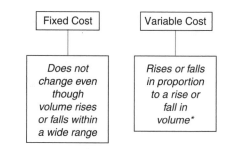

*Examples of volume: Number of procedures or patient days

Figure 15–4 Fixed Versus Variable Costs.

BUILDING AN OPERATING BUDGET: PREPARATION

Appropriate preparation is an important stage in building an operating budget. It is often difficult for the manager to allow adequate time for budget preparation, because this effort is above and beyond his or her daily responsibilities. Understanding the usual stages, or sequence, of budget construction as listed here assists in predicting how much time will be required.

Construction Stages

Operating budget construction stages include the following:

- Plan
- Gather information

Exhibit 15–1 Fixed and Variable Cost Examples

Operating Expenses	Fixed	Variable
Labor		
Gross Salaries	X	
Employers' Payroll Taxes	X	
Other Employee Benefits	X	
Part-Time Temporary Contract Labor		X
Other Expenses		
Drugs and Medical Supplies		X
Rent	X	
Insurance	X	
Five-Year Equipment Lease	X	

- Prepare input
- Construct and submit draft version of budget
- Make required revisions to draft
- Present preliminary budget
- Make required revisions to preliminary budget
- Submit final budget

Input includes both assumptions and calculations; required revisions to the draft version would occur after upper-level management has reviewed the draft. Additional revisions will typically be required after the preliminary budget has been presented. (The preliminary budget almost never becomes the final version without some degree of revision.)

Construction Elements

What will your budget look like? Will it follow guidelines from last year, or will it take on a new form? What will be expected of you, the manager? Understanding the budget construction elements will help you create a budget that is a useful tool.

As part of the preparation process, you should determine the following:

- Format to be used
- Budget scope
- Available resources
- Levels of review
- Time frame

As to format, will templates be available for use? And if so, will they be required? As to budget scope, will your budget become a segment only, to be combined and consolidated in a later stage? If this is so, you may lose some of your line items as you lose control of the final product. Necessary resources made available to you could include, for example, special data processing runs or extra staff assistance to locate required information. The levels of review, along with how many versions of the budget will be required, depend upon the structure and expectations of the particular healthcare organization.

BUILDING AN OPERATING BUDGET: CONSTRUCTION

Budget information sources, assumptions, and computations are all vital to proper operating budget construction.

Budget Information Sources

Three primary sources of operating budget information are illustrated in **Figure 15–5**. They include the Operating Revenue Forecast and the Staffing Plan or Forecast, along with a plan or forecast of other operating expenses. As Figure 15–1 illustrated earlier in this chapter, the manager who is responsible for both costs and revenues would require the revenue forecast. If, however, the manager is responsible only for costs (and not for revenues), the revenue forecast would not become part of his or her responsibility.

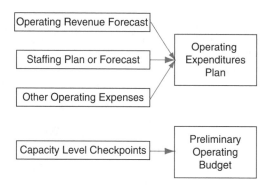

Figure 15–5 Operating Budget Inputs.

When the preliminary operating budget is under construction, the capacity-level checkpoints (discussed in a previous chapter) should also be taken into consideration. (This step may be undertaken at a different level and thus may not be your own responsibility.)

Budget Assumptions and Computations

Budget assumptions and computations are somewhat intertwined.

Assumptions

Building a budget means making a series of assumptions. The budget process should begin with a review of strategy and objectives.

Forecasting workload is a critical part of building a budget. The workload should tie into expected volume for the new budget period. Good information is necessary to forecast workload. For example, **Table 15–1** presents total nursing hours by unit. But there is not enough detail in this report to use because it does not indicate, among other things, hours by type of staff and/or staff level. Sufficient information at the proper level of detail is essential in creating a budget.

Another critical assumption in building a budget is whether special projects are going to use resources during the new budget period. Still another factor to consider is whether operations are going to be placed under some type of unusual or inconvenient

Table 15–1 Nursing Hours Report

Unit		Nursing Hours	
No.	Description	Regular	Overtime
620	S-MED-SURG DIV 5	72,509	6,042
630	N-MED-SURG DIV B	40,248	3,354
640	N-MED SURG DIV D	42,182	3,515
645	N-INTENSIVE CARE UNIT	55,952	4,663
655	S-INTENSIVE CARE UNIT	52,000	4,333
660	S-SURG ICU	21,840	1,820
665	S-STEPDOWN	52,208	4,351

circumstances during the new budget period. A good example would be renovation of the work area.

Computations

Computations should be supported by their assumptions and should be replicable; that is, another individual should be able to reproduce your computations when using the same assumptions. Computations must also be comparable; that is, the same type of computation must be used by each unit or each department. Thus, when the departmental budgets are combined, they will all be stated on the same basis.

An example of computations that must be comparable is contained in **Figure 15–6**. Recall information about preparation of the Staffing Forecast (an input to the operating budget), which has been described in the preceding chapter about staffing. Now costs must be attached to the forecast for budget purposes. As shown in Figure 15–6, the forecast should first contain annual FTEs and Total Paid Days Required. When cost is attached to the cost of Annual Paid Days Required, that cost should include Gross Salaries and Employee Benefit Costs. If one department defines total employee benefit cost one way and another department defines it more broadly, then the resulting combined budget's staffing dollars will not have been computed on a comparable basis. That budget will be flawed.

Finalize and Implement the Budget

The final budget is approved for use after multiple reviews and adjustments of the preliminary budget drafts. The final step is then to implement the new budget. It is important to explain the contents to all involved personnel. It may also be necessary to provide training for new report formats or similar issues.

WORKING WITH STATIC BUDGETS AND FLEXIBLE BUDGETS

Both static budgets and flexible budgets can be useful tools if wielded by a manager who understands both their strengths and their weaknesses.

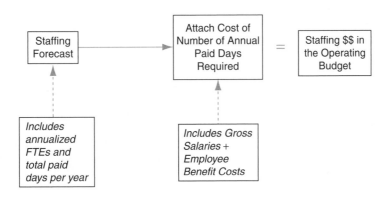

Figure 15–6 Staffing Money in the Operating Budget.

Definitions and Uses

Definitions and uses of the static budget and the flexible budget are included in this section.

Static Budget

A static budget is essentially based on a single level of operations. After a static budget has been approved and finalized, that single level of operations (volume) is never adjusted. Budgets are measured by how they differ from actual results. Thus, a variance is the difference between an actual result and a budgeted amount when the budgeted amount is a financial variable reported by the accounting system. The variance may or may not be a standard amount, and it may or may not be a benchmark amount.[2]

The computation of a static budget variance only requires one calculation, as follows:

$$\frac{\text{Actual}}{\text{Results}} - \frac{\text{Static Budget}}{\text{Amount}} = \frac{\text{Static Budget}}{\text{Variance}}$$

The basic thing to understand is that static budgeted expense amounts never change, when volume actually changes during the year. In the case of health care, we can use patient days as an example of level of volume, or output. Assume that the budget anticipated 400,000 patient days this year (patient days equating to output of service delivery; thus, 400,000 output units). Further assume that the revenue was budgeted for the expected 400,000 patient days and that the expenses were also budgeted at an appropriate level for the expected 400,000 patient days. Now assume that only 360,000, or 90%, of the patient days are going to actually be achieved for the year. The budgeted revenues and expenses still reflect the original expectation of 400,000 patient days. This example is a static budget; it is geared toward only one level of activity, and the original level of activity remains constant or static.

Static budgets may be used to plan. When utilized in this way, these budget figures represent a goal for the budget period. **Table 15–2** illustrates this concept. The table shows a goal of 100 procedures to be performed during the budget period, along with the revenues and expenses that support that goal.

Table 15–2 Static Budget: Can Be Used to Plan (a Goal)

	Static Budget Assumptions per Procedure	Static Budget Totals
# Procedures Performed		100
Net Revenue ($200 @)	$200 per procedure =	$20,000
Expenses	[various]	15,000
Operating Income		$5,000

Note: Dollar amounts shown for illustration only.

Flexible Budget

A flexible budget is one that is created using budgeted revenue and/or budgeted cost amounts. A flexible budget is adjusted, or flexed, to the actual level of output achieved (or perhaps expected to be achieved) during the budget period.[3] A flexible budget thus looks toward a range of activity or volume (versus only one level in the static budget).

Flexible budgets became important to health care when diagnosis-related groups (DRGs) were established in hospitals in the 1980s. The development of a flexible budget requires more time and effort than does the development of a static budget. If the organization is budgeting with workload standards, for example, the static budget projects expenses at a single normative level of workload activity, whereas the flexible budget projects expenses at various levels of workload activity.[4]

The concept of the flexible budget addresses workloads, control, and planning. The budget checklists contained in Appendix A are especially applicable to the flexible budget approach.

To build a flexible budget that looks toward a range of volume, or activity, instead of a single static amount, one must first determine the relevant range of volume, or activity:

- Thus, the outer limits of fluctuations are determined by defining the relevant range.
- Next, one must analyze the patterns of the costs expected to occur during the budget period.
- Third, one must separate the costs by behavior (fixed or variable).

Finally, one can prepare the flexible budget—a budget capable of projecting what costs will be incurred at different levels of volume, or activity.

Flexible budgets can readily be used to review the prior performance of the unit, the department, or the organization. When utilized for this purpose, these budget figures will typically include the volume range (for example, a range of number of procedures or number of patient days) discussed above. **Table 15–3** illustrates this concept. The table shows

Table 15–3   Flexible Budget—Used to Review Prior Performance

	(1)	(2)	(3)	(4)
	Flexible Budget Assumptions per Procedure	Range of #s of Procedures (Volume Range)		
# Procedures Performed		50	100	150
Net Revenue	$200 per procedure =	$10,000	$20,000	$30,000
Variable Expense	$150 per procedure =	7,500	15,000	22,500
Fixed Expense	[fixed total amount]	1,500	1,500	1,500
Total Expense		$9,000	$17,500	$24,000
Operating Income		$1,000	$3,500	$6,000

Note: Dollar amounts shown for illustration only.

a volume range of 50, 100, and 150 procedures to be performed during the budget period, along with the per-procedure assumptions for revenues and variable expense plus the total fixed expenses that would accompany these procedures.

Examples

Examples of both static budgets and flexible budgets appear in this section.

Static Budget Example

A static budget example for an open imaging center appears in **Table 15–4**. The net revenue is computed using a dollar amount per procedure ($400) multiplied by the budgeted total number of procedures performed (1,000 procedures). The total expenses are derived from a variety of sources.

Flexible Budget Example

A flexible budget example for an infusion center located within a physician practice appears in **Table 15–5**. The table shows a volume range of 64, 80, and 96 procedures to be performed during the budget period, along with the per-procedure assumptions for revenues and variable expense, plus the total fixed expenses that would accompany these procedures.

BUDGET CONSTRUCTION SUMMARY

There is no one right way to prepare an operating budget. The budget construction depends on factors such as the organizational structure, the reporting system, the manager's scope of responsibility and controllable costs, and so on. **Exhibit 15–2** sets out a series of questions and steps to undertake when commencing to build a budget.

Table 15–4   Static Budget Example for an Open Imaging Center

	Static Budget Assumptions per Procedure	Static Budget Totals
# Procedures Performed		1,000
Net Revenue	$400 per procedure =	$400,000
Expenses		
Salaries & Employee Benefits	[various]	$150,000
Supplies	[various]	25,000
Insurance—General	[various]	5,000
Insurance—Malpractice	[various]	10,000
Depreciation—Building	[various]	50,000
Depreciation—Equipment	[various]	100,000
Total Expenses		$340,000
Operating Income		$60,000

Note: Dollar amounts shown for illustration only.

Table 15–5 Flexible Budget Example for Infusion Center Within a Physician Practice

	(1)	(2)	(3)	(4)
	Flexible Budget Assumptions per Procedure	*Range of #s of Infusions (Volume Range)*		
# Procedures Performed		64	80	96
Net Revenue	$2,250 per infusion =	$144,000	$180,000	$216,000
Variable Expense	$1,500 per infusion =	96,000	120,000	144,000
Fixed Expense	[fixed total amount]	40,000	40,000	40,000
Total Expense		$136,000	$160,000	$184,000
Operating Income		$8,000	$20,000	$32,000

Note: Dollar amounts shown for illustration only.

It is also important to note that the budget for operations is usually part of an overall, or comprehensive, financial budget. Responsibility for the comprehensive financial budget always rests with upper-level financial officers of the organization and is beyond the scope of this chapter.

BUDGET REVIEW

The questions discussed in constructing a budget also serve to evaluate an existing budget. Issues of valid and replicable assumptions and comparability are especially essential. Comparative analysis, as examined in the preceding chapter, is an important skill to acquire. **Exhibit 15–3** sets out a series of questions and steps to undertake when commencing to review and evaluate a budget.

Exhibit 15–2 Checklist for Building a Budget

1. What is the proposed volume for the new budget period?
2. What is the appropriate inflow (revenues) and outflow (cost of services delivered) relationship?
3. What will the appropriate dollar cost be?
   (Note: this question requires a series of assumptions about the nature of the operation for the new budget period.)
3a. Forecast service-related workload.
3b. Forecast non-service-related workload.
3c. Forecast special project workload if applicable.
3d. Coordinate assumptions for proportionate share of interdepartmental projects.
4. Will additional resources be available?
5. Will this budget accomplish the appropriate managerial objectives for the organization?

Exhibit 15–3 Checklist for Reviewing a Budget

1. Is this budget static (not adjusted for volume) or flexible (adjusted for volume during the year)?
2. Are the figures designated as fixed or variable?
3. Is the budget for a defined unit of authority?
4. Are the line items within the budget all expenses (and revenues, if applicable) that are controllable by the manager?
5. Is the format of the budget comparable with that of previous periods so that several reports over time can be compared if so desired?
6. Are actual and budget for the same period?
7. Are the figures annualized?
8. Test one line-item calculation. Is the math for the dollar difference computed correctly? Is the percentage properly computed based on a percentage of the budget figure?

 INFORMATION CHECKPOINT

What is needed?	Example of variance analysis performed on a budget.
Where is it found?	Probably with the supervisor who is responsible for the budget.
How is it used?	To see what type of budget it is and to see how it is constructed.

 KEY TERMS

Capital Expenditures Budget
Flexible Budget
Operating Budget
Responsibility Center
Static Budget

 DISCUSSION QUESTIONS

1. Do you believe your organization uses one or more operating budgets? Why do you think so?
2. Do you believe your organization uses a flexible or a static budget? Why do you think so?
3. If you reviewed a budget at your workplace, do you think the major increases and decreases could be explained?
4. If so, why? If not, why not?

NOTES

1. W. O. Cleverly, *Essentials of Health Care Finance*, 4th ed. (Gaithersburg, MD: Aspen Publishers, Inc., 1997).
2. C. Horngren et al., *Cost Accounting: A Managerial Emphasis*, 9th ed. (Englewood Cliffs, NJ: Prentice Hall, 1998), 227.
3. Ibid., 228.
4. J. R. Pearson et al., "The Flexible Budget Process—A Tool for Cost Containment," *A. J. C. P.*, 84, no. 2 (1985): 202–208.

Capital Expenditure Budgets

OVERVIEW

Capital expenditures involve the acquisition of assets that are long lasting, such as equipment, buildings, and land. Therefore, capital expenditure budgets are usually intended to plan, monitor, and control long-term financial issues. Decisions must be made about the future use of funds in order to complete these types of budgets.

Operations budgets, on the other hand, generally deal with actual short-term revenues and expenses necessary to operate the facility. For example, the Great Shores Health System's operations budgets may usually be created to cover the next year only (a 12-month period), while Great Shores[1] capital expenditure budgets may be created to cover a 5-year span (a 60-month period) or even a 10-year span.

It is also important to note that the budget for capital expenditures is usually part of an overall, or comprehensive, financial budget. Responsibility for the comprehensive financial budget always rests with upper-level financial officers of the organization and is beyond the scope of this chapter.

CREATING THE CAPITAL EXPENDITURE BUDGET

The capital expenditure budget, which may sometimes be identified by another name, such as "capital spending plan," usually consists of two parts. The first part of the budget represents spending for capital assets that have already been acquired and are in place. This spending protects an existing asset; you are essentially spending in order to protect that which you already have. The sec-

Progress Notes

After completing this chapter, you should be able to

1. Recognize the reason that a capital expenditure budget is necessary.
2. Review the cash flow and the startup cost concept.
3. Understand differences between cash flow reporting methods.
4. Recognize types of capital expenditure budget proposals.
5. Understand about evaluating capital expenditure proposals.

ond part of the budget represents spending for new capital assets. In this case, you will be expending capital funds to acquire new assets such as equipment, buildings, and land.

The "existing asset" part of the budget forces planning questions about whether existing equipment and buildings should be kept in their present condition (which can involve repair and maintenance expenses), renovated, or replaced. Renovating equipment or buildings implies a large expenditure that would be capitalized. (To be capitalized means the expenditure would be placed on the balance sheet as an additional capital cost that is recognized as an asset.)

The "new capital asset" part of the budget forces more planning questions. In this case, the questions are about new assets. The reasons for new asset spending may involve the following:

- Expansion of capacity in a department or program
- Creation of a new facility, department, or program
- New equipment to improve productivity
- New equipment or space to comply with federal or state requirements

It should also be noted that acquiring new assets results in additional capital costs that will be placed on the balance sheet as assets. For more information, refer to the chapter about assets, liabilities, and net worth.

BUDGET CONSTRUCTION TOOLS

How the capital expenditure budget is constructed may be predetermined by requirements of the organization. Your facility or practice may have a template that must be used. This takes the decision out of your hands. Otherwise, you will have to decide which tool will be most effective to build your capital expenditure budget.

One important tool is net cash flow reporting. The concept of cash flow analysis, usually an important part of the capital expenditure budget, is described later. But how will the cash flow be reported? Four methods are discussed in this section.

Cash Flow Concept

As its title implies, a cash flow analysis illustrates how the project's cash is expected to move over a period of time. Many analyses concentrate only on the cash expenditure for the equipment. (This is, after all, a "capital expenditure" budget.) Other analyses, however, will also take revenue earned into account.

In any case, it is always important to report the net cash flow. While most line items will usually be expenditures, called cash outflow, sometimes there will also be cash receipts, called cash inflow. For example, if a new piece of equipment will replace an old one, and the old replaced equipment will be sold for cash, the cash received from the sale will represent a cash receipt.

Cash flow must also be reported as cumulative. This means the accumulated effect of cash inflows and cash outflows must be added and/or subtracted to show the overall net accumulated result. In our example mentioned previously: where the old equipment might be sold, the cumulative cash flow is illustrated in **Table 16–1**. As you can see, the initial expenditure or cash spent (outflow) is decreased by the cash received (inflow) to produce a net cumulative result.

Table 16–1   Illustration of Cumulative Cash Flow

Line Number		Cash Spent (Outflow)	Cash Received (Inflow)	Cumulative Cash Flow
1	Buy new equipment	(50,000)	—	(50,000)
2	Sell old equipment that is being replaced	—	+6,000	(44,000)

Cash Flow Reporting Methods

Cash flow is typically reported using one of four methods. They include the following:

- Payback method
- Accounting rate of return
- Net present value
- Internal rate of return

A previous chapter of this book has explained and illustrated each of the four methods. Their advantages and disadvantages, for purposes of capital expenditure budgeting, are summarized later.

Payback Method

The payback method is based on cash flow. This method recognizes the cash flows that are necessary to recover the initial cash invested. The payback method is advantageous because it is easy to understand and highlights risks. However, it does not take either profitability or the time value of money into account.

Accounting Rate of Return

The accounting rate of return is based on profitability. However, it does not take the time value of money into account.

Net Present Value

Net present value, or NPV, is a discounted cash flow method. It is based on cash flows in that it takes all the cash (incoming and outgoing) into account over the life of the equipment (or, if applicable, over the life of the relevant project). Although the NPV is based on cash flows, it also takes profitability and the time value of money into account.

Internal Rate of Return

Internal rate of return, or IRR, is also a discounted cash flow method that takes all incoming and outgoing cash into account over the life of the equipment (or the project). It also takes profitability and the time value of money into account.

The use of net present value, the internal rate of return, and so forth, is the vocabulary of capital budgeting. It is also an important part of the language of finance. Therefore, it is important to understand the differences between the four methods. Review the chapter about the time value of money for more detail. for more detail. Appendix 16-A at the end of this chapter presents a step-by-step method for net present value computation that assists in this understanding.

Budget Inputs

Capital expenditure budget inputs may have to be taken into consideration if the operating budget requires additional capital equipment or space renovations. **Figure 16–1** illustrates these potential inputs.

Startup Cost Concept

If the proposal for capital expenditures incorporates operational expenses, the concept of startup costs must also be taken into consideration. In these cases, management believes the cost of starting up a new service line or a new program should be included as part of the original investment. Although such operational costs do not fall into a strict definition of capital expenditure budgeting, the requirement is common enough to warrant discussion.

FUNDING REQUESTS

This section discusses the process of requesting capital expenditure funds and the types of proposals that might be submitted for consideration.

The Process of Requesting Capital Expenditure Funds

Different departments or divisions often have to compete for capital expenditure funding. The hospital's radiology department director may want new equipment, but so does

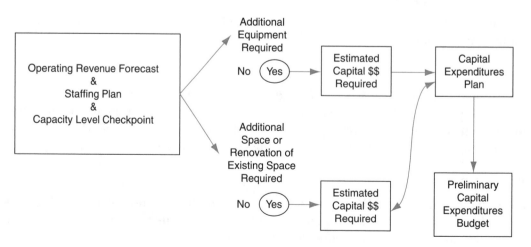

Figure 16–1 Capital Expenditures Budget Inputs.

the surgery department director, and so on. The various requests for funding are often collected and subjected to a review process in order to make decisions about where, and to whom, the available capital expenditure funds will go. While the upper levels of management make overall decisions about future use of funds, the departmental funding requests represent the first step in the overall process.

The process involved for capital expenditure funding requests varies according to the organization. Size plays a part. Due to its sheer size, we would expect a giant hospital to have a more complex process than, say, a two-physician practice. The corporate culture of the organization plays a part, too. Some organizations are extremely structured, while others are more flexible in their management principles. And in some facilities, politics may also play a part in the process of making and reviewing funding requests.

Types of Capital Expenditure Proposals

The type of proposal affects its size and scope. Proposal types commonly include the following types of requests:

- Acquiring new equipment
- Upgrading existing equipment
- Replacing existing equipment with new equipment
- Funding new programs
- Funding expansion of existing programs
- Acquiring capital assets for future use

Certain of these types may sometimes be paired as either/or choices in capital expenditure proposals. All six types of proposals are discussed in this section.

Acquiring New Equipment

The reason why new equipment is needed must be clearly stated. The acquisition cost must be a reasonable figure that contains all appropriate specifications. The number of years of useful life that can be reasonably expected from the equipment is also an important assumption.

Upgrading Existing Equipment

The reason why an upgrade is necessary must be clearly stated. What is the impact? What will the outcomes be from the upgrade? The upgrade costs must be a reasonable figure that also contains all appropriate specifications. Will the upgrade extend the useful life of the equipment? If so, by how long?

Replacing Existing Equipment with New Equipment

The rationale for replacing existing equipment with new equipment must be clearly stated. Often a comparison may be made between upgrading and replacement in order to make a more compelling argument. The usual arguments in these comparisons revolve around improvements in technology in the new equipment that are more advanced than available upgrades to the old equipment. A favorite argument in favor of the new equipment is increased productivity and/or outcomes.

Funding New Programs

A proposal for new program capital expenditures must take startup costs into account. This type of proposal will generally be more extensive than a straightforward equipment replacement proposal because it involves a new venture without a previous history or proven outcomes.

Funding Expansion of Existing Programs

A proposal for expansion of an existing program is generally easier to prepare than a proposal for a new program. You will have statistics available from the existing program with which to make your arguments. In addition, any startup costs should be negligible for the existing program. The most difficult selling point may be comparison with other departments' funding requests.

Acquiring Capital Assets for Future Use

This type of proposal may be the most difficult to accomplish. Capital expenditures for future long-term use are often postponed by decision makers in cash-strapped organizations who must first fulfill immediate demands for funding. Consider, for example, a metropolitan hospital that is hemmed in on all sides by privately owned property. The hospital will clearly need expansion space in the future. An adjacent privately owned property comes on the market at a price less than its appraised value. Even though the expansion is not scheduled until several years in the future, it would be wise to seriously consider this acquisition of a capital asset for future use.

EVALUATING CAPITAL EXPENDITURE PROPOSALS

Management planning must involve the allocation of available financial resources for projects that promise to reap returns in the future. This applies to both for-profit and not-for-profit organizations.

Hard Choices: Rationing Available Capital

Most businesses, including those providing healthcare services and products, have only a limited amount of capital available for purposes of capital expenditure. It usually becomes necessary, then, to ration the available capital funds. Different organizations approach the rationing process in different ways. However, most organizations will consider the following factors in some fashion or other:

- Necessity for the request
- Cost of capital to the organization
- Return that could be realized on alternative investments

These three factors will probably be considered in a descending sequence of decision making. The overriding question is necessity. Necessity for the request pertains to the criticality of the need. What are the basic reasons for contemplating the capital expenditure? Are these reasons necessary? If so, how necessary?

While necessity is an overarching consideration, the cost of capital to the organization for the proposed capital expenditure is a computation of the sort we have previously discussed in this section. Although the answer to "what is the cost of capital" is provided in the form of a computation, the amount of the answer depends on the method selected to illustrate this cost.

The third element in management's decision-making sequence is what return could be realized on alternative investments of the available capital. This concept is known as "opportunity cost." The term is appropriate. Assume a rationing situation where unlimited funds are not available. Thus, when a choice is made to expend funds on capital project A, an opportunity is lost to expend those same funds on project B or project C. The choice of A thus costs the opportunity to gain benefits from B or C.

To summarize, the decision makers must apply judgment in making all these choices. Thus, the rationing of available capital becomes somewhat of a management art as well as a science.

The Review and Evaluation Process

The degree of attention paid to evaluation and the level of management responsible for making the decisions may be dictated by the overall availability of capital funding and by the amount of funds requested. Evaluation of capital expenditure budget proposals may be objective or subjective. An impartial review process is most desirable.

An objective method usually involves scoring and/or ranking the competing proposals. In scoring, the basic approach generally focuses on a single proposal and evaluates it on a fixed set of criteria. In ranking, the proposal is compared with other proposals and ranked in accordance with a looser set of criteria.

The objective review and evaluation may actually first involve scoring to eliminate the very low-scoring proposals. The remaining higher scoring proposals may then be ranked in accordance with still another set of criteria.

The criteria may, in turn, contain quantitative items such as outcomes and/or productivity and may also contain qualitative items such as whether the proposal is in accordance with the organization's core mission.

Finally, some authorities believe the source of financing the project (whether it is internal or external, for example) should not be relevant to the investment decision. Real-world management, however, has a different view. How the project will be financed may be their first question in the review and evaluation process.

 INFORMATION CHECKPOINT

What is needed?	An example of an entire capital expenditure budget or a capital expenditure proposal for a particular project or a specific piece of equipment.
Where is it found?	Probably with your manager or the director of your department or, depending on the dollar amount proposed, perhaps with someone in the finance department.
How is it used?	The use would probably be one time. Can you tell if this is so?

KEY TERMS

Accounting Rate of Return
Capital Budget
Capitalized Asset
Cash Flow Analysis
Cumulative Cash Flow
Internal Rate of Return
Net Present Value
Operations Budget
Opportunity Cost
Payback Method
Unadjusted Rate of Return

DISCUSSION QUESTIONS

1. Have you ever been involved in helping to create any part of a capital expenditure budget?
2. If so, which type of proposal was it? Was the proposal successful?
3. Do you recall whether any of the four cash flow reporting methods were used? If so, which one? Do you now think that was the best choice for the particular proposal?
4. If you were assigned to prepare a capital expenditure budget request, what two people would you most want to have on your team? Why? How would you expect to use them?

NOTE

1. S. A. Finkler, "Flexible Budget Variance Analysis Extended to Patient Acuity and DRGs," *Health Care Management Review*, 10, no. 4 (1985): 21–34.

A Further Discussion of Capital Budgeting Methods

16-A

This appendix presents a further discussion of the four methods of capital budgeting computations presented in this chapter.

ASSUMPTIONS

Item: Assume the purchase of a new piece of laboratory equipment is proposed.

Cost: The laboratory equipment will cost $70,000.

Useful life: It will last five years.

Remaining value (salvage value): The lab equipment will be sold for $10,000 (its salvage value) at the end of the five years.

Cost of capital: The estimated cost of capital for the hospital is 10%.

Cash flow: The addition of this new piece of equipment is expected to generate additional revenue. In fact, the increase of revenue over expenses is expected to amount to $20,000 per year for the five years. The cash flow is therefore expected to be as follows: Year 0 = ($70,000); year 1 = $20,000; year 2 = $20,000; year 3 = $20,000; year 4 = $20,000; year 5 = $20,000. Note that year 0 is a negative figure and years 1 through 5 are positive figures.

PAYBACK METHOD

The payback method calculates how many periods are needed to recover the equipment's initial investment of $70,000. In this case, the periods to be counted are years; thus, there are five years, or five periods as shown in **Table 16-A–1**.

The investment of $70,000 is recovered halfway between year 3 and year 4, when the remaining balance to be recovered equals zero. Therefore, the payback period is three and one-half years, expressed as 3.5 years.

Table 16-A–1 Payback Method Input

Year	Cash Flow	Balance
0	(70,000)	(70,000)
1	20,000	(50,000)
2	20,000	(30,000)
3	20,000	(10,000)
4	20,000	10,000
5	20,000	30,000

Commentary: The payback method recognizes the cash flows that are necessary to recover the initial cash invested. The payback method is advantageous because it is easy to understand and highlights risks. However, it does not take either profitability or the time value of money into account.

UNADJUSTED RATE OF RETURN (AKA ACCOUNTANT'S RATE OF RETURN)

The unadjusted, or accountant's, rate of return is based on averages. The average accounting income is divided by the average level of investment to arrive at the accounting rate of return. Step 1 computes the average accounting income, Step 2 computes the average level of investment, and Step 3 then calculates the accounting rate of return.

Step 1: In this example, the average accounting income is calculated by deducting depreciation (a non-cash amount) from the annual cash flow.

Step 1.1: First, we must calculate the annual depreciation amount. In this example the depreciation is computed on a straight-line basis, which means the total amount of depreciation will equal the equipment's cost minus its salvage value.

   The equipment's cost is $70,000 and its salvage value at the end of its five-year life is estimated to be $10,000. Therefore, the total amount to be depreciated is the difference, or $60,000. To arrive at annual depreciation, the $60,000 is divided by the number of years of useful life, which is five years in this example. Therefore, the annual amount of depreciation is $60,000 divided by five years, or $12,000 per year.

Step 1.2: Next, we must use the depreciation amount to calculate the accounting income per year. In this example, the accounting income represents the cash flow per year of $20,000 as previously computed less the depreciation expense per year of $12,000. The remaining balance net of depreciation is $8,000 as shown in **Table 16-A–2**.

Step 2: In this example, the average level of investment is determined by calculating the average investment represented by the equipment. We determine the average investment by computing its midpoint as follows:

Step 2.1: Determine the total investment by adding the initial investment of $70,000 and the salvage value of $10,000, for a total of $80,000.

Step 2.2: Now divide the total investment of $80,000 by 2. The answer of $40,000 indicates the midpoint of the investment and is considered the average investment over the five-year period of its useful life.

Step 3: The unadjusted or accounting rate of return is now calculated by dividing the average income (Step 1) by the average investment (Step 2). In this example, the unadjusted

Table 16-A–2 Accounting Income Input

Year	Cash Flow	Less Depreciation	Balance Net of Depreciation
1	20,000	12,000	8,000
2	20,000	12,000	8,000
3	20,000	12,000	8,000
4	20,000	12,000	8,000
5	20,000	12,000	8,000

or accounting rate of return amounts to $80,000 average income divided by $40,000 average investment, or a 20% rate of return.

Commentary: While the accounting rate of return is based on profitability, it does not take the time value of money into account. That is why it is known as the "unadjusted" rate of return. This method is used by many capital expenditure budget decision makers.

NET PRESENT VALUE

Net present value, or NPV, is a discounted cash flow method. It is based on cash flows in that it takes all the cash (incoming and outgoing) into account over the life of the equipment. **Table 16-A–3** shows the individual steps involved in the computation as follows:

Step 1: Enter the net cash flow on the table. (For this example, the net cash flow has already been calculated; see the middle column of Table 16-A–1. Also enter the salvage value.)

Step 2: Determine the cost of capital (which is 10% in this example). Look up the present value factor for 10% for each period. Also, include the present value factor for the salvage value.

Step 3: Multiply the present value factor for each period times the period's net cash flow.

Step 4: Compute the net present value by first adding the present value answers for each operating period (Years 1 through 5 plus the salvage value) and then by subtracting the initial cash expenditure of $70,000 in Year 0 from the sum of the present value computations. In this example, 70,000 is subtracted from a total of 81,980 to arrive at the net present value of $11,980 as shown in Table 16-A–3.

Commentary: Net present value takes all the cash (incoming and outgoing) into account over the life of the equipment. Even though the net present value is based on cash flow, it also takes profitability and the time value of money into account.

INTERNAL RATE OF RETURN

Internal rate of return, or IRR, computes the actual rate of return that is expected, or assumed, from an investment. The internal rate of return reflects the discount rate at which the investment's net present value equals zero.

Table 16-A–3 Net Present Value Computations

	Year 0	Year 1	Year 2	Year 3	Year 4	Year 5	Salvage Value
Net Cash Flow	(70,000)	20,000	20,000	20,000	20,000	20,000	10,000
Present value factor (10% cost of capital)	n/a	0.909	0.826	0.751	0.683	0.620	0.620
Present value answers	(70,000)	18,180	16,520	15,020	13,660	12,400	6,200
Net present value = 11,980							

The IRR computation will be compared against the cost of capital. In our example the cost of capital is 10%, as set out in our initial assumptions.

The IRR seeks the rate of return that allows the net present value of the project to equal zero. The IRR expresses the rate of return that the organization can expect to earn when investing in the equipment (or the project, as the case may be).

The actual rate of return is determined by trial and error. The authorities say to "guess" and work forward from your initial guess. An easier method to arrive at IRR is to use a business calculator or a computer program and let it perform the computation for you. It is cumbersome, but possible, to arrive at the appropriate IRR by hand. An example follows.

This example solves for an initial investment of $70,000 and a positive cash flow of $20,000 per year for five years. Because the annual amount of $20,000 is the same for each of the five years, we can use the "Present Value of an Annuity of $1" presented in Appendix 12-C for this purpose.

The computation is approached in two steps as follows:

Step 1: Initial investment ($70,000) divided by the annual net cash inflow ($20,000) equals the annuity present value (PV) factor for five periods. We compute 70,000 divided by 20,000 and arrive at a PV factor of 3.5.

Step 2: Now we refer to Appendix 12-C, the "Present Value of an Annuity of $1." We look across the "5" row (because that is the number of periods in our example). We are looking for the column that most closely resembles our PV factor of 3.5. On our table we find 3.605 in the 12% column and 3.433 in the 14% column. Obviously 3.5 will fall somewhere between these amounts. To find what 15% would be, we add the 3.605 to the 3.433 and divide by 2. The answer is 3.519 (3.605 + 3.433 = 7.038; 7.038 divided by 2 = 3.519). Thus we have found, by trial and error, that the rate of return in our example is approximately 15%.

As we have previously stated, an easier method to arrive at IRR is to use a business calculator or a computer program and let it perform the computation for you. The business calculator or computer program will quickly give you a precise answer.

Many capital expenditure budget proposals also compare the rate of return to the organization's cost of capital. In our example, the cost of capital is 10%, so the 15% IRR is clearly greater.

Commentary: Internal rate of return is also a discounted cash flow method that takes all incoming and outgoing cash into account over the life of the equipment (or the project). It, too, takes profitability and the time value of money into account.

Tools to Plan, Monitor, and Control Financial Status

Variance Analysis and Sensitivity Analysis

VARIANCE ANALYSIS OVERVIEW

A variance is, basically, the difference between standard and actual prices and quantities. Variance analysis analyzes these differences. This discussion assumes a flexible budget prepared in accordance with the steps described in the chapters about budgeting.

Flexible budgeting variance analysis was conceived by industry and subsequently discovered by health care. It provides a method to get more information about the composition of departmental expenses.

THREE TYPES OF FLEXIBLE BUDGET VARIANCE

The method subdivides total variance into three types.

Volume Variance

The volume variance is the portion of the overall variance caused by a difference between the expected workload and the actual workload and is calculated as the difference between the total budgeted cost based on a predetermined, expected workload level and the amount that would have been budgeted had the actual workload been known in advance.[1]

Quantity (or Use) Variance

The quantity variance is also known as the use variance or the efficiency variance. It is the portion of the overall variance that is caused by a difference between the budgeted and actual quantity of input needed per unit of

After completing this chapter, you should be able to

1. Understand the three types of flexible budget variance.
2. Perform budget variance.
3. Compute a contribution margin.
4. Perform sensitivity analysis.

output, and is calculated as the difference between the actual quantity of inputs used per unit of output multiplied by the actual output level and the budgeted unit price.

Price (or Spending) Variance

The price variance is also known as the spending or rate variance. This variance is the portion of the overall variance caused by a difference between the actual and expected price of an input and is calculated as the difference between the actual and budgeted unit price, or hourly rate, multiplied by the actual quantity of goods, or labor, consumed per unit of output, and by the actual output level.

TWO-VARIANCE ANALYSIS AND THREE-VARIANCE ANALYSIS COMPARED

Variance analysis can be performed as a two- or a three-variance analysis. (There is also a five-variance analysis that is beyond the scope of this discussion.) The two-variance analysis involves the volume variance as compared with budgeted costs (defined as standard hours for actual production). The three-variance analysis involves the three types of variances defined above. **Figure 17–1** illustrates these elements.

Composition Compared

The makeup of the two-variance analysis is compared with the three-variance analysis in **Figure 17–2**. As is shown, two elements (A and B) remain the same in both methods. The third element (C) is a single amount in the two-variance method but splits into two amounts (C-1 and C-2) in the three-variance method.

Computation Compared

Actual computation is illustrated in **Figure 17–3** for two-variance analysis and **Figure 17–4** for three-variance analysis. The A, B, C, C-1, and C-2 designations are carried forward from

---

Elements of **Two-Variance Analysis** **1** Volume Variance (Activity Variance) **2** Budget Variance	**Elements of** **Three-Variance Analysis** **1** Volume Variance (Activity Variance) **2** Quantity Variance (Use Variance, Efficiency Variance) **3** Price Variance (Spending Variance, Rate Variance)

Figure 17–1 Elements of Variance Analysis.

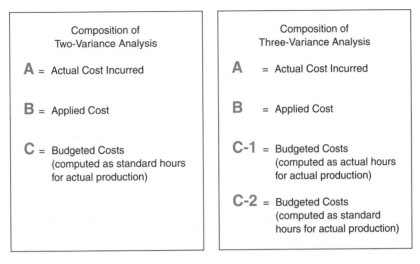

Figure 17–2 Composition of Two- and Three-Variance Analysis.

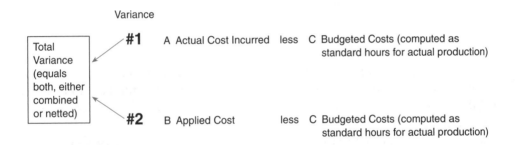

Figure 17–3 A Calculation of Two-Variance Analysis.

Figure 17–2. In Figure 17–3, the two-variance calculation is illustrated, and a proof total computation is supplied at the bottom of the illustration. In Figure 17–4, the three-variance calculation is likewise illustrated, and a proof total computation is also supplied at the bottom of the illustration. This set of three illustrations deserves study. If the manager understands the concept presented here, then he or she understands the theory of variance analysis.

Different Names for the Three Variable Cost Elements

Another oddity in variance analysis that contributes to confusion is this: all three variable cost elements—that is, direct materials, direct labor, and variable overhead—can have a price variance and a quantity variance computed. But the variance is not known by the same name in all instances. **Exhibit 17–1** sets out the different names. Even though the names

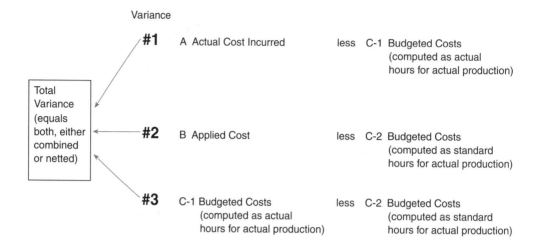

Figure 17–4 Calculation of Three-Variance Analysis.

differ, the calculation for all three is the same. Note, too, that variance analysis is primarily a matter of input–output analysis. The inputs represent actual quantities of direct materials, direct labor, and variable overhead used. The outputs represent the services or products delivered (e.g., produced) for the applicable time period, expressed in terms of standard quantity (in the case of materials) or of standard hours (in the case of labor). In other words, the standard quantity or standard hours equates to what should have been used (the standard) rather than what was actually used. This is an important point to remember.

THREE EXAMPLES OF VARIANCE ANALYSIS

This section provides three useful examples of variance analysis. The Hospital Rehab Services example is a flexible budget with all the variances expressed in Therapy Minutes (TMs). (Therapy Minutes thus serve as uniform units of measure regarding rehab services.) One of

Exhibit 17–1 Different Names for Materials, Labor, and Overhead Variances

Price or Spending Variance = Materials Price Variance	[for direct materials]
Price or Spending Variance = Labor Rate Variance	[for direct labor]
Price or Spending Variance = Overhead Spending Variance	[for variable overhead]

the two examples that follow it is a static budget variance analysis, and the other is a flexible budget example—both are carried forward from examples originating in the chapter about operating budgets.

Example 1: Hospital Rehab Services Variance Analysis

An example of variance analysis in a hospital system is given in **Exhibit 17–2**. It deals with price or spending variance and quantity or use variance. The price variance is expressed in Therapy Minutes (TMs). The quantity variance is broken out into four subtypes—physical, occupation, speech, and recreational therapy—all of which are expressed in Therapy Minutes. Finally, it is assumed that the budgeted activity level is equal to the standard activity level for purposes of this example.

Exhibit 17–2 Variance Analysis for Hospital Rehab Services

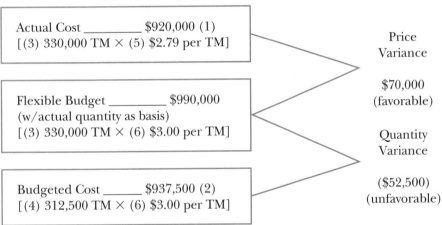

KEY TO ASSUMPTIONS
Division: Rehab Services
(Physical, Occupational, Speech, and Recreational Therapy)
Cost Driver: Therapy Minutes (TM)

	Overhead Cost	divided by	# Therapy Minutes (Activity Level)	equals	Cost per Therapy Minute
Actual	(1) $920,000		(3) 330,000		(5) $2.79
Budgeted	(2) $937,500		(4) 312,500		(6) $3.00

Computation Proof Totals
Budgeted Cost $937,500 less Actual Cost $920,000 = +$17,500
versus
Favorable Price Variance $70,000 less Unfavorable Quantity Variance ($52,500) = +$17,500

Courtesy of J.J. Baker and R.W. Baker, Dallas, Texas.

The flexible budget calculation ($990,000) is based on actual quantity. When the $990,000 is compared with the actual cost of $920,000 for this activity center, a favorable price variance of $70,000 is realized. When the $990,000 is compared with the budgeted cost of $937,500 for this activity center, an unfavorable quantity variance of ($52,500) is realized. Exhibit 17–2 also illustrates the computation of a net proof total amounting to $17,500.

Example 2: Static Budget Variance Analysis for an Open Imaging Center

An example of static budget variance analysis for an open imaging center is given in **Table 17–1**. As shown, the static budget's number of procedures performed totaled 1,000, while the actual number totaled 1,100. The revenue per procedure is $400 for both budget and actual. The net revenue variance is favorable in the amount of $40,000 ($440,000 less $400,000).

The salaries and employee benefits expense line item exceeded budget by an unfavorable balance of $20,000. Likewise, the supplies expense line item exceeded budget by an unfavorable balance of $15,000. The remaining expenses did not vary; thus the total expense variance is an unfavorable $35,000. The operating income variance equals a favorable $5,000 (the net difference between $40,000 favorable and $35,000 unfavorable).

Example 3: Flexible Budget Variance Analysis for an Infusion Center Within a Physician Practice

An example of flexible budget variance using different terminology is given for an infusion center within a physician practice in **Table 17–2**. Assumptions for revenue, variable

---

Table 17–1 Static Budget Variance Analysis for an Open Imaging Center

	Actual Amounts Incurred	Static Budget Totals	Static Budget Variance
# Procedures Performed	1,100	1,000	—
Net Revenue ($400/procedure)	$440,000	$400,000	$40,000 F
Expenses			
Salaries & Employee Benefits	$170,000	$150,000	$20,000 U
Supplies	40,000	25,000	15,000 U
Insurance—General	5,000	5,000	-0-
Insurance—Malpractice	10,000	10,000	-0-
Depreciation—Building	50,000	50,000	-0-
Depreciation—Equipment	100,000	100,000	-0-
Total Expenses	$375,000	$340,000	$35,000 U
Operating Income	$65,000	$60,000	$5,000 F

Key: "F" = "Favorable" variance, while "U" = "Unfavorable" variance.
Note: Dollar amounts shown for illustration only.

Table 17–2 Flexible Budget Variance Analysis for Infusion Center Within a Physician Practice

	(A)	(B)	(C)	(D)	(E)
	Actual Amounts at Actual Prices	Flexible Budget Variance	Flexible Budget for Actual Volume	Sales Volume Variance	Static Planning (Master) Budget
# Procedures					
1 Performed	96	—	96	16 F	80
2 Net Revenue	$216,000	—	$216,000	$36,000 F	$180,000
3 Variable Expense	$151,200	$6,000 U	$144,000	$25,200 U	120,000
4 Fixed Expense	44,000	4,000 U	40,000	—	40,000
5 Total Expense	$195,200	$10,000 U	$184,000	$25,200 U	$160,000
6 Operating Income	$20,800	$10,000 U	$32,000	$10,800 F	$20,000

Flexible Budget Variance = $11,200 U

Sales Volume Variance = $12,000 F

Static Budget Variance = $800 F

Assumptions:
Revenue per procedure = $2,250 per static budget and per actual amounts (no increase).
Variable expense (drugs) = $1,500 per static budget; increase to $1,575 actual amounts.
Fixed expense = $40,000 total per static budget; increase in total to $44,000.

Key: "F" = "Favorable" variance, while "U" = "Unfavorable" variance.
Note: Dollar amounts shown for illustration only.

expense, and fixed expense are set out below the table itself. An explanation of the computations in Table 17–2 follows.

As to Line 1, Number of Procedures:

Line 1 presents the number of planned procedures (80) and the number of actual procedures (96). Thus the procedures sales volume difference is 16 (96 less 80), and is favorable.

As to Line 2, Net Revenue:

1. Eighty planned budget procedures at $2,250 revenue apiece totals line 2 column E $180,000, while 96 actual procedures at $2,250 apiece totals line 2 column C $216,000.
2. The sales volume difference in column D totals $36,000 ($216,000 less $180,000).
3. To prove this figure, multiply the excess 16 procedures at the top of column D times $2,250 apiece equals the $36,000.

As to Line 3, Variable Expense:

1. The budgeted variable expense for drugs was $1,500 per procedure. Thus, 80 planned budget procedures times $1,500 drug expense apiece totals line 3 column E $120,000. The 96 actual procedures times the planned budget expense of $1,500

apiece totals line 3 column C $144,000. The 96 actual procedures times the actual increased variable drug expense of $1,575 apiece totals line 3 column A $151,200.

2. The total variable expense difference is $31,200 (line 3 column A $151,200 less line 3 column E $120,000).

3. Of this difference, the sales volume difference is line 3 column D $25,200. It is represented by the 16 extra procedures (96 minus 80 equals the 16 extra) times the $1,575 actual variable expense ($1,575 times 16 equals $25,200).

4. The remaining difference is line 3 column B $6,000. It is represented by the rise in expense attributed to the 80 planned budget procedures, or line 3 column B 80 procedures times $75 apiece (the difference between $1,500 and $1,575) equals $6,000. Note that line 3 column B accounts for only the rise in expense for the planned procedures (80), while line 3 column D accounts for the entire variable expense for the increase in sales volume of the extra 16 procedures.

5. Proof total is as follows: the column B $6,000 and the column D $25,200 equals the entire variable expense difference of $31,200 ($151,200 less $120,000 equals $31,200).

As to Line 4, Fixed Expense:

1. The entire $4,000 increase in line 4 fixed expense is attributed to the flexible budget variance, as it does not relate to sales volume.

2. The $4,000 excess expense is an unfavorable variance.

As to Line 5, Total Expense:

Total expenses on line 5 represents, of course, the total of variable and fixed expenses.

As to Line 6, Operating Income:

1. The entire operating income variance amounts to a favorable $800 (line 6 column E static budget of $20,000 minus line 6 column A actual of $20,800 equals $800). The $800 represents the Static Budget Variance.

2. The Flexible Budget Variance equals an unfavorable $11,200 (line 6 column C $32,000 flexible budget for actual volume minus line 6 column A actual $20,800 equals the unfavorable variance of $11,200).

3. The Sales Volume Variance equals a favorable $12,000 (line 6 column C $32,000 less line 6 column E $20,000 equals the favorable variance of $12,000).

4. Proof total is as follows: favorable $12,000 variance less unfavorable variance $11,200 equals the overall static budget variance of $800.

SUMMARY

In closing, when should variances be investigated? Variances will fluctuate within some type of normal range. The trick is to separate normal randomness from those factors requiring correction. The manager would be well advised to calculate the cost–benefit of performing a variance analysis before commencing the analysis.

SENSITIVITY ANALYSIS OVERVIEW

Sensitivity analysis is a "what if" proposition. It answers questions about what may happen if major assumptions change or if certain predicted events do not occur. The "what if" feature allows the manager to plan for a variety of possibilities in different scenarios.

Forecasts almost always should be subjected to sensitivity analysis. As previously defined, a forecast is a view of the organization's future events. Because the future cannot be predicted with absolute precision, forecasts will always contain a degree of uncertainty. Thus "what if" analyses become important to the manager's decision making. For example, "*What* will the radiology department's operating income be *if* the department's revenue is 10% greater than expected?" Or, conversely, "*What* will the radiology department's operating income be *if* the department's revenue is 10% less than expected?"

A common example of sensitivity analysis is computing three levels of forecast revenue: the basic, or most likely level, which is the planned goal; a high (best case) level; and a low (worst case) level. A chart illustrating this three-level concept for revenue appears in **Figure 17–5**.

SENSITIVITY ANALYSIS TOOLS

Manager's tools involving sensitivity analysis that are described in this section include the contribution margin and the contribution income statement; target operating income using the contribution margin method; and finding the break-even point using the contribution margin method.

Contribution Margin and the Contribution Income Statement

The contribution income statement specifically identifies the contribution margin within the income statement format. You will recall that the contribution margin is the difference between revenue and variable costs. The remaining difference is available for fixed costs and operating income.

For example, assume 100 units are sold at $50 each for a total of $5,000 revenue. Further, assume variable costs amount to $30 per unit. One hundred units have been sold, so variable costs amount to $3,000

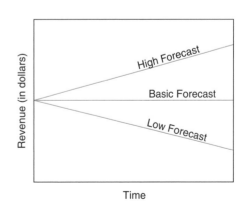

Figure 17–5 Three-Level Revenue Forecast (Sensitivity Analysis).

(100 times $30/unit = $3,000). The contribution margin equals $2,000 ($5,000 revenue less $3,000 variable costs). (For a further discussion of the contribution margin, refer to the chapter about cost behavior and break-even analysis.) Now further assume that fixed costs in this example amount to $1,200. Therefore, the operating income will amount to $800 ($2,000 contribution margin less $1,200 equals $800). The format of a contribution margin income statement will appear as follows:

Revenue	$5,000
Variable costs	3,000
Contribution margin	$2,000
Fixed costs	1,200
Operating income	$800

Target Operating Income Using the Contribution Margin Method

A target operating income computation allows the manager to determine how many units must be sold in order to yield a particular operating income. We will describe the contribution margin method of computing target operating income. This method is particularly useful to the manager because it is easily understood and can be applied in many circumstances. The formula for the contribution margin method of determining target operating income is as follows:

$$N = \frac{\text{Fixed Costs} + \text{Target Operating Income}}{\text{Contribution Margin per Unit}}$$

The necessary inputs for this formula include the following:

- Desired (target) operating income amount
- Unit price for sales
- Variable cost per unit
- Total fixed cost

Let us consider an example:

- Desired (target) operating income amount = $1,600
- Unit price for sales = $100
- Variable cost per unit = $60
- Total fixed cost = $2,000

The contribution margin per unit therefore amounts to $40 ($100 sales price per unit less $60 variable cost per unit), and the formula will appear as follows:

$$N = \frac{\$2,000 + \$1,600}{\$40}$$

$40N = $3,600

  N = $3,600 divided by $40 = 90 units

Therefore: 90 units times $100 unit price for sales = $9,000 required revenue.

  We can then create a contribution income statement to prove the formula results, as follows:

Revenue $100/unit × 90 units =	$9,000
Variable costs $60/unit × 90 units =	5,400
Contribution margin	$3,600
Fixed costs	2,000
Desired (target) operating income =	$1,600

  In summary, note that this formula is one type of cost-volume-profit (CVP) equation. (For a further discussion of the CVP concept, refer to the chapter about cost behavior and break-even analysis.)

Worksheet Example

Julie Smith is the Metropolis Health System's Director of Community Relations. She has been informed that the Health System will participate in the first area Wellness Gala, to be held at the city convention center. The gala is an annual fundraising event in which a variety of nonprofit organizations each have an opportunity to earn dollars for their cause. Individuals attending the gala will be prepared to, and are expected to, purchase items from the various booths. Julie's boss wants their proceeds to go to the Health System's auxiliary.

  It is now Julie's responsibility to make the financial arrangements and to coordinate the Health System's participation in the event. Last year the booth expense was $1,000, and Julie uses this figure as her assumption of fixed cost for the coming year's event. She finds a local vendor who assembles unique gift baskets. Her wholesale cost per basket will be $30 apiece, if she can place the order within 10 days (otherwise, the cost rises after the 10 days expires).

  Julie believes the gift baskets will sell at the gala for a sales price of $50 apiece. She prepares a worksheet to determine what dollar amount of sales would be required to earn three ranges of operating income: $5,000, $6,250, and $7,500. **Exhibit 17–3** illustrates Julie's worksheet. Line number 1 contains her first set of assumptions: $1,000 fixed cost for the booth rental and $30 variable cost for each basket.

  The convention center representative now e-mails Julie with news: due to a recent renovation of the convention center, booth rental fees have increased. It will cost Julie $1,500 for the booth. She then adds line 2 to her worksheet with a second set of assumptions: $1,500 fixed cost for the booth rental and the same $30 variable cost for each basket. She is now prepared to discuss her findings with her boss.

Break-Even Point Using the Contribution Margin Method

You will recall that the break-even point is the point at which operating revenues and costs equal each other and operating income is zero. There is a graph method to illustrate the

Exhibit 17–3 Target Operating Income Worksheet

	Fixed Cost	Variable Cost per Unit	(A)	(B)	(C)
			At $50 Sales Price per Unit, $$ Sales Required to Earn Operating Income of:		
(1)	$1,000	$30	$5,000	$6,250	$7,500
(2)	$1,500	$30	$6,250	$7,500	$8,750

break-even point (which was previously discussed in the chapter about cost behavior and break-even analysis). In this sensitivity analysis section we will describe another method to determine the break-even point. It is called the "contribution margin method." The advantage of this method is its transparency. The manager can easily explain his or her results, because the computations can be easily seen and understood.

It is understood that operating income is zero at the break-even point. It follows, then, that the number of units at break-even point can be computed. The formula is as follows:

$$\text{Break-Even Number of Units} = \frac{\text{Fixed Costs}}{\text{Contribution Margin per Unit}}$$

To compute the contribution margin per unit, subtract the variable costs per unit from the sales price per unit. In the Target Operating Income formula inputs as previously described, the sales price per unit was $100 and the variable costs per unit were $60. Thus the contribution margin per unit is $40 ($100 less $60 equals $40).

Using the same inputs, our break-even formula will now appear as follows:

$$\text{Break-Even Number of Units} = \frac{\$2,000}{\$40}$$

Thus the break-even number of units will equal $2,000 divided by $40 = 50 units.

We can create a contribution income statement to prove this formula's results, as follows:

Revenue $100/unit × 50 units = $5,000
Variable costs $60/unit × 50 units = 3,000
Contribution margin $2,000
Fixed costs   2,000
Operating income at break even = $-0-

SUMMARY

Sensitivity analysis, in its various forms, is a useful and flexible tool for planning purposes.

INFORMATION CHECKPOINT

What is needed?	Example of variance analysis performed on a budget.
Where is it found?	Possibly with the supervisor responsible for the budget. More likely, it will be found in the office of the strategic planner or financial analyst charged with actually performing the analysis.
How is it used?	To find where and how variances have occurred during the budget period, in order to manage better in the future.

KEY TERMS

Contribution Income Statement
Contribution Margin
Target Operating Income
Three-Variance Method
Two-Variance Method
Variance Analysis

DISCUSSION QUESTIONS

1. Do you believe variance analysis (or a better variance analysis) would be a good idea at your workplace? If so, why? If not, why not?
2. Are any of the reports you receive in the course of your work ever in a format that includes a contribution margin? If so, what were the circumstances?
3. Have you ever had to compute target operating income? If so, what were the circumstances?

NOTE

1. S. A. Finkler, "Flexible Budget Variance Analysis Extended to Patient Acuity and DRGs," *Health Care Management Review*, 10, no. 4 (1985): 21–34.

Estimates, Benchmarking, and Other Measurement Tools

ESTIMATES OVERVIEW

According to the dictionary, to estimate "… implies a judgment, considered or casual, that precedes or takes the place of actual measuring or counting or testing out."[1]

Such estimates may be of the following:

- amount
- value
- size

The first question should be, "Is it capable of being estimated?" Relying on estimates for input to reports (financial statements, forecasts, budgets, internal monthly statements, etc.) means sacrificing some degree of accuracy.

COMMON USES OF ESTIMATES

Using estimates often involves trade-offs, such as gaining a quick answer that is less accurate. Four common uses of estimates are described here.

Timeliness Considerations

Deadlines may dictate the use of estimates because there is no time allowed to develop more accurate figures. Some managers call these "quick and dirty" results. The quick and dirty estimates may then be followed at a later date by a more detailed report.

Cost/Benefit Considerations

Estimates may be purposely used instead of a more formal forecasting process discussed in a preceding chapter.

215

Situations do arise where an estimate is adequate. The manager may decide upon using estimates instead of proceeding with the more formal forecasting process. After assessing the effort and time involved to gather and prepare a forecast, the manager will be making a cost–benefit decision; that is, the cost (of forecasting) equivalent to the benefit (of the more precise information)? Or will estimates adequately serve the purpose? Of course, this manager's decision will depend upon the intended purpose.

Lack of Data

Estimates may also be used out of necessity when there is not enough information available to prepare a full forecast. In this case, there is no choice but to use estimates as an alternative.

Internal Monthly Statements

Estimates may be commonly used in the preparation of short-term financial statements. For example, the monthly statements that managers receive often contain a number of estimated figures that are derived from various ratios and percentages. These estimates will probably have a historical basis because they are typically based on the organization's prior years' operating history. Thus, if bad debts for the last two years averaged 2%, the monthly statements for the current year may estimate bad debts at the same 2%.

EXAMPLE: ESTIMATING THE ENDING PHARMACY INVENTORY

Certain healthcare organizations (or departments) require accounting for inventory. The most common example in health care, of course, is the pharmacy. Internal monthly statements of the pharmacy are not usually expected to reflect the results of an actual physical inventory (unless your organization has an electronic inventory program—and that is another story). So what to do? **Figure 18–1** illustrates the solution.

The computations contained in Figure 18–1 are described as follows:

1. We first add net drug purchases for the period to the beginning drug inventory, thus arriving at the cost of goods (drugs) available for sale. So far, the steps are the same and the result would be the same as that in a preceding chapter, where Figure 8–1 illustrated how to record inventory.
2. But now we will compute an estimated cost of goods (drugs) sold. To do this:

    First, find the amount of net sales (sales after allowances, discounts, rebates, etc.) for the period.

    Then find the percent of net sales that represents cost of goods (drugs) sold in a prior period. This percentage figure is your estimated assumption and it will probably come from the last year's financial report. (For example, $1,000,000 net sales and $800,000 cost of goods [drugs] sold equals 80% cost of goods sold [drugs] for last year. The 80% is your estimated assumption for this calculation.)

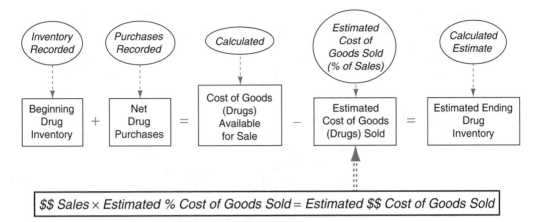

Figure 18–1 Estimating the Ending Pharmacy Inventory.

Apply this estimated assumption to the net sales for the period. (For example, if the month's drug sales amounted to $70,000, multiply the $70,000 by 80% to arrive at $56,000 for the estimated cost of goods [drugs] sold this month.)

3. Finally, we will compute the estimated ending drug inventory. We subtract the cost of goods (drugs) sold (per Step 2 above) from the cost of goods (drugs) available for sale (per Step 1 above) to arrive at the "Estimated Ending Drug Inventory" for the monthly internal report.

EXAMPLE: ESTIMATED ECONOMIC IMPACT OF A NEW SPECIALTY IN A PHYSICIAN PRACTICE

Estimates can be extremely general, or they can reflect considerable judgment, with line-item detail that has been well thought out. **Figure 18—2** illustrates an example of a general estimate and its subsequent impact.

In this case we have a four-doctor physician practice. The four MDs decide to bring another doctor into the practice. He is a pulmonary specialist. The county is growing rapidly, economically speaking, and the local hospital has just expanded. The doctors determine there is a sufficient demand within this growing area to support the services of a pulmonary specialist. They want him to join their practice, even though they have not previously had such a specialty within this practice.

One morning, the senior doctor asks the practice manager to estimate the expense involved in adding the pulmonary specialist to the practice. He wants the report for their four o'clock meeting that afternoon. They must make a decision quickly because the specialist has had another offer.

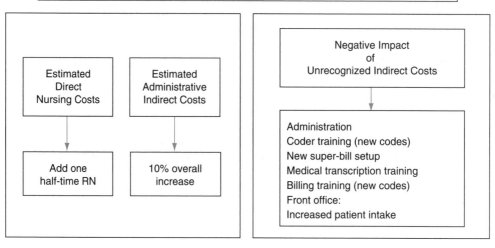

Figure 18–2 Estimated Economic Impact of a New Specialist in a Physician Practice.

The practice manager is trying to close the books for the month, but makes some time to produce an estimate. The doctors already know the amount that the specialist wants as a guaranteed salary for the first year, and they have already projected what revenue he should produce for the first year. There is an empty office available that was acquired in the initial lease for purposes of future expansion. Thus, the practice manager needs to estimate the impact on basic practice operational costs. His "quick and dirty" estimate is in two parts.

Part 1: Add one half-time RN for direct support. Assume existing nursing staff can take up any slack.

Part 2: Assume an overall 10% increase in practice administration operating costs. He has no specific basis for the 10% estimate. Instead, he knows that labor is the greatest part of practice administration costs. As a result of his "back of the envelope" calculation he thinks that administrative staff is not overworked at present and can handle tasks imposed by an additional physician. Since he disregards adding any administrative staff, he feels estimating an overall 10% increase for administrative expenses of the practice is adequate.

Three months after the pulmonary specialist has arrived and joined the practice, the senior doctor meets with the practice manager to complain. Operational costs to absorb the new specialist have far exceeded the original estimate. The doctors want an explanation from the practice manager for their meeting the next afternoon.

The practice manager realizes that his estimate did not allow for start-up costs. He composes a memo explaining that the administrative expenses were impacted by start-up costs such as coder training for the new pulmonary codes, the consultants' fees for the new super-bill setup in the office software, training about pulmonary services for the medical records transcriptionist, and training for the office biller regarding the new codes. He also notes the front office problems arising from increased patient intake, which had been underestimated. The original estimates and the negative impact of unrecognized indirect costs are illustrated in Figure 18–2.

OTHER ESTIMATES

Other commonly used computations are actually estimates. The weighted average inventory method is a good example. Weighted average cost is determined by dividing the cost of goods available for sale by the number of units available as described in the preceding chapter about inventory. The resulting average cost of inventory is in fact an estimate.

IMPORTANCE OF A VARIETY OF PERFORMANCE MEASURES

If operations are to be managed most effectively, a variety of performance measures must be in place for the organization. Generally, a broad variety of such measures are available, and different organizations tend to lean toward using one type over another. One healthcare organization, for example, may rely heavily on one type of measure, whereas another organization may rely on a very different measurement profile. Generally speaking, a wider variety of performance measures are evident in organizations that have adopted total quality improvement (TQI).

ADJUSTED PERFORMANCE MEASURES OVER TIME

We have previously discussed how measures over time are very effective when evaluating the use of money. The example given in **Figure 18–3** now combines these measures over

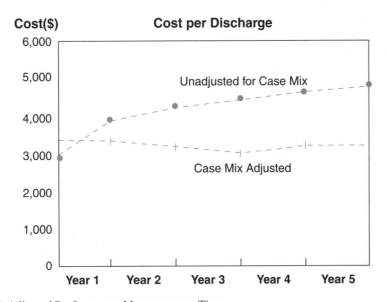

Figure 18–3 Adjusted Performance Measures over Time.

time with a two-part case mix adjustment. (*Case mix adjustment* refers to adjusting for the acuity level of the patient. It may also refer to the level of resources required to provide care for the patient with the acuity level.) In this case, the desired measure is cost per discharge. The vertical axis is cost in dollars. The horizontal axis is time, a five-year span in this case. Two lines are plotted: the first is unadjusted for case mix, and the second is case mix adjusted. The unadjusted line rises over the five-year period. However, when the case mix adjustment is taken into account, the plotted line flattens out over time.

BENCHMARKING

Benchmarking is the continuous process of measuring products, services, and activities against the best levels of performance. These best levels may be found inside the organization or outside it. Benchmarks are used to measure performance gaps.

There are three types of benchmarks:

1. A financial variable reported in an accounting system
2. A financial variable not reported in an accounting system
3. A nonfinancial variable

How to Benchmark

The benchmarking method is predicated on the assumption that an exemplary process, similar to the process being examined, can be identified and examined to establish criteria for excellence. Benchmarking can be accomplished in one of several ways, including (1) studying the methods and end results of your prime competitors, (2) examining the analogous process of noncompetitors with a world-class reputation, or (3) analyzing processes within your own organization (or health system) that are worthy of being emulated. In any of these three cases, the necessary analysis will rely on one or both of the following methods: parametric analysis or process analysis. In parametric analysis, the characteristics or attributes of similar services or products are examined. In process analysis, the process that serves as a standard for comparison is examined in detail to learn how and why it performs the way it does.

Benchmarking is used for opportunity assessment. Opportunity assessment, used for strategic planning and for process engineering, provides information about the way things should or possibly could be. Benchmarking is a primary information-gathering approach for opportunity assessment when it is used in this way.

Benchmarking in Health Care

Financial benchmarking compares financial measures among benchmarking groups. This is the most common type of "peer group" healthcare benchmarking in use. An example of a healthcare financial benchmarking report is provided in **Table 18–1**. The computation of ratios included in this report has been discussed in preceding chapters. The computation of quartiles is described later in this chapter.

Table 18–1 Financial Benchmark Example

Indicator	Total	Upper Quartile	Mid Quartile	Low Quartile
No. of hospitals	500.0	105.0	305.0	90.0
Total margin (%)	4.1	11.0	4.5	−6.0
Occupancy (%)	64.5	65.7	64.0	56.1
Deductions from GPR (%)	29.0	28.5	29.2	31.3
Medicare (%GPR)	53.0	55.1	52.2	50.4
Medicaid (%GPR)	10.0	8.4	9.7	13.7
Self-pay (%GPR)	7.0	8.5	7.1	6.4
Managed care plans (%GPR)*	16.0	13.0	17.0	17.5
Other third party (%GPR)	14.0	15.0	14.0	12.0
Outpatient revenue (%GPR)	22.0	25.0	21.8	17.7
No. of days in accounts receivable	75.0	70.0	74.0	80.0
Cash flow as a percentage of total debt	30.0	60.0	27.0	−0.5
Long-term debt as a percentage of total assets	35.0	26.0	36.0	42.0
Change in admissions (2003–2007, %)	−7.0	−3.7	−6.3	−15.8
Change in inpatient days (2003–2007, %)	−6.0	−1.8	−6.5	−11.1

*Note: Managed care plans other than Title XVIII or Title XIX. All amounts are fictitious.
Adapted from J.J. Baker, *Activity-Based Costing and Activity-Based Management for Health Care*, p. 140, © 1998, Aspen Publishers, Inc.

Statistical benchmarking is a related method of benchmarking. In this case, the statistics of utilization and service delivery, on which inflow and outflow are based, are compared with those of certain other hospitals.

In summary, benchmarking is a comparative method that allows an overview of the individual organization's indicators. Objective measurement criteria are always required for best practices purposes.

ECONOMIC MEASURES

Other performance measures may be made outside the actual confines of the facility. A good example of a widespread performance measure would be the role of community hospitals in the performance of local economies. Nonprofit organizations in particular are concerned about their ability to measure such performance. This case study gives a specific direction for such measurement efforts.

MEASUREMENT TOOLS

Pareto Analysis

Creating benchmarks, especially in an organization committed to continuous quality improvement, ultimately leads managers to explore how to improve some step in a process. Pareto analysis is an analytical tool that employs the Pareto principle and helps in this exploration. Pareto was a 19th-century economist who was a pioneer in applying mathematics to economic theory. His Pareto principle states that 80% of an organization's problems, for example, are caused by 20% of the possible causes: thus the "80/20 Rule."

The usual way to display a Pareto analysis is through the construction of a Pareto diagram. A Pareto diagram displays the important causes of variation, as reflected in data collected on the causes of such variation. **Figure 18–4** presents an example of a Pareto diagram. This example reinforces the idea behind the Pareto analysis: that the majority of problems are due to a small number of identifiable causes.

The chief financial officer of XYZZ Hospital believes that the billing and collection department is inefficient—or, to be more specific, that the process is probably inefficient. An activity analysis is conducted. It shows that billing personnel are spending too much time on unproductive work. This Pareto diagram displays the activities involved in resubmitting denied bills. (Resubmitting denied bills is an inefficient and nonproductive activity, as we have discussed in a preceding chapter.)

Constructing a Pareto diagram is really simple. The first step is to prepare a table that shows the activities recorded, the number of times the activities were observed, and the percentage of the total number of times represented by each count. In Figure 18–4, the total number of times these activities were observed is 43. The number of times that processing denied bills for resubmission (coded as PDB) was observed is 22. Thus, 100 (22/43) = 51%. Similar calculations complete the table. The table of observations is shown in its entirety within the figure.

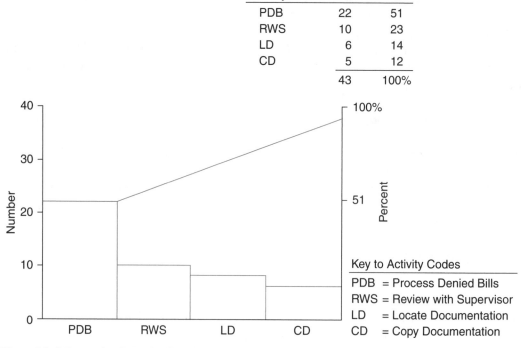

Activity	No.	%
PDB	22	51
RWS	10	23
LD	6	14
CD	5	12
	43	100%

Key to Activity Codes

PDB = Process Denied Bills
RWS = Review with Supervisor
LD   = Locate Documentation
CD   = Copy Documentation

Figure 18–4 Pareto Analysis of Billing Department Data.

The Pareto diagram has two vertical axes, the left one corresponding to the "No." column in the table, the right one corresponding to the "%" column in the table. On the horizontal axis, the activities are listed, creating bases of equal length for the rectangles shown in the diagram. The activities are listed in decreasing order of occurrence. Constructing the diagram in this manner means that the most frequently observed activity lies on the left extreme of the diagram and the least frequently observed activity on the right extreme. The heights of the rectangles are drawn to show the frequencies of the activities, and then the sides of the rectangle are drawn.

The next step is to locate the cumulative percentage of the activities, using the right-hand axis. The cumulative percent for the first rectangle, labeled *PDB*, is 51%. (The calculation of the 51% was previously explained.) For the second rectangle from the left, labeled *RWS*, the cumulative percentage is 51 + 23 = 74%. The 74% is plotted over the right-hand side of the rectangle labeled *RWS*. The next cumulative percentage, for the third rectangle from the left, labeled *LD*, is 51 + 23 + 14 = 88%. The 88% is plotted over the right-hand side of the rectangle labeled *LD*. The last cumulative percentage is, of course, 100% (51 + 23 + 14 + 12 = 100%), and it is plotted over the right-hand side of the last rectangle on the right, labeled *CD*.

Now draw straight lines between the plotted cumulative percentages as shown in Figure 18–4. The next step is to label the axes and add a title to the diagram. In Figure 18–4, the tallest rectangle could be lightly shaded to highlight the most frequent activity, suggesting the one that may deserve first priority in problem solving.

In general, the activities requiring priority attention—the "vital few"—will appear on the left of the diagram where the slope of the curve is steepest. Pareto diagrams are often constructed before and after improvement efforts for comparative purposes. When comparing before and after, if the improvement measures are effective, either the order of the bars will change or the curve will be much flatter.

In conclusion, note that many authorities recommend that Pareto analysis take the costs of the activities into account. The concern is that a very frequent problem may nevertheless imply less overall cost than a relatively rare but disastrous problem. Also, before basing a Pareto analysis on frequencies, as this example does, the analyst needs to decide that the seriousness of the problem is roughly proportional to the frequency. If seriousness fails to satisfy this criterion, then activities should be measured in some other way. Figure 18–4 underlines the importance of judging the relevance of the measurements used in a Pareto analysis.

Quartile Computation

Reporting by quartiles is an effective way to show ranges of either financial or statistical results. Quartiles represent a distribution into four classes, each of which contains one-quarter of the whole. Each of the four classes is a quartile. Quartile computation is not very complicated, although several steps are involved. We can use the outpatient revenue line item in Table 18–1 to illustrate the computation of quartile data. (Outpatient revenue, expressed as a percentage of all revenue, is found on the tenth line down from the top in Table 18–1.) We see from the first line that 500 hospitals were in the group used for benchmarking. The median is found for the outpatient revenue of the entire group of hospitals. (Most computer spreadsheet programs offer median computation as an available function.) Then each hospital's revenue is identified as a percentage of this median. These percentages are arrayed. In the case of this report, cutoffs were then made to arrange the arrayed percentages into three groups. The percentages that were between 0 and 25% were designated as the low-quartile group. The percentages that were between 75 and 100% were designated as the upper-quartile group. The percentages that were between 25 and 75% were designated as the mid-quartile group.

The average (also known as the arithmetic mean) of each quartile group is then presented in this report. Thus, the outpatient revenue (expressed as a percentage of gross revenue) for the upper-quartile group in the report is 25.0; for the mid-quartile group, 21.8; and for the low-quartile group, 17.7. (A grand total of the entire 500 hospitals is also computed and presented in the left-hand column; the grand total amounts to 22%.) In summary, quartiles are based on a quantitative method of computation and are an effective way to illustrate a variety of performance measures.

 INFORMATION CHECKPOINT

What is needed?   An example of estimates, either used in some way in your work, or published.

Where is it found?   In your own files or from a public source.

How is it used?   Use the example to examine how the estimate was determined, if possible.

 KEY TERMS

Benchmarking
Case Mix Adjusted
Estimates
Pareto Analysis
Performance
Performance Measures
Quartiles

 DISCUSSION QUESTIONS

1. Have you, in the course of your work, had to estimate items for reports? If so, what type of items? How did you go about estimating?
2. Does your organization use measurements such as the case mix adjustment over time? If not, do you believe they should? Why?
3. Does your organization use financial benchmarking? Would you use it if you had a chance to do so? Why?

NOTE

1. *Merriam Webster's Collegiate Dictionary*, 10th ed., s.v. "Estimate."

# PART VIII

Financial Terms, Costs, and Choices

Understanding Investment Terms

OVERVIEW

The language of investment is an integral part of the finance world. Being knowledgeable about the meaning that lies behind investment terms allows you a wider view of finance transactions. This chapter concerns a selection of common investment terms. We will briefly explore investment terminology and related meanings for cash equivalents, long-term investments in bonds, investments in stocks, and company ownership (public or private) in the context of investing, along with investment indicators.

Investments should be recorded as either current assets or long-term assets on the balance sheet of the organization. You will recall from a previous chapter that current assets involve cash and cash equivalents, along with short-term securities (those that will mature in one year or less). These items should all appear as current assets on the balance sheet. Long-term investments, on the other hand, involve longer-term securities that will mature in more than one year. These investments should appear as long-term items on the balance sheet.

CASH EQUIVALENTS

Cash equivalents are termed liquid assets; that is, they can be liquidated and turned into cash on short notice when needed. Healthcare organizations need to keep operating monies on hand. But it is not usually practical to hold those monies in a non-interest-bearing checking account. Instead, the chief financial officer will probably decide to temporarily place the monies in some type of liquid asset (a cash equivalent) in order to earn a little interest.

After completing this chapter, you should be able to

1. Define cash equivalents.
2. Understand what the FDIC does and does not insure.
3. Understand the difference between municipal bonds and mortgage bonds.
4. Understand the difference between privately held companies and public companies.
5. Define Gross Domestic Product (GDP).

Actual cash includes not just currency (the dollar bills in your wallet), but also monies held in bank checking accounts and savings accounts, plus coins, checks, and money orders. Cash equivalents include the following:

- certificates of deposit (CDs) from banks
- government securities (including both Treasury bills and Treasury notes)
- money market funds

All of these short-term investments should be not only very liquid, but low-risk. (A prudent chief financial officer should, of course, seek low-risk investments.)

Certificates of deposit can be purchased for various short periods of time (30 days, 60 days, 90 days, etc.). The certificates earn interest and can be withdrawn (cashed) after the short period, or term, expires, without paying a penalty.

Government securities that rank as cash equivalents include both Treasury bills and Treasury notes. Treasury bills are typically issued with maturities of 3, 6, or 12 months. There is a minimum dollar amount to purchase. A Treasury bill pays the full amount invested if redeemed at maturity. If the bill is redeemed prior to maturity, however, the amount received may be either higher or lower than your cost, depending upon the current market.

Treasury notes are typically issued with longer maturities—years instead of months. The shortest maturity period for a Treasury note is one year. A one-year note would be classified as short-term and could be recorded as a current asset.

Money market funds are supposed to invest in conservative instruments such as commercial bank CDs and Treasury bills. A money market fund should invest in an assortment of such conservative instruments. Portfolio managers, who are expected to manage responsibly and thus select only low-risk investments, manage these funds. Money market funds are somewhat of a hybrid, as these funds typically allow check-writing privileges. Thus, the investor is able to withdraw funds by writing what is actually a draft against the fund, although most everyone thinks of this draft as a check.

GOVERNMENTAL GUARANTOR: THE FDIC

In the United States, the Federal Deposit Insurance Corporation (FDIC) "preserves and promotes public confidence in the U.S. financial system by insuring deposits in banks and thrift institutions ... by identifying and monitoring and addressing risks to the deposit insurance funds; and by limiting the effect on the economy and the financial system when a bank or thrift institution fails."[1] The FDIC insured deposits in banks and thrift institutions for at least $250,000 through December 31, 2009. However, this was supposed to be a temporary increase and the FDIC deposit insurance was supposed to be restored to its usual limit of $100,000 after that date. Savings, checking, and other deposit accounts are combined to reach the deposit insurance limit. "Deposits held in different categories of ownership—such as single or joint accounts—may be separately insured. Also, the FDIC generally provides separate coverage for retirement accounts, such as individual retirement accounts (IRAs) and Keoghs."[2] It is important to note that

Exhibit 19–1 The FDIC: Insured or Not Insured?

FDIC-Insured
- Checking Accounts (including money market deposit accounts)
- Savings Accounts (including passbook accounts)
- Certificates of Deposit

Not FDIC-Insured
- Investments in mutual funds (stock, bond, or money market mutual funds), whether purchased from a bank, brokerage, or dealer
- Annuities (underwritten by insurance companies, but sold at some banks)
- Stocks, bonds, Treasury securities or other investment products, whether purchased through a bank or a broker/dealer

Reproduced from the Federal Deposit Insurance Corporation. "The FDIC: Insured or Not Insured?: A Guide To What Is And Is Not Protected" (April 2011).

---

not all institutions—and thus all funds—are insured by the FDIC. **Exhibit 19–1** sets out these facts.

LONG-TERM INVESTMENTS IN BONDS

A bond is a long-term debt instrument under which a borrower agrees to make payments of interest and principal on particular dates to the holder of the debt (the bond). We have titled this section "long-term investments in bonds," but in actuality the bondholder is a creditor, because bonds are liabilities to the issuing company.

Because these are long-term contracts, bonds typically mature in 20 to 30 years, although there are exceptions. In general, interest is paid throughout the term, or life, of the bonds, and the principal is paid at maturity. (Although there are exceptions to this rule of thumb, too.) Three types of bonds are discussed below.

Municipal Bonds

Municipal bonds are long-term obligations that are typically used to finance capital projects. Municipal bonds are issued by states and also by political subdivisions. The political subdivision might be, for example, a county, a bridge authority, or the authority for a toll road project.

General Obligation Bonds

General obligation bonds are backed, or secured, by the "full faith and credit" of the municipality that issues them. This means the bonds are backed by the full taxing authority of the municipality that issues them.

Revenue Bonds

Revenue bonds, as their name implies, are backed, or secured, by revenues of their particular project. Eligible healthcare organizations that are not-for-profit can sometimes issue revenue bonds through a local healthcare financing authority.

Mortgage Bonds

Mortgage bonds, as their name implies, are backed, or secured, by certain real property. When first mortgage bonds are issued, this means the first mortgage bondholders have first claim to the real property that has been pledged to secure the mortgage. If second mortgage bonds are also issued, this means the second mortgage bondholders will not have a claim against the real property until the claims of the first mortgage bondholders have been paid.

Debentures

Debentures are bonds that are unsecured. Instead of being backed by real property, debentures are backed by revenues that the issuing organization can earn. Unlike bondholders, holders of debentures are unsecured. Subordinated debentures are even further unsecured, in that these debentures cannot be paid until any and all debt obligations that are senior to the subordinated debentures have been paid.

INVESTMENTS IN STOCKS

Stocks represent equity, or net worth, in a company. This is in contrast to bonds. Generally speaking, a bondholder is a creditor, because bonds are liabilities to the issuing company. On the other hand, an individual or organization that buys stock in that company becomes an investor, not a creditor.

Common Stock

A purchaser of common stock expects to receive a portion of net income of the company who issues the stock. The proportionate share of net income will be paid out as a dividend. (Note that start-up companies that do not pay dividends are not part of this discussion about investments in stocks.)

Preferred Stock

Preferred stock, as its name implies, has preference over common stock in certain issues such as payment of dividends. In actual fact, preferred stock is a type of hybrid, in that it generally has a fixed-rate dividend payment, much like a bond's interest payment. But like common stock, it also expects to receive a portion of net income of the company who issues the stock, up to the amount of the fixed-rate dividend payment. (Also note that the preferred stock dividends are paid before the common stock dividends.)

Convertible preferred stock is a type of preferred stock that can be exchanged for common shares. The exchange is usually at a particular time and price, and the exchange ratio of preferred-to-common is also stipulated.

Stock Warrants

Stock warrants allow the owner of the warrant to purchase additional shares of stock in the company, generally at a particular price and prior to an expiration date. Warrants do not pay dividends. They are often part of the compensation package awarded to executives.

PRIVATELY HELD COMPANIES VERSUS PUBLIC COMPANIES

Whether a stock is listed on a stock exchange or not is a function of ownership and size of the organization. These distinctions are described here.

Privately Held Companies

A small company with common stock that is not traded is known as a "privately held" company. Its stock is termed "closely held" stock.

Public Companies

Companies with publicly owned common stock are known as "public companies." The stocks of many larger public companies may be listed on one of several stock exchanges. Stock exchanges exist to trade the stock of publicly held companies. At the time of this writing, besides multiple regional exchanges such as the Chicago Stock Exchange, there is the American Stock Exchange, known as AMEX, along with the New York Stock Exchange, known as the NYSE. (At the time of this writing it is probable that the New York Stock Exchange will be acquired by the IntercontinentalExchange [ICE]. If so, the NYSE acronym may be changed to reflect the new ownership.)[3]

Smaller public companies, however, may not be listed on a stock exchange. The stock of these companies is considered to be unlisted; instead, their stock is traded "over the counter," or OTC. The National Association of Securities Dealers (NASD), oversees this market. The OTC stock market uses a computerized trading network called NASDAQ, which stands for the "NASD Automated Quotation system."

Published stock tables typically reflect the composite regular trading on the stock exchanges as of closing. A stock table will generally contain four columns: the first column is an abbreviation of the public company's name, the second column is the company's symbol (an alpha symbol), the third column is the stock's price as of closing for that day, and the fourth column is the net change of the stock price when compared to close of the previous day. Using healthcare organizations as examples, Johnson & Johnson's symbol is "JNJ," while Humana, Inc.'s symbol is "HUM."

Governmental Agency as Overseer

At the time of this writing, the overseer of the stock market in the United States is the U.S. Securities and Exchange Commission (SEC). (It is possible that in the future the SEC may be reorganized as a somewhat different entity with somewhat different responsibilities.) The mission of the SEC is to "protect investors, maintain fair, orderly, and efficient markets, and facilitate capital formation."[4] The SEC oversees "the key participants in the securities world, including securities exchanges, securities brokers and dealers, investment advisors, and mutual funds. Here, the SEC is concerned primarily with promoting the disclosure of important market-related information, maintaining fair dealing, and protecting against fraud."[5]

INVESTMENT INDICATORS

The annual rate of inflation (or deflation) is a typical investment indicator, as is the gross domestic product measure. Both are discussed here.

Inflation Versus Deflation

Inflation means "an increase in the volume of money and credit relative to available goods and services resulting in a continuing rise in the general price level."[6]

"Indexed to inflation" means these monies will rise in accordance with an inflationary increase. For example, Social Security payments are indexed to inflation. Excessive inflation is feared because it reduces or devalues the spending power of the dollars you possess.

Deflation, on the other hand, means "a contraction in the volume of available money and credit that results in a general decline in prices."[7] Deflation is feared because the contraction in volume of available money and credit generally results in a fall in prices that limits and/or reduces the country's economic activity.

Gross Domestic Product (GDP)

The GDP measures "the output of goods and services produced by labor and property located in the United States."[8] Investors watch the GDP because this measure is considered to be the "gold standard" measure of the country's overall economic fitness. The Bureau of Economic Analysis (BEA), located within the U.S. Department of Commerce, releases quarterly estimates of the GDP. The BEA is also responsible for the price index for gross domestic purchases. The price index measures "prices paid by U.S. residents,"[9] and is also released on a quarterly basis.

 INFORMATION CHECKPOINT

What is needed?	A copy of the *Wall Street Journal*.
Where is it found?	At a newsstand or possibly within the offices of your own organization.
How is it used?	Locate the "Stock Tables" section of the *Journal*. Review the column headings in the tables and locate the names of various stock exchanges that are included in the findings.

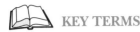 KEY TERMS

Common Stock
Debentures
Deflation
Federal Deposit Insurance Corporation (FDIC)
Gross Domestic Product (GDP)
Inflation
Money Market Funds
Municipal Bonds
Preferred Stock
Securities and Exchange Commission (SEC)
Stock Warrants

 DISCUSSION QUESTIONS

1. Do you know if your own monies on deposit are FDIC insured? If you do not know, how would you go about finding out?
2. Do you know of a healthcare company whose stock is publicly held? If you do not know, how would you go about finding out?
3. Do you know if any healthcare company that you have worked for (now or previously) had issued revenue bonds that were purchased by investors? If you do not know, how would you go about finding out?

NOTES

1. Federal Deposit Insurance Corporation, "Who Is the FDIC?" Federal Deposit Insurance Corporation. http://www.fdic.gov/about/index.html.
2. Ibid.
3. Wall Street Journal Opinion, "ICE Buys NYSE," *Wall Street Journal*, 21 December, 2012, A18.
4. U.S. Securities and Exchange Commission, "The Investor's Advocate: How the SEC Protects Investors, Maintains Market Integrity, and Facilitates Capital Formation." www.sec.gov/about/whatwedo.shtml.
5. Ibid.
6. *Merriam Webster's Collegiate Dictionary*, 10th ed., s.v. "Inflation."
7. Ibid., 303.
8. U.S. Department of Commerce, Bureau of Economic Analysis (BEA). News Release: Gross Domestic Product: Fourth Quarter 2008 (Final). http://bea.gov/newsreleases /national/gdp/gdpnewsrelease.htm.
9. Ibid.

Business Loans and Financing Costs

Business loans, as the term implies, represent debts incurred to assist in running a business. Whether to take on debt and how much to take on are common and necessary parts of financial planning. This type of planning involves the organization's capital structure, as discussed in the following section.

OVERVIEW OF CAPITAL STRUCTURE

"Capital" represents the financial resources of the organization and is generally considered to be a combination of debt and equity.

"Capital structure" means the proportion of debt versus equity within the organization. The phrase "capital structure" actually refers to the debt–equity relationship. For example, if a physician practice partnership owed $500,000 in debt and also had $500,000 in partner's equity, the partnership capital structure, or debt–equity relationship, would be 50–50.

Different industries typically have different debt–equity relationships. In the case of health care, the chief financial officer of the organization is usually responsible for guiding decisions about the proportion of debt. The chief financial officer will take into account various sources of capital, as discussed in the next section.

SOURCES OF CAPITAL

Sources of capital traditionally include four methods of obtaining funds:

- Borrowing from a lending institution
- Borrowing from investors

After completing this chapter, you should be able to

1. Understand what capital structure means.
2. Recognize four sources of capital.
3. Explain an amortization schedule.
4. Understand loan costs.

- Retaining the excess of revenues over expenses
- Selling an additional interest in the organization

Borrowing from a lending institution is generally classified by the length of the loan. Short-term borrowing is commonly expected to be repaid within a 12-month period. Long-term borrowing is usually to finance land, buildings, and/or equipment. Long-term borrowing for these purposes is usually accomplished by obtaining a mortgage from the lending institution.

Borrowing from investors assumes the organization is big enough and has the proper legal structure to do so. A common example of borrowing from investors is that of selling bonds. Bonds represent the company's promise to pay at a future date. When bonds are sold, the purchaser expects to receive a certain amount of annual interest and also expects that the bonds will be redeemed on a certain date, several years in the future.

Retaining the excess of revenues over expenses represents retaining operating profits to a proprietary, or for-profit, company. (Of course this assumes there is an excess of funds to retain.) A not-for-profit organization may be bound by legal limitations on the retention of its funds. However, the not-for-profit organization can also sometimes rely on a different income stream. Church-affiliated not-for-profits, for example, may be able to solicit donations. This example represents a unique method of raising capital.

Selling an additional interest in the organization depends on its legal structure. Typically, this method involves a for-profit corporation selling additional shares of common stock to raise funds. Not-for-profit organizations are bound by legal limitations and may not be able to follow this route.

THE COSTS OF FINANCING

Financing costs typically involve interest expense and usually also involve loan costs, as described in this section.

Interest Expense

Payments on a business loan typically consist of two parts: principal and interest expense. The principal portion of the loan payment reduces the loan itself, while the rest of the payment is made up of interest on the remaining balance due on the loan.

The amount of principal and the amount of interest contained in each payment are illustrated in an "amortization schedule." For example, assume the purchase of equipment for $60,000. Monthly payments will be made over a 3-year period, and the annual, or per-year, interest rate will be 12%. The first 6 months of the amortization schedule for this loan is illustrated in **Table 20–1**. The entire 36-month amortization schedule is found in Appendix 20-A at the end of this chapter.

The interest expense for each monthly payment is computed on the principal balance remaining after the principal portion of the previous payment has been subtracted. The "Remaining Principal Balance" column shows the declining balance of the principal. Now refer to the "Remaining Principal Balance" column and compare it with the "Interest Expense Portion of Payment" column. Remember that the 12% annual interest rate in

Table 20–1 Loan Amortization Schedule

Payment Number	Total Payment	Principal Portion of Payment	Interest Expense Portion of Payment	Remaining Principal Balance
Beginning balance = $60,000.00				
1	$1,992.86	$1,392.86	$600.00	$58,607.14
2	1,992.86	1,406.79	586.07	57,200.35
3	1,992.86	1,435.07	572.00	55,779.49
4	1,992.86	1,449.42	557.79	54,344.42
5	1,992.86	1,463.91	543.44	52,895.00
6	1,992.86	1,478.55	528.95	51,431.09

this example amounts to 1% per month. You can see how 10% of $60,000.00 amounts to a $600.00 interest payment for month 1; 10% of $58,607.14 amounts to a $586.07 interest payment for month 2; and so on. The remainder of the payment amount—after interest expense—is then deducted from the principal amount due, as shown in Table 20–1. Thus, of the $1,992.86 monthly payment 1, if $600.00 is interest, then $1,392.86 is the principal portion, and of the $1,992.86 monthly payment 2, if $586.07 is interest, then $1,406.79 is the principal portion, and so on.

Not all amortization schedules are set up in the same configuration. The columns that are shown can vary. For example, the entire 36-month amortization schedule for the Table 20–1 loan is contained in Appendix 20-A. Refer to this appendix to see how the columns are different from Table 20–1. While the basic information necessary for computation is shown, the layout of the schedule is different.

Loan Costs

The term "loan costs" covers expenses necessary to close the loan. Loan closing costs generally include some expenses that would be reported in the current year and some other expenses that should be spread over several years.

Suppose, for example, the Great Lakes Home Health Agency bought a tract of land for expansion purposes. The home health agency paid a 20% down payment and obtained mortgage financing from a local bank for the remainder of the purchase price. When the loan was closed, meaning the transaction was completed, the statement that lists closing costs included prorated real estate taxes and "points" on the loan. Points represent a certain percentage of the loan amount paid, in this case to the bank, to cover costs of the financing.

The prorated real estate taxes represent an expense to be reported in the current year by the HHA. The points, however, would be spread over several years. How would this multiple-year reporting be handled? The total would first be placed on the balance sheet as an amount not yet recognized as expense. Each year a certain portion of that amount would be charged to current operations as an "amortized expense." Amortization expense is a noncash expense that is assigned to multiple reporting periods. It works much the same way as depreciation expense.

MANAGEMENT CONSIDERATIONS ABOUT REAL ESTATE FINANCING

Real estate financing typically occurs in the form of real estate mortgages. Management must take several important considerations into account when contemplating a real estate purchase that involves a mortgage. These considerations include the following:

- What would the return on investment (ROI) be for this purchase?
- What is the cost of money (i.e., the interest rate) for this mortgage?
- What would the return of capital (equity) computation amount to?
- What is the liquidity prospect (i.e., the ability to sell this property)?
- What is the potential risk factor (if any) involved in the purchase and/or the mortgage financing?
- Is there an income tax factor to be considered? If so, what is the impact?

Repayment of a mortgage is typically a long-term liability, and this fact is yet another element in management's decision-making process.

MANAGEMENT DECISIONS ABOUT BUSINESS LOANS

Decisions concerning how to obtain capital are an important part of financial management decision making. The chapter on capital expenditures budgets discussed how new capital often has to be rationed within an organization. Repaying long-term loan obligations will impact the facility's cash flow for years to come, and decisions to undertake a large debt load should not be made lightly. Therefore, most institutions and/or companies have put a formal approval process into place that generally begins with the chief financial officer and his or her staff and progresses upward all the way to board of trustees' approval, depending on the amount of the debt proposed.

Because of the implications, management decisions about business loans are often interwoven with strategic planning.

 INFORMATION CHECKPOINT

What is needed?	An example of the details of a loan.
Where is it found?	In the department responsible for the organization's finances.
How is it used?	Loan information is used by your financial decision makers.

 KEY TERMS

Amortization Schedule
Bonds
Capital
Capital Structure
Equity Ratio

Loan Costs
Long-Term Borrowing
Short-Term Borrowing

 DISCUSSION QUESTIONS

1. Have you ever been informed of details about business loans in your unit or division?
2. If so, did you receive the information in the context of a new project (a new business loan that was made for purposes of the new project)?
3. Do the operating reports you receive contain information about loan costs, such as interest expense?
4. If so, do you think the interest expense seems reasonable for the operation? Why?

Sample Amortization Schedule 20-A

Principal borrowed: $60,000.00

Annual payments: 12

Total payments: 36

Annual interest rate: 12.00%

Periodic interest rate: 1.0000%

Regular payment amount: $1,992.86*

Final balloon payment: $0.00

The following results are estimates that do not account for values being rounded to the nearest cent. See the amortization schedule for more accurate values.

Total repaid: $71,742.96**

Total interest paid: $11,742.96

Interest as percentage of principal: 19.572%

---

*Take any line item on the next page. If you add the amount in the principal column and the amount in the interest column together, the total will amount a payment of $1,992.86.
**($60,000 principal plus $11,742.96 equals $71,742.96.)

Table 20-A–1 36-Month Sample Amortization Schedule

Payment Number	Principal	Interest	Cumulative Principal	Cumulative Interest	Principal Balance
1	$1,392.86	$600.00	$1,392.86	$600.00	$58,607.14
2	$1,406.79	$586.07	$2,799.65	$1,186.07	$57,200.35
3	$1,420.86	$572.00	$4,220.51	$1,758.07	$55,779.49
4	$1,435.07	$557.79	$5,655.58	$2,315.86	$54,344.42
5	$1,449.42	$543.44	$7,105.00	$2,859.30	$52,895.00
6	$1,463.91	$528.95	$8,568.91	$3,388.25	$51,431.09
7	$1,478.55	$514.31	$10,047.46	$3,902.56	$49,952.54
8	$1,493.33	$499.53	$11,540.79	$4,402.09	$48,459.21
9	$1,508.27	$484.59	$13,049.06	$4,886.68	$46,950.94
10	$1,523.35	$469.51	$14,572.41	$5,356.19	$45,427.59
11	$1,538.58	$454.28	$16,110.99	$5,810.47	$43,889.01
12	$1,553.97	$438.89	$17,664.96	$6,249.36	$42,335.04
13	$1,569.51	$423.35	$19,234.47	$6,672.71	$40,765.53
14	$1,585.20	$407.66	$20,819.67	$7,080.37	$39,180.33
15	$1,601.06	$391.80	$22,420.73	$7,472.17	$37,579.27
16	$1,617.07	$375.79	$24,037.80	$7,847.96	$35,962.20
17	$1,633.24	$359.62	$25,671.04	$8,207.58	$34,328.96
18	$1,649.57	$343.29	$27,320.61	$8,550.87	$32,679.39
19	$1,666.07	$326.79	$28,986.68	$8,877.66	$31,013.32
20	$1,682.73	$310.13	$30,669.41	$9,187.79	$29,330.59
21	$1,699.55	$293.31	$32,368.96	$9,481.10	$27,631.04
22	$1,716.55	$276.31	$34,085.51	$9,757.41	$25,914.49
23	$1,733.72	$259.14	$35,819.23	$10,016.55	$24,180.77
24	$1,751.05	$241.81	$37,570.28	$10,258.36	$22,429.72
25	$1,768.56	$224.30	$39,338.84	$10,482.66	$20,661.16
26	$1,786.25	$206.61	$41,125.09	$10,689.27	$18,874.91
27	$1,804.11	$188.75	$42,929.20	$10,878.02	$17,070.80
28	$1,822.15	$170.71	$44,751.35	$11,048.73	$15,248.65
29	$1,840.37	$152.49	$46,591.72	$11,201.22	$13,408.28
30	$1,858.78	$134.08	$48,450.50	$11,335.30	$11,549.50
31	$1,877.37	$115.49	$50,327.87	$11,450.79	$9,672.13
32	$1,896.14	$96.72	$52,224.01	$11,547.51	$7,775.99
33	$1,915.10	$77.76	$54,139.11	$11,625.27	$5,860.89
34	$1,934.25	$58.61	$56,073.36	$11,683.88	$3,926.64
35	$1,953.59	$39.27	$58,026.95	$11,723.15	$1,973.05
36	*$1,973.05	$19.73	$60,000.00	$11,742.88	$0.00

*The final payment has been adjusted to account for payments having been rounded to the nearest cent.

Choices: Owning Versus Leasing Equipment

PURCHASING EQUIPMENT

Purchasing equipment means taking title to, or assuming ownership of, the item. In this case, the asset representing the equipment is recorded on the organization's balance sheet. The purchase could take place by paying cash from the organization's cash reserves, or the organization could finance all or part of the purchase. If financing occurs, the resulting liability is also recorded on the balance sheet.

LEASING EQUIPMENT

When is a lease not a lease? When it is a lease-purchase, also known as a financial lease. This is a very real question that affects business decisions. The financial lease is described in the next section, and it is followed by a description of the operating lease.

Financial Lease

The lease-purchase is a formal agreement that may be called a lease, but it is really a contract to purchase. This contract-to-purchase transaction is also called a financial lease. The important difference is this: the equipment must be recorded on the books of the organization as a purchase. This process is called "capitalizing" the lease.

A financial lease is considered a contract to purchase. Generally speaking, a lease must be capitalized and thus placed on the balance sheet as an asset, with a corresponding liability, if the lease contract meets any one of the following criteria:

1. The lessee can buy the asset at the end of the lease term for a bargain price.

Progress Notes

After completing this chapter, you should be able to

1. Understand what purchasing equipment involves.
2. Understand what leasing equipment involves.
3. Recognize a for-profit organization.
4. Recognize a not-for-profit organization.

2. The lease transfers ownership to the lessee before the lease expires.
3. The lease lasts for 75% or more of the asset's estimated useful life.
4. The present value of the lease payments is 90% or more of the asset's value.

Operating Lease

The cost of an operating lease is considered an operating expense. It does not have to be capitalized and placed on the balance sheet because it does not meet the criteria just described.

An operating lease is treated as an expense of current operations. This is in contrast to the financial lease just described that is treated as an asset and a liability. A payment on an operating lease becomes an operating expense within the time period when the payment is made.

BUY-OR-LEASE MANAGEMENT DECISIONS

Leasing is an alternative to other means of financing. When analyzing lease-versus-purchase decisions, it is usually assumed that the money to purchase the equipment will be borrowed. In some cases, however, this is not true. The organization might decide to use cash from its own funds to make the purchase. This decision would, of course, change certain assumptions in the comparative analysis.

Another differential in comparative analysis concerns service agreements. Sometimes the service contracts or service agreements (to service and/or repair the equipment) are made a part of the lease agreement. This feature would need to be deleted from the total agreement before the comparison between leasing and purchasing can occur. Why? Because the service agreement would be an expense, regardless of whether the equipment would be leased or purchased.

An Example

The question for our example is whether a clinic should purchase or lease equipment. We examine two clinics: Northside Clinic, a for-profit corporation, and Southside Clinic, a not-for-profit corporation.

For both Northside and Southside, assume that the equipment's cost will be $50,000 if it is purchased. Likewise, assume for both Northside and Southside that if the equipment is leased, the lease will amount to $11,000 per year for five years.

We also need to make assumptions about depreciation expense for the purchased equipment. We further assume straight-line depreciation in the amount of $10,000 for years 2 through 4. For the initial year of acquisition (year 0), we assume the half-year method of depreciation, whereby the amount will be one-half of $10,000, or $5,000. We will further assume the purchased equipment will be sold for its salvage value of 10%, or $5,000, on the first day of year 5. (Therefore, the full amount of [prior] year 4's depreciation can be taken.)

The difference between the for-profit Northside and the not-for-profit Southside is that the for-profit is subject to income tax. We assume the federal and state income taxes will amount to a total of 25%. Thus, the depreciation taken as an expense results in a tax savings amounting to one-quarter of the total expense in each year. The depreciation expense and its equivalent tax savings are shown by year in **Table 21-1**. Also, the same rationale is applicable for the leasing expense in the for-profit organization.

In the following section, we compare two financial situations that affect the way the analysis is performed: a for-profit, or proprietary, clinic and a not-for-profit clinic. For purposes of this analysis, what is the major difference? As we have previously stated, the for-profit practice realizes tax savings on expense items such as depreciation. The not-for-profit clinic does not realize such tax savings because it does not pay taxes. Consequently, one analysis later here (the for-profit) includes the effect of tax savings on depreciation, and the other analysis (the not-for-profit) does not.

Computing the Comparative Net Cash Flow Effects of Owning Versus Leasing

This description results in computation of the net cash flow for owned equipment versus leased equipment in a for-profit organization compared with that of a not-for-profit organization. **Table 21-2-A.1** and **Table 21-2-A.2** first illustrate the comparative net cash flow effects of owning versus leasing in a for-profit organization. Table 21-2-A.1 illustrates the cost of owning. The equipment purchase price of $50,000 in year 0 (line 1) and the salvage value of $5,000 in year 5 (line 3) are shown. The for-profit's net cash flow is also affected by tax savings from depreciation expense, as was previously explained and as is shown on line 2. The resulting net cash flow by year is shown on line 4.

Table 21-2-A.2 illustrates the cost of leasing in the for-profit organization. The equipment lease or rental payments are shown on line 5. The for-profit's net cash flow is affected by tax savings from the lease payments, as is shown on line 6. The resulting net cash flow by year is shown on line 7.

Table 21-2-B.1 and **Table 21-2-B.2** now illustrate the comparative net cash flow effects of owning versus leasing for the not-for-profit organization. Table 21-2-B.1 illustrates the cost of owning. The equipment purchase price of $50,000 in year 0 (line 8) and the salvage value of $5,000 in year 5 (line 10) are shown. The not-for-profit's net cash flow is not affected by tax savings from depreciation expense because it is exempt from such income taxes. Therefore, the depreciation expense tax savings entry on line 9 is shown as not applicable, or "n/a." The resulting net cash flow by year is then shown on line 11.

Table 21-2-B.2 illustrates the cost of leasing in the not-for-profit organization. The equipment lease or rental payments are shown on line 12. The not-for-profit's net cash flow is

---

Table 21–1 Depreciation Expense Computation

	Year 0	Year 1	Year 2	Year 3	Year 4	Year 5
Depreciation expense	$5,000	$10,000	$10,000	$10,000	$10,000	—
Depreciation expense tax savings	$1,250	$2,500	$2,500	$2,500	$2,500	—

Table 21–2–A.1 Cost of Owning—Northside Clinic (For-Profit)—Comparative Cash Flow

Line Number		Year 0	Year 1	Year 2	Year 3	Year 4	Year 5
1	Equipment purchase price	($50,000)					
2	Depreciation expense tax savings	$1,250	$2,500	$2,500	$2,500	$2,500	—
3	Salvage value	—	—	—	—	—	$5,000
4	Net cash flow	($48,750)	$2,500	$2,500	$2,500	$2,500	$5,000

Table 21–2–A.2 Cost of Leasing—Northside Clinic (For-Profit)—Comparative Cash Flow

Line Number		Year 0	Year 1	Year 2	Year 3	Year 4	Year 5
5	Equipment lease (rental) payments	($11,000)	($11,000)	($11,000)	($11,000)	($11,000)	—
6	Lease expense tax savings	$2,750	$2,750	$2,750	$2,750	$2,750	—
7	Net cash flow	($8,250)	($8,250)	($8,250)	($8,250)	($8,250)	—

Table 21–2–B.1 Cost of Owning—Southside Clinic (Not-for-Profit)—Comparative Cash Flow

Line Number		Year 0	Year 1	Year 2	Year 3	Year 4	Year 5
8	Equipment purchase price	($50,000)					
9	Depreciation expense tax savings	n/a	n/a	n/a	n/a	n/a	—
10	Salvage value	—	—	—	—	—	$5,000
11	Net cash flow	($50,000)	—	—	—	—	$5,000

Table 21–2–B.2 Cost of Leasing—Southside Clinic (Not-for-Profit)—Comparative Cash Flow

Line Number		Year 0	Year 1	Year 2	Year 3	Year 4	Year 5
12	Equipment lease (rental) payments	($11,000)	($11,000)	($11,000)	($11,000)	($11,000)	—
13	Lease expense tax savings	n/a	n/a	n/a	n/a	n/a	—
14	Net cash flow	($11,000)	($11,000)	($11,000)	($11,000)	($11,000)	—

not affected by tax savings from the lease payments because it is exempt from such income taxes. Therefore, the lease expense tax savings entry on line 13 is shown as not applicable, or "n/a." The resulting net cash flow by year is then shown on line 14.

Computing the Comparative Present Value Cost of Owning Versus Cost of Leasing

This continuing description results in computation of the present value cost of owning versus leasing equipment in a for-profit organization compared with that of a not-for-profit organization.

Table 21-2-C.1 and **Table 21-2-C.2** now illustrate the present value cost of owning versus leasing for the for-profit organization. Table 21-2-C.1 first carries forward (on line 15) the net cash flow computed on line 4. Line 16 then shows the present value factor for each year at 8%, which is the assumed cost of capital in this example. Line 17 contains the present value answers, which result from multiplying line 15 times line 16. The overall present value cost of owning (derived by adding all items on line 17) is shown on line 18.

Table 21-2-C.2 illustrates the present value cost of leasing in the for-profit organization. Table 21-2-C.2 first carries forward (on line 19) the net cash flow computed on line 7. Line 20 then shows the present value factor for each year at 8%, which is the assumed cost of capital in this example. Line 21 contains the present value answers, which result from multiplying line 19 times line 20. The overall present value cost of owning (derived by adding all items on line 21) is shown on line 22.

Finally, **Table 21-2-C.3** compares the for-profit organization's cost of owning to its cost of leasing. In the case of the for-profit, the net advantage is to leasing by a net amount of

---

Table 21–2–C.1 Cost of Owning—Northside Clinic (For-Profit)—Comparative Present Value

Line Number	For-Profit Cost of Owning	Year 0	Year 1	Year 2	Year 3	Year 4	Year 5
15	Net cash flow (from line 4)	($48,750)	$2,500	$2,500	$2,500	$2,500	$5,000
16	Present value factor (at 8%)	n/a	0.926	0.857	0.794	0.735	0.681
17	Present value answers =	($48,750)	$2,315	$2,143	$1,985	$1,838	$3,405
18	Present value cost of owning = ($37,064)						

Table 21–2–C.2 Cost of Leasing—Northside Clinic (For-Profit)—Comparative Present Value

Line Number	For-Profit Cost of Leasing	Year 0	Year 1	Year 2	Year 3	Year 4	Year 5
19	Net cash flow (from line 7)	($8,250)	($8,250)	($8,250)	($8,250)	($8,250)	—
20	Present value factor (at 8%)	n/a	0.926	0.857	0.794	0.735	—
21	Present value answers =	($8,250)	($7,640)	($7,070)	($6,551)	($6,064)	—
22	Present value cost of leasing = ($35,575)						

Table 21–2–C.3 Comparison of Costs—Northside Clinic (For-Profit)

Line Number	Computation of Difference
23 Net advantage to leasing = $1,489	(37,064) (line 18) less (35,575) (line 22) equals 1,489

$1,489. The tables now illustrate the present value cost of owning versus leasing for the not-for-profit organization. **Table 21-2-D.1** illustrates the present value cost of owning. It first carries forward (on line 24) the net cash flow computed on line 11. Line 25 then shows the present value factor for each year at 8%, which is the assumed cost of capital in this example. Line 26 contains the present value answers, which result from multiplying line 24 times line 25. The overall present value cost of owning (derived by adding all items on line 26) is shown on line 27.

    Table 21-2-D.2 illustrates the present value cost of leasing in the not-for-profit organization. It first carries forward (on line 28) the net cash flow computed on line 14. Line 29 then shows the present value factor for each year at 8%, which is the assumed cost of capital in this example. Line 30 contains the present value answers, which result from multiplying line 28 times line 29. The overall present value cost of owning (derived by adding all items on line 30) is shown on line 31.

    Finally, **Table 21-2-D.3** compares the not-for-profit organization's cost of owning to its cost of leasing. In the case of the not-for-profit, the net advantage is to owning by a net

Table 21–2–D.1 Cost of Owning—Southside Clinic (Not-for-Profit)—Comparative Present Value

Line Number	Not-for-Profit Cost of Owning	Year 0	Year 1	Year 2	Year 3	Year 4	Year 5
24	Net cash flow (from line 11)	($50,000)	—	—	—	—	$5,000
25	Present value factor (at 8%)	n/a	—	—	—	—	0.681
26	Present value answer =	($50,000)	—	—	—	—	$3,405
27	Present value cost of owning =	($46,595)					

Table 21–2–D.2 Cost of Leasing—Southside Clinic (Not-for-Profit)—Comparative Present Value

Line Number	Not-for-Profit Cost of Leasing	Year 0	Year 1	Year 2	Year 3	Year 4	Year 5
28	Net cash flow (from line 14)	($11,000)	($11,000)	($11,000)	($11,000)	($11,000)	—
29	Present value factor (at 8%)	n/a	0.926	0.857	0.794	0.735	
30	Present value answer =	($11,000)	($10,186)	($9,427)	($8,573)	($8,085)	—
31	Present value cost of leasing =	($47,271)					

Table 21–2–D.3 Comparison of Costs—Southside Clinic (Not-for-Profit)

Line Number	Computation of Difference
32 Net Advantage to Owning = $676	(47,271) (line 31) less (46,595) (line 27) equals 676

amount of $676. It might be noted that the net difference of $676 is so small that it might be disregarded and considered as a nearly neutral comparison between the two methods of financing.

In summary, the tax effect on cash flow of for-profit versus not-for-profit will generally (but not always) be taken into account in comparative proposals for funding.

ACCOUNTING PRINCIPLES REGARDING LEASES

As previously explained, financial statements used for external purposes in the United States must follow generally accepted accounting principles, or GAAP. The treatment of equipment leases for such accounting purposes would, of course, fall under GAAP, and the technical aspects of such reporting are beyond the scope of this text. Be aware, however, that sometime in the near future U.S. publicly held companies may be required to adopt certain international accounting standards as produced by the International Accounting Standards Board (IASB).[1] The treatment of leases is a particular issue within these potential adoption requirements and is, of course, beyond the scope of this text.

 INFORMATION CHECKPOINT

What is needed?	An example of a buy-or-lease management decision analysis.
Where is it found?	Probably with your manager or your departmental director.
How is it used?	Study the way the analysis is laid out and the method of comparison used.

 KEY TERMS

Buy-or-Lease Decisions
Depreciation
Equipment Purchase
Financial Lease
For-Profit Organization
Lease-Purchase
Not-for-Profit Organization
Operating Lease
Present Value

DISCUSSION QUESTIONS

1. In the examples given in the chapter, there is not much monetary difference between owning versus leasing. In these circumstances, which method would you recommend? Why?
2. Have you ever been involved in a lease-or-buy decision in business? In your personal life?
3. If so, was the decision made in a formal reporting format, or as an informal decision?
4. Do you think this was the best way to make the decision? If not, what would you change? Why?

NOTE

1. K. Tysiac, "Still in Flux: Future of IFRS in U.S. Remains Unclear After SEC report," *Journal of Accountancy*, p.4 (September 2012). Source: www.journalofaccountancy .com/Issues/2012/Sep/20126059.htm

Strategic Planning: A Powerful Tool

Strategic Planning and the Healthcare Financial Manager

MAJOR COMPONENTS OF THE STRATEGIC PLAN: OVERVIEW

This chapter will cover the six major components of planning and their process flows, along with various examples of mission, value, and vision statement types. A federal governmental agency planning example will be presented. The chapter also discusses strategic planning tools, including situational analysis and financial projections.

INTRODUCTION

Strategic planning is vital for any organization. There are multiple approaches to accomplish such planning, and there is often confusion about the terminology used in these different approaches. In this section we will describe the typical components of strategic planning. We will also discuss the confusion about differences in approach and related terminology.

SIX MAJOR COMPONENTS

The ultimate result of strategic planning is an actual plan, presented in report form. The major components of a strategic plan include the following:

- Mission Statement
- Vision Statement
- Organizational Values
- Goals
- Objectives
- Action Plans and/or Performance Plans and/or Initiatives

Progress Notes

After completing this chapter, you should be able to

1. Describe the six major components of strategic planning.
2. Understand the purpose and relationship between mission, vision, and value statements.
3. Describe the strategic planning cycle and its process flow.
4. Understand why the governmental planning requirements are important.
5. Identify the four components of a SWOT analysis.
6. Recognize the difference between a financial forecast and a financial projection.

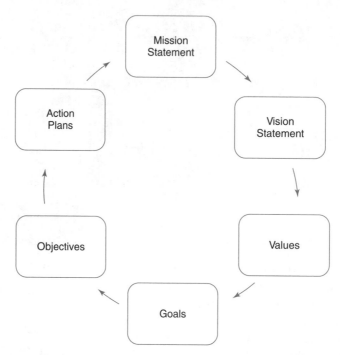

Figure 22–1 The Six Major Components of Strategic Planning.
Courtesy of J.J. Baker and R.W. Baker, Dallas, Texas.

These components are illustrated in **Figure 22–1** and are further described as follows.

Mission Statement

The mission statement explains the purpose of the organization. In other words, it explains "what we are now." Generally speaking, the mission statement will cover a near-future period, usually three to five years.

Vision Statement

The vision statement explains "what we want to be" or perhaps "what we aspire to be." It is a look further into the future, perhaps 10 years from now. Not all organizations publicize a vision statement.

Organizational Values

Values express the philosophy of the organization. There seems to be two approaches to expressing values: either they are summarized into just a few meaningful phrases or they are quite lengthy and "wordy."

Goals

A goal is "…a statement of aim or purpose included in a strategic plan."[1] Goals support the mission statement. While strategic goals are necessarily broad in nature, nevertheless each goal should tie directly into an element of the mission statement. Every goal should be considered an outcome that can be accomplished in the future.

Objectives

A strategic objective further defines intended outcomes in order to achieve a goal. Each objective must support—and thus tie directly into—a particular strategic goal. There are typically several objectives associated with each goal.

Action Plans

An Action Plan is a detailed plan of operations that shows how one part of a particular objective will be accomplished. It supports a subcomponent of the overall objective. It is a short-term plan that provides details (actions) about how a specific area of a particular objective will be carried out. Action plans are often called by other names, such as "Operational Plans," "Performance Plans" or "Initiatives." They may also be called "Targets."

VARIED APPROACHES TO STRATEGIC PLANNING

How strategic planning is approached may be affected by the organization type and/or the program or project type.

Governmental Versus Nongovernmental

Governmental entities are guided by regulatory restrictions. Among these restrictions are federal regulations that mandate strategic planning. These regulations apply to federal governmental organizations and specify the format, contents, and timing of the required strategic plans. On the other hand, nongovernmental entities are not covered under these mandated requirements.

For-Profit Versus Not-For-Profit

A for-profit company is in business to make a profit (supposedly, anyway) and is answerable to its owners. Its owner may be shareholders (for corporations) or partners (for partnerships) or possibly sole proprietors. This company's mission will generally be proprietary in nature.

A not-for-profit organization, on the other hand, is expected to have a mission that is broadly charitable in nature. It is typically answerable to the stakeholders who are impacted in one way or another by its mission.

Specific Programs or Projects

In some cases the type of program or project or initiative will define the basic approach to strategic planning. Funding sources and/or regulations may also make such demands. For example, in some states construction of healthcare facilities is controlled by a regulatory Certificate of Need process. In these states, then, strategic planning for a new facility would be a specific project. The outcome would be uncertain—because there is competition, success would be unknown—so the project would be specially treated within the plan.

EXAMPLES OF MISSION, VISION, AND VALUE STATEMENTS

This section introduces various types of mission, vision, and value statements. The organization and the length of statements can vary. Their terminology and their emphasis can also vary. One set of examples that follow recognizes a special status or focus, another recognizes a financial emphasis, and a third shows how the message is relayed.

RECOGNIZING A SPECIAL STATUS OR FOCUS WITHIN THE STATEMENTS

The following five examples each recognize a special status or focus within the statements.

Recognizing Non-Profit Status: Sutter Health

Sutter Health is a network of doctors and hospitals located in Northern California. Sutter's mission statement specifically points out its not-for-profit commitment.

Mission

We enhance the well-being of people in the communities we serve through a not-for-profit commitment to compassion and excellence in health care services.

Vision

Sutter Health leads the transformation of health care to achieve the highest levels of quality, access and affordability.

Values

- Excellence and Quality
- Innovation
- Affordability
- Teamwork
- Compassion and Caring
- Community
- Honesty and Integrity[2]

[Note: Sutter's values are arranged in a circular graphic, with "Honesty & Integrity" in the middle of the circle.]

Recognizing For-Profit Status: Tenet Healthcare Corporation

Tenant Healthcare Corporation is a publicly held corporation that is listed on the New York Stock Exchange (NYSE:THC). As a for-profit corporation operating a healthcare delivery system, Tenant specifically mentions providing a return to its shareholders.

Mission

At Tenet, our business is health care. Our mission is to improve the quality of life of every patient who enters our doors. Our approach makes us unique and defines our future.

Values

As we seek to improve the quality of our patients' lives, to serve our communities, to provide an exceptional environment for our employees and affiliated physicians and provide an attractive return to our shareholders, we are guided by five core values.[3]

Recognizing Hospital Taxing-District Status: Parkland Hospital

Parkland Hospital is the tax-supported hospital serving Dallas County, Texas. As such, Parkland first states its mandate from the taxpayers.

Mandate

To furnish medical aid and hospital care to indigent and needy persons residing in the hospital district.

Mission

Dedicated to the health and well-being of individuals and communities entrusted to our care.

Vision

By our actions, we will define the standards of excellence for public academic health systems.

Guiding Principles

Our values and principles reflect our shared responsibility to achieve health care excellence for our patients and communities.[4]

Recognizing the Vision and Intent of Their Founders: Mayo Clinic

The Mayo Clinic, a large nonprofit organization with a long history, provides medical care, research, and education at locations including the Midwest, Arizona, and Florida. The Mayo Clinic is research oriented and is known for treating difficult cases.

Mission

To inspire hope and contribute to health and well-being by providing the best care to every patient through integrated clinical practice, education and research.

Primary Value

The needs of the patient come first.

Value Statements

These values, which guide Mayo Clinic's mission to this day, are an expression of the vision and intent of our founders, the original Mayo physicians and the Sisters of Saint Francis.[5]

Recognizing Patient and Community Commitment: Regions Hospital

Regions Hospital is a private not-for-profit hospital in St. Paul, Minnesota, that is over 100 years old. Regions' commitment to both patients and community is very clear.

Mission

Our mission is to improve the health of our patients and community by providing high quality health care which meets the needs of all people.

Vision

Our vision is to be the patient-centered hospital of choice of our community.[6]

FINANCIAL EMPHASIS WITHIN THE STATEMENTS

This section presents two examples of financial emphasis within the statements, as follows.

A Foundation's Financial Responsibility: Saint Barnabas Medical Center Foundation

A healthcare foundation typically exists to receive and manage charitable gifts. This foundation exists to support a specific hospital: Saint Barnabas Medical Center, a major teaching hospital located in Livingston, New Jersey.

Mission

The Saint Barnabas Medical Center Foundation is a charitable organization dedicated to nurturing philanthropic support for the programs and services of Saint Barnabas Medical Center.

These programs provide the communities we serve with the highest quality, most compassionate healthcare. To accomplish our mission, the Foundation will:

- Ensure that charitable gifts are used effectively, responsibly, and as directed by the donor; and
- Carefully manage the endowed funds entrusted to us.[7]

A Medical Practice Network Emphasizes Financial Structure: Texas Oncology

Texas Oncology specializes in oncology patients through a network of physicians that covers the state of Texas. This organization places its vision first and mission second, as follows. Note also that evidence-based, or scientific, care is contained within the mission statement.

Vision

To be the first choice for cancer care.

Mission

To provide excellent, evidence-based care for each patient we serve, while advancing cancer care for tomorrow.

Texas Oncology has three Core Values, consisting of Patient Care, Culture, and Business. The Business Core Value is of particular interest to us. At the time of this writing, it reads as follows: Business—Our practice values professional management that:

- Promotes convenient access at rural and urban sites.
- Provides leadership in efficient care delivery and improves all aspects of cancer care.
- Provides a financial structure to expand services to our patients.
- Is competitive in all aspects of our business.[8]

These values clearly recognize the fact that an organization must have the financial structure and resources to endure and to succeed.

RELAYING THE MESSAGE

The results of strategic planning as expressed in the mission statement, vision, and values are of little use unless people know about them and what they say. This section focuses upon relaying that message.

Introducing the Message

This section presents three examples of introducing the message within the statements, as follows.

An Overall Title for the Message: Aetna Insurance Company

Aetna is a national insurance company over 150 years old that offers health insurance plans. This company has wrapped their mission, values, and goals together under one overall title called The Aetna Way, as follows:

Our company's mission, values and goals are expressed through The Aetna Way. The Aetna Way, comprising the elements below, encompasses our shared sense of purpose and provides clarity as we pursue our operational and strategic goals.[9]

Emphasizing Areas of Focus: American Medical Association

The American Medical Association (AMA) is, according to its website, "…the largest physician organization in the nation."[10] It provides a wide variety of resources and support for its members.

The AMA has created a five-year strategic plan, "…which aims to ensure that enhancements to health care in the United States are physician-led, advance the physician-patient relationship, and ensure that health care costs can be prudently managed."[11]

This plan places emphasis on three particular "core areas of focus," which include the following:

- Improving health outcomes
- Accelerating change in medical education
- Enhancing physician satisfaction and practice sustainability by shaping delivery and payment models[12]

The plan was posted electronically, and an AMA member could click on any of the three focus areas to read more. The AMA also provided a members-only feedback form in order to receive input.

Explaining the Terms: Good Samaritan Society

The Good Samaritan Society is the largest not-for-profit provider of senior care and services in the United States.

There is an important paragraph that appears before Good Samaritan's Strategic statements. That paragraph explains the purpose of each term contained with the statements, as follows:

- Our Mission states why the Society exists.
- Our Vision defines the desired outcome of our work.
- Our Strategic Direction defines where we want to be as an organization.
- And our Hallmark Values and related Core Principles identify the values that we strive to integrate into all aspects of our work.[13]

Mission Expressed as a Motto

Mottos are an effective way to communicate the organization's mission. However, composing such a short [piece] is much more difficult than it seems at first. Two examples follow.

A Six-Word Motto: Good Samaritan Society

The Good Samaritan Society has also created a pithy concise motto consisting of only six words.

Grounded in Mission
Centered in Values[14]

A Three-Phrase Motto: Providence Healthcare Network

Providence Healthcare Network is a member of Ascension Health, "…the nation's largest Catholic and largest nonprofit health system."
A mission of compassion.
Compassion is perfected by excellence.

Because excellence goes beyond the will to help others by providing the determination and tools to succeed where the heart takes you.[15]

The Message Available as Website Downloads

Website downloads make the information available to anyone who has access to a computer. This section presents two examples of making the message available as a website download.

Downloadable Summaries from Duke Medicine

The umbrella term "Duke Medicine" actually covers three components—the Duke University Health System, the Duke University School of Medicine, and the Duke University School of Nursing, all based in the Raleigh-Durham, North Carolina area. Duke Medicine has created both a mission and a vision that encompasses all these components. Then each component also has its own strategic plan that feeds in turn into the combined plan.

At the time of this writing an overview of these plans was available in booklet form. The booklet, entitled "Thinking Big" could be downloaded from the Duke Medicine website as a PDF file.[16] Summaries of each strategic plan could also be downloaded. Thus Duke provides transparency and useful summaries in a readily accessible electronic format.

Downloadable Visuals from Johns Hopkins Medicine

Johns Hopkins also uses a single name—John Hopkins Medicine—for its overall medical enterprise. This enterprise, based in Baltimore, Maryland, includes the Johns Hopkins Health System along with the John Hopkins University School of Medicine.

Johns Hopkins Medicine has created a mission, vision, and core values for the entire enterprise. At the time of this writing it was possible to download and print out the Johns Hopkins Medicine mission, vision, and core values in one of three ways:

- A Wall-Mounted Poster (large)—24" × 36"
- A Framed Desk-top Poster (small)—8" × 10"
- A Pocket Card—2.5" × 3.5" [17]

Thus the message is definitely relayed, and in three possible forms, for three different display purposes. It keeps the message visible as a reminder.

THE STRATEGIC PLANNING CYCLE AND ITS PROCESS FLOW

The basic elements of strategic planning can be visualized as a series of process flows. Thus by visualizing the process involved, the planning function can be broken into its various manageable components.

PROCESS FLOW FOR CREATING GOALS, OBJECTIVES, AND ACTION PLANS

Figure 22–2 illustrates these initial three components of the strategic plan.

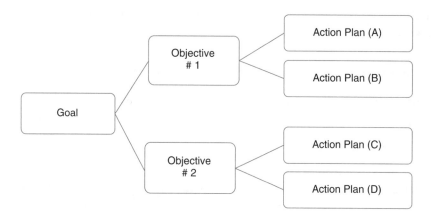

Figure 22–2 Process Flow for Creating Goals, Objectives, and Action Plans.
Courtesy of J.J. Baker and R.W. Baker, Dallas, Texas.

Establishing Goals

You will recall that a goal is a statement of aim or purpose. In order to establish such a goal, it is important to define how it will accomplish a particular segment of the mission statement. Establishing the actual goal involves the following:

- Define the goal.
- Determine that there is a clear and distinct connection to the mission statement.
- Decide how long it will take to accomplish this goal; that is, will it take one year, two years, three years?
- Compose and condense final wording of the goal to properly express it in a concise manner.

Broad Goals Become Narrower Objectives

A strategic objective further defines a particular strategic goal. Thus a single broad goal is segmented into several narrower and more defined objectives, as illustrated in Figure 22–2.

Narrower Objectives Become Detailed Action Plans

You will also recall that an action plan provides a detailed plan of operations that shows how to achieve one part of a particular objective. Thus a single defined objective is segmented into a number of even more detailed action plans. This step shows how part of the objective will actually be accomplished. The action plan's relationship to objectives and to goals is also illustrated in Figure 22–2.

PROCESS FLOW FOR CREATING ACTION PLANS AND THEIR PERFORMANCE MEASURES

Figure 22–3 illustrates the multiple performance measures that make each action plan operational.

The Action Plan Must Relate to Its Objective

As previously discussed, an action plan should always directly relate to the relevant component of its specific strategic objective. Details will be organized into subcomponents

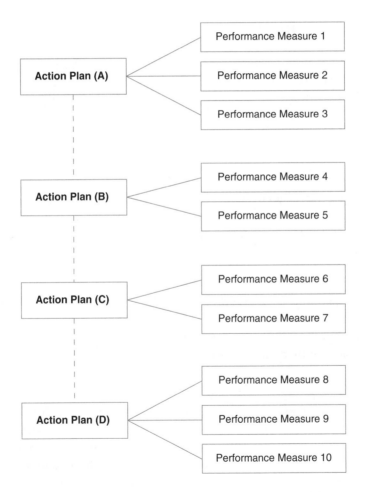

Figure 22–3 Process Flow for Creating Action Plans and Their Performance Measures.
Courtesy of J.J. Baker and R.W. Baker, Dallas, Texas.

as necessary and, as its title implies, the action plan will demonstrate how actions will be accomplished.

Detailed Action Plans Will Contain Multiple Performance Measures

So how will the action plan demonstrate that its actions will be accomplished? The required actions, or operations, will be linked to a series of performance measures, as illustrated in Figure 22–3. The performance measures provide accountability.

When these measures are properly designed, performance can be reported as outcomes. This achieves desired accountability and one cycle of the planning process flow is thus complete.

THE PLANNING CYCLE OVER TIME

We visualize the ideal strategic planning cycle itself as a never-ending process. In other words, a completed plan is not set in stone, never to change. Instead, there should be a "refresh and renew" approach to such planning. Incidentally, planning cycle segments may be called by different names, but they are still in a cycle. Look past the names to see the "skeleton" of the overall process.

Goals, Objectives, and Action Plans Interact and Repeat

The interaction of goals, objectives, and action plans should take feedback into account. This feedback should be obtained as is appropriate from all levels of management within the organization. However, internal managers are not the only stakeholders involved with the strategic plan.

Planning Revisions and Updates Are Necessary

The capability for planning revisions and updates should ideally be built into the plan itself. Unanticipated events can occur—both internally and externally—that require major revisions if the plan is to be kept operational. Updates, on the other hand, are to be expected and allowance should be made for them in order to keep the plan.

Stakeholders Provide Input Within the Cycle

Stakeholders can be both internal and external. In order to maintain a manageable planning cycle, questions need to be answered. For example, how many external stakeholders need input into the plan? Who, specifically are they? How will they provide this input?

Likewise, how many internal stakeholders need to provide input and/or feedback to the plan? Who, specifically, are they? What departments or divisions do they represent within the organization? Is this representation a good balance? And how will they provide this input?

Programming and Budgets Support the Planning Cycle

It makes sense that planning should be supported by budgets and the related funding. It is also logical that programming should in turn support these budgets. We can then ask: "What goal and what objective does this particular program and this budget support?"

Financial Aspects of the Plan

A plan must, above all, be operational. And to be operational, it must have financial support. How will this financial support be provided? Will another division or project be cut in order for this to happen? Can the consequences be predicted? If so, what will they be?

Related Timeframes

Necessary timeframes are appropriate for the particular portion of strategic planning. For example, the plan itself typically covers a period of 4 to 5 years. If there is a vision statement, it should be much further into the future, perhaps out to 10 years. Yet the managers' accountability should be at least annually, and in fact may be quarterly.

MANAGERS' RESPONSIBILITIES

Responsibility for the various segments can be assigned. The manager's responsibility will generally rest in one of three management areas as follows.

Planning

The manager may contribute to planning by gathering data or by analyzing the data to provide specific information that is desired and necessary for the plan. In other words, the manager is participating in the planning function by doing his/her part in the preliminary segment of the process.

Decision Making

The manager may or may not be able to participate in the actual decision making for the plan, depending upon his/her staff level within the organization. However, he/she may be assigned to work on a planning committee or a task force that contributes directly to the decision makers in the organization. This type of assignment is an important responsibility.

Providing Accountability

The manager can definitely contribute in suggesting criteria for performance measures. The action plan will require performance measures in order to provide the necessary accountability. And the manager is the best person to understand what measures are needed within his/her department or division.

A well-designed planning process will also include milestones. The milestones signify the completion of plan segments within a designated timeframe for completion of the entire plan. The manager can and should be responsible for assisting in reaching certain milestones on a timely basis. This function (one hospital CEO called it "ramrodding") is another type of accountability responsibility.

FEDERAL GOVERNMENTAL AGENCIES MUST PREPARE STRATEGIC PLANS

Agencies in the federal government are required by law to prepare strategic plans. They are also required by law to provide reports on performance that tie to the strategic plans. This section explains the importance of the federal planning cycle and describes its planning and performance requirements. It also provides an example of an agency strategic planning cycle.

WHY ARE FEDERAL PLANNING REQUIREMENTS IMPORTANT TO US?

The federal government's planning requirements are important to us because they provide guidance in the form of well-thought-out and time-tested regulated concepts and a framework for strategic planning.

INTRODUCTION: REQUIREMENTS, PLANS, AND PERFORMANCE

Legislative requirements for strategic planning and related performance reporting are discussed as follows.

Legislative Requirements: Overview

Congress has enacted a law that provided for the establishment of strategic planning and performance measurement in the federal government. This law, known as the Government Performance and Results Act (GPRA) of 1993, required each agency of the federal government to prepare a strategic plan for program activities. These strategic plans were then to be submitted to Congress and to the Director of the Office of Management and Budget (OMB).[18]

Legislative Requirements for Strategic Planning

Each agency's strategic plan must contain the following:

- A comprehensive mission statement
- General goals and objectives for major functions and operations
- A description of how these goals and objectives are to be achieved
- Key factors external to the agency and beyond its control that might significantly affect achieving these goals and objectives[19]

Strategic Plan Timeframes

The original 1993 Act required that the strategic plan cover a period of not less than five years forward from the fiscal year in which it would be submitted. (You will recall that the federal government's fiscal year is not a calendar year. Instead it begins on October 1st and ends on September 30th.) In addition the plan was to be updated and revised at least every three years.[20]

The plan's timeframe has been subsequently revised to four years by the GPRA Modernization Act of 2010. At the time of this writing the specific requirement is as follows: "…The plan shall cover a period of not less than four years following the fiscal year in which the plan is submitted."[21]

Plans' Impacts on Budgets and Funding

Governmental managers must reconcile their budget requests with their applicable part of the strategic plan. The projects for which they are responsible can't (usually) be funded if they are not approved in the budget.

A common problem involves maintaining a project's carry forward over sequential annual budgets. In other words, a multi-year project will need to be recognized for funding in each annual budget as the project progresses. This can be a real problem, considering the multiple levels of bureaucracy within the government that hinder the approval process.

We can also turn the concept of "impact" around the other way. Instead of asking "What is the impact of the plan on budgets and funding," we can ask the opposite questions. They include "Does the intent of the plan actually get funded? And stay funded?"

How Agency Strategic Plans Are Tied to Performance

This section describes performance reporting requirements for federal agencies.

Legislative Requirements for Performance Reporting

The 1993 Act actually had three elements: besides requiring strategic plans that covered multiple years, it also required that performance plans and program performance reports be submitted. These requirements actually make the strategic plan itself operational because they hold the agencies accountable.

Agency Performance Plans Are Required

The GPRA Modernization Act of 2010 legislation requires the agency performance plans to be submitted annually. The performance plans are to be posted on the Agency's website.[22]

Agency Performance Reports Are Also Required

The Agency is also required to prepare an update report that compares actual performance achieved with performance goals as established in the performance plan. This report is also to be posted on the Agency's website.[23]

Unmet Goals May Require a Performance Improvement Plan

Each fiscal year the Office of Management and Budget (OMB) is supposed to determine whether the Agency has met the performance goals and objectives of the performance plan. The OMB produces a review report. If goals are not met according to the OMB report, the Agency must then prepare and submit a Performance Improvement Plan to increase program effectiveness for each unmet goal. The plan must include measurable milestones.[24]

Strategic Mission Statements: Two Federal Departmental Examples

Two departmental examples of governmental strategic mission statement appear in this section. The first example belongs to the Department of Health and Human Services (HHS). This mission statement is of interest because the Centers for Medicare and Medicaid Services (CMS) is an agency within the HHS department. The Medicare and Medicaid programs administered by CMS are frequent subjects of interest in this book.

The second example belongs to the Department of Veterans Affairs (VA). We include this example as background information because the VA's Office of Information Technology is the subject of the governmental planning cycle example that appears in the next section of this chapter. Note the necessarily broad wording within both of these departmental mission statements.

Department of Health and Human Services (HHS)

The Department of Health and Human Services (HHS) is "...the United States government's principal agency for protecting the health of all Americans and providing essential human services, especially for those who are least able to help themselves."[25]

There are more than 300 programs within HHS, including both the Medicare and the Medicaid programs.

Department of Health and Human Services (HHS) Mission Statement

The mission of the U.S. Department of Health and Human Services (HHS) is to enhance the health and well-being of Americans by providing for effective health and human services and by fostering sound, sustained advances in the sciences underlying medicine, public health, and social services.

HHS accomplishes its mission through several hundred programs and initiatives that cover a wide spectrum of activities, serving the American public at every stage of life.[26]

Department of Veterans Affairs (VA)

The Department of Veterans Affairs (VA) oversees benefits and services, including health care, for the nation's veterans. There are three VA sub-agencies within the Department as follows. The Veterans Health Administration (VHA) manages veterans' health care and services. The Veterans Benefits Administration (VBA) manages veterans' benefits, including life insurance and pensions. The National Cemetery Administration (NCA) oversees both burials and memorials for veterans.[27]

Department of Veterans Affairs (VA) Mission Statement

"Our mission at VA is to serve Veterans by increasing their access to our benefits and services, to provide them the highest quality of health care available, and to control costs to the best of our abilities."[28]

AN EXAMPLE: THE VA OFFICE OF INFORMATION TECHNOLOGY IT STRATEGIC PLANNING CYCLE

This section contains a governmental planning cycle example. Elements of the cycle are then defined and discussed. The section concludes with a summary of management responsibilities.

INTRODUCTION

You will recall that federal planning requirements are especially important to us because these requirements provide guidance through a time-tested and regulated framework for strategic planning. We are about to provide a real-life illustration of the planning cycle.

We present the illustrated cycle as an excellent example of the planning process. This example is drawn from a VA Directive concerning strategic planning. The entire scope of the Directive's requirements is, of course, well beyond the scope of this text. We have had to generalize the required process in order to provide this example. In generalizing we are forced to disregard additional explanations, terminology, and background details contained in the Directive. Please refer to it as a source for further details.

The elements within this VA illustrated example include components that we have described earlier in this chapter. The components include the following:

- Set Broad Goals and Narrower Objectives for Programs
- Set Performance Measures to Achieve the Goals and the Objectives
- Determine External Key Factors that are Significant
- Prepare Annual Performance Plan
- Prepare Periodic Performance Reports
- Revise and Update As Needed

THE VA OFFICE OF INFORMATION TECHNOLOGY IT STRATEGIC PLANNING CYCLE: AN EXAMPLE

Figure 22–4 illustrates the planning cycle in accordance with VA Directive 6052. The Directive's version used here is dated 2009. While there will inevitably be future updates and revisions, this example of the planning cycle process serves our purpose very well.[29]

THE VA PLANNING CYCLE'S PROCESS FLOW

Figure 22–4 shows the overall VA Strategic Plan and Goals at the top of the visual. This overall plan and its goals then flow to four "administrative strategic plans." The four plans include one apiece for the three subagencies (VHA, VBA, and NCA), plus a fourth plan for the VA Staff Office.

Each of the four plans flow to, and relate to, VA key business priorities, goals, and objects. The Information Technology (IT) Strategic Plan contains IT goals, objectives, and strategies. Its multi-year planning cycle (shown on Figure 22–4 as a five-year cycle) flows back in and out of the four Administrative Strategic Plans, as indicated by the two-way arrows.

Program and Operational Plans that support the IT Strategic Plan are the responsibility of the Deputy Assistant Secretary (DAS), the Deputy Chief Information Officers (DCIOs) and the Executive Directors. These plans are shown on a three-year planning cycle.

IT Performance Plans and their related Performance Measures are an outgrowth of the Program and Operational Plans. They are on a shorter cycle that we interpret as the base year plus one target.

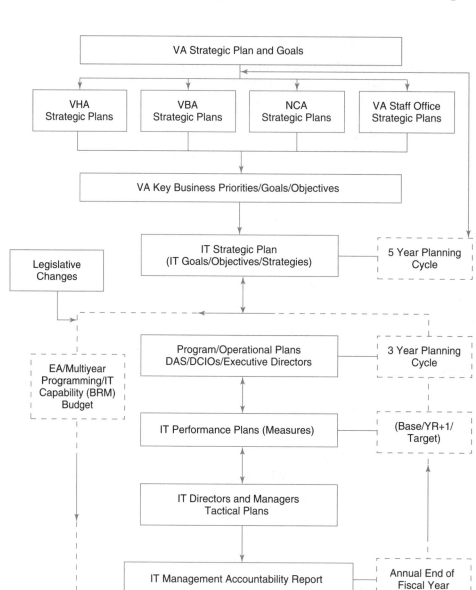

Figure 22–4 VA Office of Information Technology IT Strategic Planning Cycle.
Reproduced from the Department of Veterans Affairs. VA Directive 6052 Appendix A (April 23, 2009).

The Tactical Plans that will carry out the Performance Plans are the responsibility of the IT Directors and Managers. Finally, an IT Management Accountability Report is required annually at the end of each fiscal year.

The Legislative Changes (an external factor that influences the process) are shown in a box on the left-hand side of the visual. Their influence feeds into and impacts the overall process.

Finally, the box on the dotted line to the left reads "EA/Multiyear Programming/IT Capability (BRM) Budget." We understand this is a budget that contains multi-year programming. We further understand it references IT Capability. The remaining portion of the acronym references the "One VA EA Business Reference Model," or BRM. The BRM was developed in part to provide a common set of process definitions. It thus assists in making "…the complex integration between business processes transparent."[30]

PLANNING CYCLE DEFINITIONS FOR THIS EXAMPLE

The following definitions are contained in the Office of Information Technology IT Planning Directive. While they are specific to the Directive's purpose, they provide greater depth to an overall understanding of the illustrated cycle and its process flow.

Strategic Planning

Strategic planning is a continuous process by which IT determines direction and operational focus over the next three to five years consistent with priorities established by the Secretary of Veterans Affairs as expressed in the Departmental Strategic Plan. There is one IT Strategic Plan; however, strategic planning involves all parts of VA Administrations and Staff Offices.

IT Mission

A mission statement is brief, defines the basic purpose of the organization, and corresponds directly with the organization's core programs and activities. An organization's program goals should flow from the mission statement. The mission defines the approach and means IT will take to fulfill the mission of VA as a whole.

IT Vision

The vision defines the ideal state for IT. (It is) what an organization desires to accomplish in the future.

IT Strategic Goals

A goal is a statement of aim or purpose included in a strategic plan (required under GPRA). The strategic goal defines how an agency will carry out a major segment of its mission over a period of time. The goal is expressed in a manner that allows a future assessment to be made of whether the goal was or is being achieved. Most strategic goals will be outcomes and are long-term in nature. IT goals define the forward-thinking and transformational outcomes IT pursues to achieve its mission over a period of time.

IT Strategic Objectives

Strategic objectives are strategy components or continuous improvement activities that are needed to create value for the customers. IT objectives further define intended program outcomes to achieve IT goals.

Program Plans

A program plan consists of planned activities or related projects managed in a coordinated way to include an element of ongoing work products or projects. A program plan is designed to accomplish a predetermined objective or set of objectives.

Operational Plans

An operational plan is a detailed action plan to accomplish the specific objectives. The plan is a derivative of the strategic plan describing short-term business strategies, showing how the strategic plan will be put into operation and serving as a basis for an annual operating budget. An operational plan may comprise a three-year rolling plan to be completed by a small subgroup of people with expertise and/or a stake relating to a major goal.

Performance Measures

Performance measures are valid and reliable metrics for evaluating the extent to which goals and objectives are achieved. The measures should be SMART (Specific, Measurable, Achievable, Results-oriented, Time-limited).

IT Management Accountability Report (IT MAR)

The IT MAR is an annual report that provides OI&T performance information (i.e., strategic goals, objectives, fiscal year performance goals, and outcomes). The IT MAR is a management tool that will provide a basis for assessing the organization's effectiveness.

Environmental Scan: Feedback and Assessment

An environment scan is an ongoing internal and external customer feedback and assessment process conducted at all levels of the organization for use in developing vision, goals, and objectives.[31]

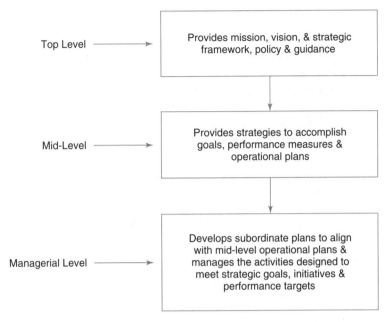

Figure 22–5 Primary Planning Responsibilities by Management Levels.

MANAGEMENT RESPONSIBILITIES WITHIN THE PLANNING CYCLE

This section concludes with a generalized view of planning responsibilities by three levels of management. **Figure 22–5** illustrates the three levels. Any planning cycle should reflect these levels, as does the previous example.

Upper-Level Responsibilities

Top-level management represents those individuals at the top of the organization chart. These upper-level individuals should provide overall direction for the organization's mission, vision, and strategic framework. They should be responsible for policymaking and supervisory guidance issues.

Mid-Level Responsibilities

Mid-level individuals are basically accountable to those above, while they operate in a supervisory mode to those below them in the organization chart. Mid-level management should typically provide the strategies to accomplish goals, performance measures, and operational plans.

Managerial-Level Responsibilities

The managers, meanwhile, are accountable to all those above them on the organization chart. The managerial level should typically develop the subordinate plans that will align with mid-level operational plans. Other responsibilities include managing the activities that are designed to meet strategic goals, initiatives, and performance targets.

TOOLS FOR STRATEGIC PLANNING: SITUATIONAL ANALYSIS AND FINANCIAL PROJECTIONS

Situational analysis and feasibility studies are discussed in this section, with an emphasis on their roles in strategic planning.

SITUATIONAL ANALYSIS (SWOT)

This section defines situational analysis and discusses its components.

Definition

A situational analysis does two things. It reviews the organization's internal operations for strengths and weaknesses and it explores the organization's external environment for opportunities and threats. (Thus SWOT: strengths-weaknesses-opportunities-threats.) A situational analysis allows management to, literally, analyze the organization's situation.

SWOT Analysis as a Strategic Tool

A SWOT analysis, properly performed, can be an excellent strategic tool. The four components of a SWOT analysis include the following:

- Strengths
- Weaknesses
- Opportunities
- Threats

The basic SWOT analysis format is illustrated in **Figure 22–6**. Here we see that the "Strengths" and "Weaknesses" sectors of the matrix are labeled "Internal," while the "Opportunities" and "Threats" sectors are labeled "External."

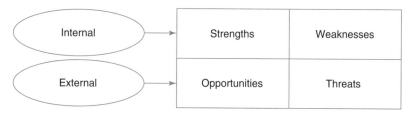

Figure 22–6   Basic SWOT Analysis Format.

Sample SWOT Worksheets Are Contained in the Appendix

The Appendix to this chapter contains Sample SWOT Worksheets. The worksheets and their supplemental Question Guides concern Electronic Health Records (EHR) adoption and implementation. These worksheets can, however, be easily adopted for other purposes.

The Appendix contains three "Internal Worksheets" for analyzing strengths and weaknesses, and an "External Worksheet" for analyzing external opportunities and threats. Supplemental Question Guides are also included for each worksheet. A Scoring Summary Sheet is included to complete the analysis.

Sequential Steps in the SWOT Analysis Project

The following steps pertain to both the internal and external components of the analysis:

1. First, decide if the sample worksheets and the supplemental question guides need to be customized; if so, do so.
2. Gather necessary information.
3. Fill in the worksheets, utilizing the question guides as needed.
4. Reach agreement, or consensus, on the final score for each line item on the worksheets.
5. Summarize the scores.
6. Enter the final net scores on the Scoring Summary Sheet.
7. Report the results.

Commencing the SWOT Analysis Project Process

In order to commence the SWOT analysis project's process, a number of decisions must be made. They include the following:

1. What type of task force or committee does the project need?
2. Who will be appointed to this task force?
3. What types of data/information should be gathered for this project?
4. Who will gather the information that is needed?
5. Will the scoring process be subjective or objective? (This may depend on the amount and type of available data.)
6. Will the same task force members that are involved in recording the worksheet information also be involved in the scoring process, or will a separate group be appointed to carry out the scoring function?
7. Who prepares the final report?
8. Who receives the report?
9. Who is responsible for taking appropriate action after the analysis and its report are completed?

Conclusion

Situational analysis is particularly appropriate for the analysis of electronic records implementation because such implementation requires the collaboration of multiple knowledge areas. A meeting of the minds can better occur with the discipline that a situational analysis can impose. It is a powerful tool when properly applied.

We should also acknowledge that there are a variety of approaches to performing a situational analysis, and this brief discussion features only a single approach. No matter what approach is utilized, the results of the situational analysis are what count.

FINANCIAL PROJECTIONS FOR STRATEGIC PLANNING

The type of financial projection that we discuss is this section is produced internally. These projections are intended for internal use during the planning process, and are thus not intended for any use outside the organization.

Definition

Projections are views into the future. We "project" future events, projects, or operations using a set of presumed, or hypothetical, assumptions.

Projections are different than forecasts, although both are considered to be "prospective" (thus "future") financial statements. Forecasts are based on assumptions that are expected to exist, and that reflect actions that are expected to occur.[32]

Projections, on the other hand, are often prepared to answer a "what-if" question, such as "what if … this service/program/initiative were to be adopted?" In these "what-if" situations several projections may be prepared, each based on a different set of hypothetical assumptions and each reflecting the actions that might occur, based on such assumptions.[33]

Build a Planner's Projection

An eight-step process for building a financial projection to be used internally for planning purposes is described as follows. The process is also illustrated in **Figure 22–7**.

1) Determine the future time frame

2) Determine the focus

3) Gather enough information

4) Make reasonable assumptions

5) Document the assumptions

6) Prepare the projected statements

7) Review for reasonableness

8) Create alternative scenarios

Figure 22–7   Build a Planner's Financial Projection. Courtesy of J.J. Baker and R.W. Baker, Dallas, Texas.

Determine the Future timeframe

What should the future start and end dates be for this projection? Is the time period to be covered long enough? Or is it too long for reasonable assumptions to be made?

Determine the Focus

Focus on what the plan (or planner) needs to know in order to go forward. Let that focus determine the direction your search for information will take. (Also note that sometimes a different agenda can redirect the focus.)

Gather Enough Information

You will need enough information to make informed decisions about your projection. The range of subjects may vary, but the information should be as up-to-date as possible.

Make Reasonable Assumptions

By "reasonable assumptions" we mean no wildly unattainable assumptions. For example, in most instances "we will increase revenue by 200% in the fourth quarter of next year" is an assumption that will not be accomplished thus is not reasonable.

Document the Assumptions

Assumptions used for the projection are key to its success. Documenting the assumptions is an indication of a well-constructed projection. The documentation adds validity to the final product. It also provides a record of the overall process of information-gathering that underlies the assumptions themselves.

Prepare the Projected Statements

Projected financial statements are then assembled using the documented assumptions. In accountant's terminology this is known as "compiling" the projections.

Review for Reasonableness

For example, ask: "Is this assumption reasonable for an organization of my type and size?" This type of review may be subjective, but it is a logical part of the process. Appropriate members of the organization may also perform a review in order to highlight any weak spots within the assumptions.

Create Alternative Scenarios

It is often helpful to produce multiple versions of the projections ("Model A," "Model B," etc.). In this case certain key assumptions are changed for each model. Thus the "what if" question is answered in several different ways.

Financial Projections as Strategic Tools

These internal planning projects may be used to better make informed decisions. If properly constructed, they can provide information that is laid out in a logical format, supported by assumptions that are properly explained for the knowledgeable reader. To summarize, projections can be an important tool to inform and support the planning process.

CASE STUDY: STRATEGIC FINANCIAL PLANNING IN LONG-TERM CARE

Chapter 27, "Case Study: Strategic Financial Planning in Long-Term Care" later in this volume involves a case study about strategic financial planning in long-term care. The case study is authored by Dr. Neil R. Dworkin, Emeritus Associate Professor of Management at Western Connecticut State University. His case study merits your close attention, as it will utilize planning concepts that have been discussed within this chapter.

APPENDIX 22-A: SAMPLE SWOT WORKSHEETS AND QUESTION GUIDES

Appendix 22-A contains four Sample SWOT Worksheets (three internal and one external) concerning EHR adoption and implementation, along with a Scoring Summary Sheet. A Question Guide is also included for each Worksheet. Electronic medical records adoption is a good subject for situational analysis. The sample worksheets in this Appendix can assist in beginning such a project.

 INFORMATION CHECKPOINT

What is needed?	A "set" of an organization's mission statement, vision statement, and values.
Where is it found?	In the planning and policy division or within the administration office.
How is it used?	These documents are used to guide the organization.

 KEY TERMS

Action Plan
Financial Forecast
Financial Projection
Goal
Innovation
Mission Statement
Situational Analysis
Strategic Objective
SWOT Analysis
Values Statement
Vision Statement

 DISCUSSION QUESTIONS

1. Do you know if your organization has a mission statement and a vision statement? If so, how are they communicated? Are they printed, posted on a website, or available in some other format? Please describe.
2. Have you ever been involved in a strategic planning session? If so, please describe how the group and the session were structured (but without revealing proprietary information).
3. Have you ever been involved in (or have observed) the process of a situational analysis (SWOT)? If so, please describe how the group went about performing the analysis (but again without revealing proprietary information).

NOTES

1. Department of Veterans Affairs (VA), VA Directive 6052 Appendix A (April 23, 2009).
2. www.sutterhealth.org/about/mission (accessed May 31, 2012).
3. www.tenethealth.com/about/pages/missionandvalues.aspx (accessed July 30, 2012).

4. www.parklandhospital.com/whoweare/mission_vision.html (accessed June 7, 2012).

5. www.mayoclinic.org/about/missionvalues.html (accessed July 30, 2012).

6. www.regionshospital.com/rh/about/index.html (accessed May 31, 2012).

7. www.saintbarnabasfoundation.org/about/mission.html (accessed July 30, 2012).

8. www.texasoncology.com/about-txo/vision-mission-history.aspx (accessed December 3, 2012).

9. www.aetna.com/about-aetna-insurance/aetna-corporate-profile/aetna_mission_statement (accessed July 30, 2012).

10. AMA Press Release November 26, 2012 from www.ama-assn.org (accessed January 16, 2013).

11. www.ama-assn.org/ana/pub/about-ama/strategic-focus.page? (accessed October 17, 2012).

12. Ibid.

13. www.good-sam.com/index.php/about_us/ (accessed July 30, 2012).

14. Ibid.

15. http://www.providence.net/about/ (accessed January 16, 2013).

16. www.dukemedicine.org/AboutUs (accessed July 30, 2012).

17. www.hopkinsmedicine.org/se/util/display_mod.cfm?MODULE=/se-server/mod/mod (accessed July 30, 2012).

18. Public Law 103-62. 103 P.L. 62; 107 Stat. 285 – Section 3(a) The language of the Act says "every agency", but in fact certain Executive agencies were excluded, including the Central Intelligence Agency, the General Accounting Office, the Panama Canal Commission, the United States Postal Service, and the Postal Rate Commission. [See 103 P.L. 62 Section 3(f).].

19. P.L. 62 – Section 3(a) (1), (2), (3), (5).

20. P.L. 62 – Section 3(a) (6b).

21. P.L.111-352 Section 2(b).

22. Ibid. Section 3(b)(1).

23. Ibid. Section 4(b).

24. Ibid. Section 4(g).

25. http://www.hhs.gov/about/whatwedo.html (accessed December 4, 2012).

26. http://www.hhs.gov/secretary/about/introduction.html (accessed May 25, 2012).

27. www.administrativelawreview.org/publicresources/index.php?option=com_content&view=article&id=21&Itemid=28 (accessed February 2, 2013).

28. www.va.gov/VA_2011-2015_Strategic_Plan_Refresh_wv.pdf.

29. Department of Veterans Affairs (VA), "VA Directive 6052, Appendix A" (April 23, 2009), http://www.itstrategy.oit.va.gov/docs/directive_6052.pdf p. 6 (accessed December 4, 2012).

30. www.mpoweredstrategies.com/news/2011/12/one-va-ea-business-reference-model/ (accessed February 2, 2013).

31. www.mpoweredstrategies.com/news/2011/12/one-va-ea-business-reference-model/ (accessed February 2, 2013).

32. American Institute of Certified Public Accountants (AICPA), "Financial Forecasts and Projections" AT Section 301 (c)(d), http://www.aicpa.org/Research/Standards/AuditAttest/DownloadableDocuments/AT-00301.pdf

33. Ibid. AT Section 301 (d)(f).

Sample SWOT Worksheets and Question Guides 22-A

The following Sample SWOT Worksheets and their supplemental Question Guides concern Electronic Health Records (EHR) adoption and implementation. However, the worksheets and question guides can be readily adapted for other purposes.

INTRODUCTION

Situational analysis explores an organization's internal operation for strengths and weakness and observes the organization's external environment for opportunities and threats. The analysis process is often called "SWOT," for strengths-weaknesses-opportunities-threats. To be effective, the analysis must be objective and realistic.

Electronic medical records adoption is a good subject for situational analysis. The sample worksheets in this Appendix provide assistance in commencing such a project.

This Appendix contains four Sample SWOT Worksheets (three internal and one external) concerning EHR adoption and implementation, along with a Scoring Summary Sheet. A Question Guide is also included for each Worksheet. The Guides are intended to commence the process of analysis. Other questions may be added to customize the analysis for a particular process, situation, or department.

SCORING SUMMARY SHEET FOR EHR ADOPTION AND IMPLEMENTATION

Exhibit 22-A–1 collects and summarizes the SWOT analysis scores. Both the internal and external worksheets are to be scored for each item appearing on that particular worksheet. The scores range from 1 to 5, as follows: 1 = very good; 2 = good; 3 = fair; 4 = poor; and 5 = very poor. These scores are then summarized and the final net score is entered on the Exhibit 22-A–1.

THREE INTERNAL WORKSHEETS FOR STRENGTHS AND WEAKNESSES

Three internal worksheets present the results of the SWOT strengths and weaknesses internal analysis. These worksheets represent four important subjects that are relevant to EHR. The first two worksheets concern staff members involved in some capacity with EHR. The

Exhibit 22-A–1 SWOT Scoring Summary Sheet for EHR Adoption and Implementation

	1	2	3	4	5
INTERNAL STRENGTHS SCORES					
IT Department Staff	☐	☐	☐	☐	☐
Financial, Clinical, and Administrative Staff	☐	☐	☐	☐	☐
EHR Technology	☐	☐	☐	☐	☐
Capital Funding	☐	☐	☐	☐	☐
INTERNAL WEAKNESSES SCORES					
IT Department Staff	☐	☐	☐	☐	☐
Financial, Clinical, and Administrative Staff	☐	☐	☐	☐	☐
EHR Technology	☐	☐	☐	☐	☐
Capital Funding	☐	☐	☐	☐	☐
EXTERNAL OPPORTUNITIES SCORES					
Government	☐	☐	☐	☐	☐
Economy	☐	☐	☐	☐	☐
Competition	☐	☐	☐	☐	☐
Other Funding Sources	☐	☐	☐	☐	☐
EXTERNAL THREATS SCORES					
Government	☐	☐	☐	☐	☐
Economy	☐	☐	☐	☐	☐
Competition	☐	☐	☐	☐	☐
Other Funding Sources	☐	☐	☐	☐	☐

Score 1 to 5 with 1 being very good and 5 being very poor

Courtesy of J.J. Baker and R.W. Baker, Dallas, Texas.

third worksheet addresses both technology and capital funding. These subjects are, of course, separate from the staffing issues. Each worksheet is described below.

INTERNAL WORKSHEET FOR EHR INFORMATION TECHNOLOGY (IT) STAFF

Exhibit 22-A–2 specifically addresses the information technology staffing. These staff members are the ones who must make electronic health records implementation work. The responsible staff are divided into three levels, depending upon the type of work they are expected to perform. The three levels represent "IT operations staff," who are the most directly involved; the "hands-on managers," who manage the operations staff day-to-day;

Exhibit 22-A–2 EHR Internal Operations Analysis: Worksheet for Information Technology (IT) Department Staff

IT OPERATIONS STAFF (for each type of position listed)
Overall Computer Skills
Strengths _____
Weaknesses _____

Specific EHR Skills
Strengths _____
Weaknesses _____

Staffing Capacity
Strengths _____
Weaknesses _____

HANDS-ON IT MANAGERS
Background and Experience
Strengths _____
Weaknesses _____

EHR Proficiency and Support
Strengths _____
Weaknesses _____

Coverage (Man Hours Available)
Strengths _____
Weaknesses _____

UPPER-LEVEL SUPERVISORY IT MANAGEMENT
Background and Experience
Strengths _____
Weaknesses _____

EHR Proficiency and Support
Strengths _____
Weaknesses _____

Coverage (Man Hours Available)
Strengths _____
Weaknesses _____

Attach sheets to document the additional information used for this analysis.

Courtesy of J.J. Baker and R.W. Baker, Dallas, Texas.

Exhibit 22-A–3 Question Guide for EHR Internal Operations Analysis: Information Technology (IT) Department Staff

Staff questions (Answer the questions about IT staff as appropriate for the various staff levels: IT operations staff, hands-on IT managers, and upper-level supervisory IT management.)

☐ Possess advanced computer operations concepts?
☐ Possess basic computer operations concepts?
☐ Understand EHR technical computer applications in depth?
☐ Understand basic EHR technical computer applications?
☐ Understand the concept of EHR calculations?
☐ Cooperate/support multidisciplinary EHR adoption and implementation efforts?
☐ Resist/ignore EHR process and procedures?
☐ Sufficient IT staffing for EHR implementation?
☐ Sufficient IT staffing for EHR ongoing support?
☐ Acceptable productivity for EHR implementation?

Attach sheets to document the additional information used for this analysis.

Courtesy of J.J. Baker and R.W. Baker, Dallas, Texas.

and the "upper-level supervisory IT management," who manage from afar, but who are responsible for results.

Question Guide for EHR Information Technology Staff

Exhibit 22-A–3 contains 10 questions about IT staff. The questions are to be answered as is appropriate for the various staff levels described in the preceding paragraph.

INTERNAL WORKSHEET FOR OTHER STAFF INVOLVED IN EHR

Exhibit 22-A–4 addresses responsible staff in three other departments of the organization. These staff members are the ones who must make electronic health records implementation work within their own departments. The responsible staff members in each of these three departments (financial, clinical, and administrative) are again divided into three levels, depending upon the type of work they are expected to perform. The three levels represent "Staff responsible for some aspect of EHR," who are the most directly involved; the "hands-on managers," who are responsible for some aspect of EHR; and the "upper-level supervisory management," who manage from afar, but who are responsible for results.

Exhibit 22-A-4 Worksheet for EHR Internal Operations Analysis: Financial, Clinical, and Administrative Staff

STAFF RESPONSIBLE FOR SOME ASPECT OF EHR

Overall Computer Skills

Strengths _____

Weaknesses _____

Specific EHR Skills

Strengths _____

Weaknesses _____

Staffing Capacity

Strengths _____

Weaknesses _____

HANDS-ON MANAGERS RESPONSIBLE FOR SOME ASPECT OF EHR

Background and Experience

Strengths _____

Weaknesses _____

EHR Proficiency and Support

Strengths _____

Weaknesses _____

Coverage (Man Hours Available)

Strengths _____

Weaknesses _____

UPPER-LEVEL SUPERVISORY MANAGEMENT RESPONSIBLE FOR SOME ASPECT OF EHR

Background and Experience

Strengths _____

Weaknesses _____

EHR Proficiency and Support

Strengths _____

Weaknesses _____

Coverage (Man Hours Available)

Strengths _____

Weaknesses _____

Attach sheets to document the additional information used for this analysis.

Courtesy of J.J. Baker and R.W. Baker, Dallas, Texas.

Exhibit 22-A–5 Question Guide for EHR Internal Operations Analysis: Financial, Clinical, and Administrative Staff

Staff questions (Answer the questions about staff as appropriate for the various financial, clinical, and administrative staff levels: workers; hands-on managers, and upper-level supervisory management.)

- ☐ Possess advanced financial management concepts?
- ☐ Possess basic financial management concepts?
- ☐ Possess advanced clinical management concepts?
- ☐ Possess basic clinical management concepts?
- ☐ Understand EHR technical applications in depth from the financial view?
- ☐ Understand basic EHR technical applications from the financial view?
- ☐ Understand EHR technical applications in depth from the clinical view?
- ☐ Understand basic EHR technical applications from the clinical view?
- ☐ Understand the concept of EHR calculations?
- ☐ Cooperate/support multidisciplinary EHR adoption and implementation efforts?
- ☐ Resist/ignore EHR process and procedures?
- ☐ Sufficient relevant staffing for EHR implementation?
- ☐ Sufficient relevant staffing for EHR ongoing support?
- ☐ Acceptable productivity for EHR implementation?

Attach sheets to document the additional information used for this analysis.

Courtesy of J.J. Baker and R.W. Baker, Dallas, Texas.

Question Guide for Financial, Clinical, and Administrative Staff

Exhibit 22-A–5 contains 14 questions about relevant staff members within these 3 departments. This guide and its accompanying worksheet would, of course, be reproduced with as many copies as would be necessary in order to answer these questions for each department.

INTERNAL WORKSHEET FOR TECHNOLOGY AND CAPITAL FUNDING

Exhibit 22-A–6 addresses two subjects: computer technology and capital funding resources. The computer technology section concerns hardware, software, space requirements, and vendors. The section is then divided into two parts: one for overall computer systems and one for specific EHR computer resources.

The capital funding section of the worksheet addresses both short-term and long-term funding resources. The short-term funding requirement concerns EHR transition cash flow. The long-term funding requirement concerns what fixed capital may be specified for EHR implementation. Both are important to success.

Exhibit 22-A–6 Worksheet for EHR Internal Operations Analysis: Resources Other than Staff

OVERALL COMPUTER SYSTEMS
Hardware and Software
Strengths _____

Weaknesses _____

Space Requirements
Strengths _____

Weaknesses _____

Vendor Contractual Agreements (if applicable)
Strengths _____

Weaknesses _____

Vendor Performance (if applicable)
Strengths _____

Weaknesses _____

SPECIFIC EHR COMPUTER RESOURCES
Hardware and Software
Strengths _____

Weaknesses _____

Additional Space Requirements (if applicable)
Strengths _____

Weaknesses _____

Vendor Contractual Agreements (if applicable)
Strengths _____

Weaknesses _____

Vendor Performance (if applicable)
Strengths _____

Weaknesses _____

CAPITAL FUNDING
Short-Term EHR Transition Cash Flow Requirements
Strengths _____

Weaknesses _____

Long-term Fixed Capital Specified for EHR Implementation
Strengths _____

Weaknesses _____

Attach sheets to document the additional information used for this analysis.

Courtesy of J.J. Baker and R.W. Baker, Dallas, Texas.

Exhibit 22-A–7　Question Guide for EHR Internal Operations Analysis: Resources Other than Staff

---

OVERALL COMPUTER SYSTEMS
☐ Sufficient equipment (hardware and software) for general operations?

SPECIFIC EHR COMPUTER RESOURCES
☐ Sufficient equipment (hardware and software) for EHR implementation?
☐ Sufficient equipment (hardware and software) for EHR ongoing support?
☐ Equipment operates adequately?
☐ Equipment costly to maintain? To operate?
☐ If applicable, are vendor contracts costly to maintain (updates, add-ons, etc.)?
☐ Does the equipment produce desired results? Timely results?
☐ If applicable, does the vendor produce desired results? Timely results?

CAPITAL FUNDING
☐ Have the short-term EHR transition cash flow requirements been accurately projected?
☐ Are these cash flow requirements accurately presented in the organization's budget?
☐ Are the long-term fixed capital specified for EHR implementation accurately projected?
☐ Are these long-term fixed capital requirements acknowledged in the strategic plan?

Attach sheets to document the additional information used for this analysis

Courtesy of J.J. Baker and R.W. Baker, Dallas, Texas.

Question Guide for Technology and Capital Funding Resources

Exhibit 22-A–7 contains eight questions about computer systems and four questions about capital funding resources. Additional customized questions may supplement this initial guide's content.

EXTERNAL WORKSHEET FOR OPPORTUNITIES AND THREATS

Exhibit 22-A–8 addresses four external environment subjects, including Government, Economy, Competition, and Funding Sources Other than Patient Revenue. Other subjects may, of course, be added as desired.

Exhibit 22-A–8 Worksheet for EHR External Environment Analysis

---

GOVERNMENT (EHR impact for each governmental element listed)

Medicare Program

Opportunities _____

Threats _____

Medicaid Program

Opportunities _____

Threats _____

Regulations About Electronic Standards (Version 5010 and ongoing versions)

Opportunities _____

Threats _____

Other Federal/State Regulations

Opportunities _____

Threats _____

ECONOMY (as to continuing need for and impact of EHR)

Opportunities _____

Threats _____

COMPETITION (relevant to EHR)

Opportunities _____

Threats _____

FUNDING SOURCES OTHER THAN PATIENT REVENUE (impact, if any, on EHR)

Opportunities _____

Threats _____

Attach sheets to document the additional information used for this analysis.

Courtesy of J.J. Baker and R.W. Baker, Dallas, Texas.

Question Guide for EHR External Environment Analysis

Exhibit 22-A–9 contains a total of 22 questions about various components of the external environment. This guide may also be augmented with customized questions that relate to issues within the specific organization under analysis.

Exhibit 22-A–9 Question Guide for EHR External Environment Analysis

GOVERNMENT (EHR impact for each governmental element listed)
Medicare Program

☐ What EHR implementation costs are related to this program initiative?
☐ What revenues from EHR governmental sources are related to this program initiative?
☐ What savings in work flow or processes are related to adopting EHR?
☐ Additional changes to the EHR Medicare Initiative are scheduled to occur at various points in the future. How will these initiative changes impact the organization?

Medicaid Program

☐ What EHR implementation costs are related to this program initiative?
☐ What revenues from EHR governmental sources are related to this program initiative?
☐ What savings in work flow or processes are related to adopting EHR?
☐ Additional changes to the EHR Medicaid Initiative are scheduled to occur at various points in the future. How will these initiative changes impact the organization?

Regulations About Electronic Standards (Version 5010 and ongoing versions)

☐ What EHR implementation costs are related to these requirements?
☐ What savings in work flow or processes are related to adopting these standards?
☐ Additional changes to the regulatory electronic standards are scheduled to occur at various points in the future. How will these initiative changes impact the organization?

Other Federal/State Regulations

☐ What other federal and/or state regulations affect EHR implementation?
☐ How do these regulations impact the organization?

ECONOMY (as to continuing need for and impact of EHR)

☐ Will EHR affect continuing need for medical services? If so, how?
☐ What impact is EHR implementation projected to have on the medical services economy nationally? Regionally?

COMPETITION (relevant to EHR)

☐ What are your three biggest competitors?
☐ How do the services they provide compare to your services?
☐ What do you predict the impact of EHR adoption will be on each?
☐ How have they prepared for EHR initial implementation?
☐ How does their preparation and impact affect your own organization?

OTHER FUNDING SOURCES (impact, if any, on EHR)

☐ Does your organization have such funding sources?
☐ If so, what impact, if any, will EHR adoption have on such sources?

Attach sheets to document the additional information used for this analysis.

Courtesy of J.J. Baker and R.W. Baker, Dallas, Texas.

Putting It All Together: Creating a Business Plan That Is Strategic

OVERVIEW

A business plan is a document typically prepared in order to obtain funding and/or financing. A traditional business plan typically contains information about three major elements: the proposed project's organization, marketing, and financial aspects. However, the actual business plan is generally constructed in a series of segments, each involving a particular type of information. The overall business plan is built up as these individual segments are completed. The segments are described in this chapter.

ELEMENTS OF THE BUSINESS PLAN

A traditional business plan typically contains three major elements:

- Organization plan
- Marketing plan
- Financial plan

The organization segment should describe the management team. The marketing segment should discuss who may use the service and/or product. The financial segment should contain the numbers that illustrate how the project is expected to operate over an initial period of time. We believe that it is also important to begin the business plan with an executive summary that outlines key points, plus a clear and concise description of the service and/or product that is the subject of the plan.

Progress Notes

After completing this chapter, you should be able to

1. Understand the construction of a business plan.
2. Describe the organization segment of a business plan.
3. Describe the marketing segment of a business plan.
4. Describe the financial segment of a business plan.

PREPARING TO CONSTRUCT THE BUSINESS PLAN

The planning stage will shape a business plan's content. The initial decisions, such as those shown in **Exhibit 23–1**, will determine your approach to the plan. For example, if your organization requires a certain type of format and preexisting blank spreadsheets, many of the initial decisions have already been made for you. Otherwise, the checklist contained in Exhibit 23–1 will assist you in making initial decisions for the business plan's approach.

It is important to note that the level of sophistication for the overall plan should be based on the decision makers who will be the primary audience. Another practical consideration involves creating a grid or matrix to assist in gathering all necessary information. The grid or matrix could also include which individuals are responsible for helping to create or collect the required information. Finally, it is important to create a file at the beginning of the project in which all computations, backup information, dates, and sources are kept together in an organized fashion.

Exhibit 23–1 Initial Decisions for the Business Plan

> Business Plan Initial Decisions
>
> - Outline necessary format
> - Decide on length
> - Decide on level of sophistication
> - Determine what information is needed
> - Determine who will provide each piece of information
>
> Courtesy of J.J. Baker and R.W. Baker, Dallas, Texas.

Exhibit 23–2 Basic Information for the Service or Equipment Description

> Service or Equipment Description
> - What the service specifically provides
> - Why this service is different and/or special
> - What the equipment specifically does
> - Why this equipment is different and/or special
> - Required training, if applicable
> - Regulatory requirements and/or impact, if any
>
> Courtesy of J.J. Baker and R.W. Baker, Dallas, Texas.

THE SERVICE OR EQUIPMENT DESCRIPTION

The service and/or equipment description should do a good job of describing what the heart of the business plan is about. If the business plan is for a project or a new service line, then this description would expand to include the entire project or the overall service line. Information that should always be included in the description is contained in **Exhibit 23–2**.

The test of a good description is whether an individual who has never been involved in your planning can read the description and understand it without additional questions being raised.

THE ORGANIZATION SEGMENT

The organization segment should describe the management team. But it should also describe how the proposed service or equipment fits into the organization. Who will be charged with the new budget? Who will be responsible for the controls and reporting for this proposal? It is important to provide a clear picture that informs decision makers about how the proposed acquisition will be managed. Basic facts to explain are included in **Exhibit 23–3**.

Visual depictions of the chain of authority and supervisory responsibilities provide helpful illustrations for this segment.

THE MARKETING SEGMENT

The marketing segment should describe the available market, that portion of the market your service or equipment should attract, and that portion of the market occupied by the competition. This segment should achieve a balance between describing those individuals who will be availing themselves of the service or equipment and a description of the competition. A description of who will be responsible for the marketing is also valuable information for the decision makers. Strive for a realistic and objective appraisal of the situation. Basic facts to include are illustrated in **Exhibit 23–4**.

Of all areas of the business plan, the marketing segment is most likely to be overoptimistic in its assumptions. It is wise to be conservative about estimations of physician and patient acceptance and usage. And it is equally wise to be realistic when assessing the competition and its likely impact.

THE FINANCIAL ANALYSIS SEGMENT

Exhibit 23–3 Basic Information for the Organization Segment

Organization Segment Information

- Physical location where service will be provided
- Physical location of the equipment
- The department responsible for the budget
- The division responsible for operations
- The directly responsible supervisor
- Composition of the overall management team

Courtesy of J.J. Baker and R.W. Baker, Dallas, Texas.

Exhibit 23–4 Basic Information for the Marketing Segment

Marketing Segment Information

- Physicians who will use the service or equipment
- New patients who will use the service or equipment
- Established patients who will use the service or equipment
- Estimated portion of the market to be captured
- Competition and its impact

Courtesy of J.J. Baker and R.W. Baker, Dallas, Texas.

The financial segment should contain the numbers that illustrate how the project is expected to operate over an initial period of time. Financial plans may range from a projected period of 1 year to as much as 10 years. A 1-year projection is often too short to show true outcomes, whereas a 10-year projection may be too long to meaningfully forecast. Your organization will usually have a standard length of time that is accepted for these projections. The standard forecasted periods for high-tech equipment, for example, often range from 3 to 5 years. Why? Because advances in technology may render them obsolete in 5 years or less. Therefore, the forecast is set for a realistically short time period.

The financial analysis for a business plan should contain a forecast of operations. The forecast may be simple, such as a cash flow statement, or it may be more extensive. A more extensive forecast would also require a balance sheet and an income statement.

The required statements and schedules will depend on two factors: the size and complexity of the project and the usual procedure for a business plan presentation that is expected in your organization.

The Projected Cash Flow Statement

As we have just stated, it is possible that the forecast of operations may simply consist of the cash flow statement. In any case, the statement can be complex, with many detailed line items, or it can be condensed. The condensed type of statement is most often found in a business plan. Keep in mind, however, that a detailed worksheet—the source of the information on the condensed statement—may well be filed in the supporting work papers for the project. Necessary cash flow assumptions are illustrated in **Exhibit 23–5**.

Exhibit 23–5 Basic Assumptions for Business Plan Cash Flow Statement Projections

Cash Flow Statement Assumptions

- Number of years in the future to forecast
- Capital asset purchase or lease information
- Capital asset salvage value (if any)
- Cash inflow
- Cash outflow
- Cost of capital (if applicable)

Courtesy of J.J. Baker and R.W. Baker, Dallas, Texas.

The Projected Income Statement

What income statement assumptions will your business plan's financial analysis require? The basic assumptions for a healthcare project's income statement are illustrated in **Exhibit 23–6**.

The "revenue type" in Exhibit 23–6 refers to whether, for example, the revenue is derived entirely from services or whether part of the revenue is derived from drugs and devices. The "revenue sources" refers to how many payers will pay for the service and/or drug and device, and in what proportion (such as Medicare 60%, Medicaid 15%, and commercial payers 25%). The "revenue amount" refers to how much each payer is expected to pay for the service and/or drug and device. The total amount of revenue can then be determined by multiplying each payer's expected payment rate times the percentage of the total represented by that payer.

In regard to the "expenses" in Exhibit 23–6, the labor cost will usually be determined by staffing assumptions. The required staffing should be set out by type of employee and the pay rate for each type of

Exhibit 23–6 Basic Assumptions for Business Plan Income Statement Projections

Income Statement Assumptions

- Revenue type
- Revenue source(s)
- Revenue amount
- Expenses:
  - Labor
  - Supplies
  - Cost of drug or device (if applicable)
  - Equipment
  - Space occupancy
  - Overhead

Courtesy of J.J. Baker and R.W. Baker, Dallas, Texas.

employee. The number of full-time equivalents (FTEs) for each type of employee will then be established. The FTEs will be multiplied times the assumed pay rate to arrive at the labor cost assumption.

"Supplies" refers to the necessary supplies required to perform the procedure or service. "Cost of drug or device" refers to the cost to the organization of purchasing the drug or device (if a drug or device is necessary to the service). The labor, supplies, and cost of drug or device are costs that can be directly attributed to the service that is the subject of the business plan. Likewise, the "equipment" cost refers to the annual depreciation expense of any equipment that is directly attributed to the service that is the subject of the business plan.

"Space occupancy" refers to the overall cost of occupying the space required for the service or procedure. "Space occupancy" is a catchall phrase. It includes either annual depreciation expense (if the building is owned) or annual rent expense (if the building is leased) of the square footage required for the service. Space occupancy also includes other related costs such as utilities, maintenance, housekeeping, and insurance. Security might also be included in this category. The actual forecast might group these expense items into one line item, or the forecast might show each individual expense (depreciation, housekeeping, etc.) on a separate line. If the expenses are grouped, a footnote or a supplemental schedule should show the actual detail that makes up the total amount.

"Overhead" refers to the remaining expenses of operation that are necessary to produce the service but that are not directly attributable to that service. Examples of such overhead in a physician's office might include items such as postage and copy paper. This amount of indirect overhead may be expressed as a percentage; for example, "overhead equals 10%." Whether the "space occupancy" example or the "overhead" example discussed previously here are grouped or detailed in the forecast will probably depend on how large the amount is in relation to the other expenses, or it might depend instead on the usual format that your organization expects to see in a typical business plan that is presented to management.

The Projected Balance Sheet

What balance sheet assumptions will your business plan's financial analysis require? The basic assumptions for a healthcare project's balance sheet are illustrated in **Exhibit 23–7**.

The elements of a balance sheet (assets, liabilities, and equity) are described in a previous chapter. If a full projected set of statements is required for the business plan, the balance sheet entries will in large part be a function of the income statement projections discussed in the preceding section of this chapter. For example, accounts receivable would be primarily determined by the

Exhibit 23–7 Basic Assumptions for Business Plan Balance Sheet Projections

Balance Sheet Assumptions

- Cash
- Accounts Receivable
- Inventories
- Property and Equipment
- Accounts Payable
- Accrued Current Liabilities
- Long-Term Liabilities
- Equity

Courtesy of J.J. Baker and R.W. Baker, Dallas, Texas.

revenue assumptions, while accounts payable would be primarily determined by the expense assumptions. Likewise, acquisition of equipment or other capital assets will affect capital assets (property and equipment), while their funding assumptions will affect either or both liability and equity totals on the projected balance sheet.

THE "KNOWLEDGEABLE READER" APPROACH TO YOUR BUSINESS PLAN

We believe a good business plan should answer the questions that occur to a knowledgeable reader. Thus, the information you include in the business plan should reflect the choices that you made in selecting the assumptions for your financial analysis. For instance, an example of considerations for forecasting an equipment acquisition is presented in **Exhibit 23–8**. The content of the final business plan should touch upon these points in describing your assumptions that underlie the financial analysis.

Exhibit 23–8 Considerations for Forecasting Equipment Acquisition

Considerations for Forecasting Equipment Acquisition

- Only one location?
- Equipment single purpose or multi-purpose?
- Technology: new, middle-aged, old (obsolete vs. untested)?
- Equipment compatibility?
- Medical supply cost?
- High or low capital investment?
- Buy new or used (refurbished)?
- Buy or lease?
- Lease for number of years or lease on a pay-per-procedure deal?
- How much staff training is required?
- Certification required?
- Square footage required for equipment?
- Is the required square footage available?
- Cleaning methods and equipment (and staff level required)?
- Repairs and maintenance expense (high, medium, low)?

Courtesy of J.J. Baker and R.W. Baker, Dallas, Texas.

THE EXECUTIVE SUMMARY

The executive summary should contain a well-written and concise summary of the entire plan. It should not be longer than two pages; many decision makers consider one page desirable. Some people like to write the executive summary first. They tend to use it as an outline to guide the rest of the content. Other people like to write the executive summary last, when they know what all the detailed content contains. In either instance, the executive summary should tell the entire story in a compelling manner.

ASSEMBLING THE BUSINESS PLAN

The business plan should be assembled into a suitable report format that is determined by many of your initial decisions, such as length and level of sophistication. A sample format appears in **Exhibit 23–9**.

If an appendix is desired, it should contain detail to support certain contents in the main part of the business plan. In preparing the final report, certain other logistics are important. It is expected, for example, that the pages should be numbered. (You might also want to add the date in the footer and perhaps a version number

Exhibit 23–9   Sample Format for a Business Plan

A Sample Business Plan Format

- Title Page
- Table of Contents
- Executive Summary
- Service and/or Equipment Description
- The Organizational Plan
- The Marketing Plan
- The Financial Plan
- Appendix (optional)

Courtesy of J.J. Baker and R.W. Baker, Dallas, Texas.

Exhibit 23–10   Tips on Presentation of the Business Plan

Tips on Presenting Your Business Plan

- Determine who will be attending ahead of time
- Determine how long you will have for the presentation
- Be sure you have a copy for each attendee
- Decide upon whether to use audio/visual aids
  - LCD projector and PowerPoint slides?
  - Flip chart and markers?
  - Other methods?
- Practice your presentation in advance
- Leave time for questions and for discussion

Courtesy of J.J. Baker and R.W. Baker, Dallas, Texas.

as well.) Although the report may or may not be bound, it should have all pages firmly secured.

PRESENTING THE BUSINESS PLAN

You may be asked to present more than once. Sometimes you will have to prepare a short form and a long form of the plan, depending on the audience. Tips on presenting your business plan are presented in **Exhibit 23–10**.

It is especially important to practice your presentation in advance. When you leave time for questions and for discussion, you also want to be well prepared for anticipated questions. By constructing a well-thought-out business plan, you have substantially increased your chances for a successful outcome.

STRATEGIC ASPECTS OF YOUR BUSINESS PLAN

Your business plan must fit into your organization's strategic plan. To begin to do so, you might answer the following questions:

- How does my business plan fit into the overall strategic plan (the "master plan") for my organization?
- How does my business plan specifically fit into my department or division's segment of the organization's overall strategic plan/master plan?
- Does the proposed timing of my business plan coincide with the strategic plan's time frames?
- Does the proposed funding of my business plan fit into available funding resources mentioned in the strategic plan?
- What competition will my business plan face, strategically speaking, within my organization? Does my plan provide a good defense against this competition?

- Are there external competition and or legislative aspects mentioned in my business plan that are also addressed within the strategic plan? If so, does my plan's treatment of these external aspects coordinate with that of the strategic plan? If not, have I explained why not?

The previous chapter explored Strategic Planning in some depth. Other aspects contained in that chapter may also be applicable to your business plan.

 INFORMATION CHECKPOINT

What is needed?	A sample of a business plan.
Where is it found?	Probably with your manager or the departmental director.
How is it used?	Study the way the business plan was distributed. Who received it? What did they do with it? What was the result?

 KEY TERMS

Business Plan
Overhead
Revenue Amount
Revenue Sources
Revenue Type
Space Occupancy
Supplies

 DISCUSSION QUESTIONS

1. Have you ever been involved in the creation of a business plan?
2. If so, did the plan include all three segments (organizational, marketing, and finance)? If not, why do you think one or more of the segments was missing?
3. Have you ever attended the formal presentation of a business plan? If so, was it successful in obtaining the desired funding?
4. Was the plan that was presented similar to what we have described in this chapter? What would you have changed in the presentation? Why?

Technology as a Financial and Strategic Tool

Information Technology and EHR: Adoption Requirements, Initiatives, and Management Decisions

INTRODUCTION

While this chapter has a lot of technical terms and footnotes, you need to pay close attention. Why? Because this chapter describes a major revolution that is occurring in healthcare systems right now. And if you are working in health care, you too will almost surely be affected in some way.

We are presently in a decade of significant change to the management of healthcare information. Central to this change are Electronic Health Records (EHRs).

THE BEGINNING OF ADOPTION REQUIREMENTS: ELECTRONIC DATA INTERCHANGE AND PAPERLESS PROCESSING

This section discusses the history of electronic efforts. This history leads to today's issues.

Background

Federal governmental efforts on behalf of electronic data interchange and paperless processing began in the early 1990s.[1]

At that time "Electronic Data Interchange" (EDI) was a relatively new concept. A 1994 report issued by the Office of the Inspector General (OIG) defined EDI as follows:

"Electronic Data Interchange is the electronic transfer of information, such as electronic media claims, in a standard format between trading partners. As it

Progress Notes

After completing this chapter, you should be able to

1. Identify three adoption deadlines that force management decisions.
2. Describe the HITECH EHR incentive programs.
3. Recognize HITECH incentive opportunities for hospitals and physicians.
4. Define an electronic health record (EHR).
5. Define health information technology (HIT).
6. Recognize the private sector contributions to EHR.
7. Understand the process of leadership decisions.

relates to health care, this new technology will allow entities within the healthcare system, connected by an integrated system of electronic communication networks, to exchange medical, billing and other information and process transactions in a manner which is fast and cost effective. Most of these improvements are likely to result from the significant reduction or elimination of paper transactions."[2]

Early Efforts

Another part of the history lesson: at the time of this report in 1994, the Center for Medicare and Medicaid Services (CMS) was still called the Health Care Financing Administration (HCFA). The name didn't change until 2001.[3]

According to the OIG, in January 1994 HCFA published a proposed notice that would "...require hospitals to submit all inpatient and outpatient bills electronically and to receive payments and remittance advices electronically."[4]

In order to reach this point (providers submitting bills and receiving payment electronically, with paperless processing), two major steps had to be previously accomplished as follows:

- First Step: Create a standardized claim form (a national claims format) that could be sent and received electronically.
- Second Step: Implement the ability to make Electronic Funds Transfers (EFTs) so payments could be sent and received electronically.

So what is our point in bringing up old history? It is this: we cannot consider the electronic advances discussed in this chapter if those pioneering steps had not been established.

CURRENT ADOPTION REQUIREMENTS THAT FORCE MANAGEMENT DECISIONS

This section describes adoption deadlines and legislative initiatives that force management decisions and subsequent actions.

Three Adoption Deadlines for Electronic Health Records

Healthcare organizations in the United States are now required to comply with a series of adoption rates for electronic health records. These requirements are driven by a series of financial incentives and penalties. Current adoption requirements include the following:

- Electronic health records initiated by the HITECH Act initiative
- Electronic prescribing (eRx) program
- ICD-10 codes

Management decisions are required because each of these three requirements has a deadline for compliance. The three deadlines are as follows.

Adoption Dates for the HITECH Initiative

The Health Information Technology for Economic and Clinical Health Act (HITECH), part of the American Recovery and Reinvestment Act of 2009 (ARRA), allows a range of transition dates for inpatient hospital service paid incentives. The hospital transition dates range from October 1, 2011, to 2015. The last year that physicians can adopt electronic health records under HITECH without financial penalty is 2014.[5]

Adoption Dates for the Electronic Prescribing (eRx) Program

The last year for physicians to adopt e-prescribing under the eRx program without a financial penalty was calendar year 2012.[6] While compliance dates for this program were initially set to allow for transition periods, it appears no extensions will now occur.

Adoption Date for ICD-10 Codes

The final compliance date for adoption of ICD-10-CM and ICD-10-PCS codes was initially set for October 1, 2013.[7] This final adoption date has now been moved forward by one year to October 1, 2014.[8] The Centers for Medicare and Medicaid (CMS) has stated there will be no further extensions of this date for compliance.

Further Discussion of the Three Adoption Requirements

We further describe and discuss the three programs as follows:

- Adoption of Electronic Health Records Initiated by the Health Information Technology for Economic and Clinical Health Act (HITECH): An overview of the HITECH initiative along with related management decisions is presented in this chapter, while the following chapter explores how the HITECH process of objectives, measures, and meaningful use works.
- Adoption of the Electronic Prescribing (eRx) Program: The eRx program's implementation is more fully described in the Appendix to this chapter.
- Adoption of ICD-10 Codes: The issues involved in ICD-10-CM and ICD-10-PCS adoption are briefly discussed within this chapter. A following chapter focuses entirely upon the ICD-10 transition and related strategic management issues.

WHY IS EHR ADOPTION REQUIRED THROUGH LEGISLATIVE INITIATIVES?

While adoption rates continue to lag, federal policymakers have a nationwide infrastructure vision and are willing to assist in funding it.

Adoption Rates for Electronic Health Records Have Been Historically Slow

In the past, adoption has been slow. For example, a study published in 2009 revealed that only 1.5% of U.S. hospitals have a comprehensive electronic records system (defined as a system that is present in all clinical units), and only an additional 7.6% of U.S. hospitals have a basic system (defined as a system that is present in at least one clinical unit). Furthermore, only 17% of hospitals have a computerized provider order entry system for medications. The authors of this 2009 study state that "A policy strategy focused on financial support, interoperability, and training of technical support staff may be necessary to spur adoption of electronic-records systems in U.S. hospitals."[9] The authors report that they surveyed "all acute care hospitals that are members of the American Hospital Association for the presence of specific electronic-record functionalities"[10] and achieved a 63.1% response rate.

The Federal Infrastructure Goal and Its Funding of Initiatives

Federal policymakers are working toward the "development of a nationwide health information technology infrastructure that allows for the electronic use and exchange of information" and an appointed National Coordinator (of the Office of the National Coordinator for Health Information Technology) is instructed to work toward this goal.[11]

The Health and Human Services Department (HHS) is charged with establishing programs to improve healthcare quality, safety, and efficiency through the use of the health IT infrastructure. The HITECH Act provides approximately 17 billion dollars in incentives for hospitals and physicians. A brief description of the HITECH program and its incentives follows. This description is for general information only; consult the appropriate legislation and regulations for pertinent details.

THE HITECH INITIATIVE: MEDICARE AND MEDICAID EHR INCENTIVE PROGRAMS OVERVIEW

This section contains an overview of one important initiative that is requiring many changes in healthcare information management. These changes will stretch over a period of years. We will also describe the strategic decisions that managers must make in order to participate in the incentive programs.

While this chapter focuses upon a program overview and the related management issues, the following chapter shows how meaningful use (necessary in order to collect incentive payments) is determined. That chapter also contains details about the standards and measures used to achieve meaningful use, along with further information about the associated incentive payments.

THE EHR INCENTIVE PROGRAMS: INTRODUCTION

This section provides a basic introduction to the HITECH initiative.

HITECH EHR Incentive Programs Description

CMS describes the EHR Incentive Programs in a single sentence: "The Medicare and Medicaid EHR Incentive Programs provide incentive payments to eligible professionals, eligible hospitals and critical access hospitals (CAHs) as they adopt, implement, upgrade or demonstrate meaningful use of certified EHR technology."[12]

There are differences between the two HITECH EHR programs, and CMS describes these differences as follows:

- The Medicare Program: "…provides incentive payments to EP, eligible hospitals and Critical Access Hospitals (CAHs) that demonstrate meaningful use of certified EHR technology. [The program]…can receive payments over five years."[13]
- The Medicaid Program: "…provides incentive payments to eligible professionals, eligible hospitals and CAHs as they adopt, implement, upgrade, or demonstrate meaningful use of certified EHR technology in their first year of participation and demonstrate meaningful use for up to five remaining participation years. The Medicaid program is voluntarily offered by the individual states and not all states have yet reported that they will be participating."[14]

Technically speaking, the Health Information Technology for Economic and Clinical Health Act (HITECH) is a part of the American Recovery and Reinvestment Act of 2009 (ARRA) that was signed into law on February 17, 2009. The HITECH Act promotes the adoption and use of health information technology (HIT) and electronic health records (EHRs).[15] This law impacts future healthcare information management for many years to come (up to 2021 in the case of one program).

HITECH Regulatory Authority

The HITECH Act provides the Department of Health and Human Services (HHS) with the authority to establish programs to improve healthcare quality, safety, and efficiency by promoting Health Information Technology (Health IT). The terminology "Health IT" includes both electronic health records and the exchange of private and secure electronic health information. Under HITECH, eligible healthcare professionals and eligible hospitals must:

1. adopt certified EHR technology and
2. use it to achieve particular objectives in order to qualify for Medicare or Medicaid incentive payments.[16]

CMS Responsibilities

The Center for Medicare and Medicaid Services (CMS), an HHS agency, is responsible for regulations that define the meaningful use objectives that must be met in order to qualify for incentive payments. The CMS regulations set out the requirements that providers must meet, using certified EHR technology to achieve meaningful use and thus qualify for the incentive payments.[17]

ONC Responsibilities

The Office of the National Coordinator for Health Information Technology (ONC) is responsible for regulations regarding technical capabilities required for certified EHR technology. These rules set out the Standards and Certification Criteria for the certification of EHR technology. (These criteria are required so that hospitals and eligible professionals participating in the program can rely upon the fact that the systems they adopt can actually perform the functions required by the program.)[18]

Definitions

Three definitions follow.

Electronic Health Record (EHR)

An electronic health record (EHR), according to CMS, "...allows healthcare providers to record patient information electronically instead of using paper records. However, EHRs are often capable of doing much more than just recording information. The EHR Incentive Program asks providers to use the capabilities of their EHRs to achieve benchmarks that can lead to improved patient care."[19] (Note also that an EHR might be called an "electronic medical record" [EMR] instead).

Qualified Electronic Health Record

A qualified electronic health record, according to the HITECH Act, is "an electronic record of health-related information on an individual that:

(A) includes patient demographic and clinical health information, such as medical history and problem lists; and
(B) has the capacity
   i. to provide clinical decision support;
   ii. to support physician order entry;
   iii. to capture and query information relevant to health care quality; and
   iv. to exchange electronic health information with, and integrate such information from, other sources."[20]

Health Information Technology (HIT)

Health information technology (HIT), also according to the HITECH Act, means "hardware, software, integrated technologies or related licenses, intellectual property, upgrades, or packaged solutions sold as services that are designed for, or support the use by, health care entities or patients for the electronic creation, maintenance, access, or exchange of health information."[21]

HITECH DEADLINES AND PAYMENTS

This section describes both compliance deadlines and payments for the HITECH initiative.

Adoption Deadlines

The required transition dates for hospitals represent a range of years, from October 1, 2011 to 2015. The last date to adopt without penalty for physicians,

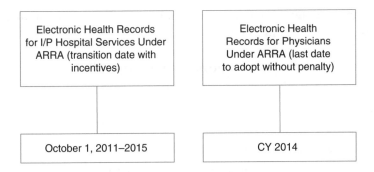

Note: Dates may subsequently move forward

Figure 24–1 Electronic Health Records Adoption Dates.
Reproduced from the American Recovery and Reinvestment Act of 2009 (ARRA) Title IV Sec. 4101.

however, is calendar year (CY) 2014. **Figure 24–1** illustrates these compliance requirements.[22]

Program Payments

Program payments are as follows at the time of this writing.

Hospital Incentives Payments

Hospital incentives payments under the HITECH Medicare program are based upon inpatient hospital services and the hospital must be a "meaningful electronic health records (EHR) user" to be eligible for payment. In general, an eligible hospital can receive a $2,000,000 base amount payment plus discharge-related payments that span a four-year period. (The discharge-related amounts are paid for 1,150 through 23,000 discharges. Thus, the 1st through the 1,149th discharges receive no payment, while discharges over 23,000 are limited by law to a maximum amount.) The eligible discharge-related amounts are paid at 100% for year 1; at 75% for year 2; at 50% for year 3; at 25% for year 4; and nothing thereafter. Payment years may begin for the fiscal year beginning October 1, 2011. If a hospital has not adopted by 2015 it will face financial penalties.[23]

Eligible Professionals Incentives Payments

These "eligible professional" incentives under the HITECH Medicare program are paid only to physicians as defined by law who are "meaningful EHR users." It is important to note that these incentive payments will not be made to hospital-based eligible professionals who might be otherwise eligible. (The determination is made on the basis of site of service.)[24]

In the Medicare incentive program, for example, the maximum amount a physician can receive decreases year by year as follows:

> Year 1 = $15,000; except if the first year is 2011 or 2012, then the year 1 payment is $18,000
> Year 2 = $12,000
> Year 3 = $ 8,000
> Year 4 = $ 4,000
> Year 5 = $ 2,000

Subsequent years = $-0-(no incentive payments after 2016).[25]

If the first payment year (year 1) is after 2014, no incentive dollars will be paid. If adoption has not occurred by 2015, the physician's fee schedule amount will be reduced by a percentage.[26]

PROGRAM ELIGIBILITY

Program eligibility for both hospitals and for eligible professionals (EPs) is discussed in this section.

The HITECH Initiative Contains Two Separate Programs

The HITECH initiative contains two programs: the Medicare program and the Medicaid program. Furthermore, the eligibility requirements differ between the two programs in the case of eligible professionals (EPs), as is described below. A discussion of additional choices between the two programs appears in a later section of this chapter.

Eligibility Requirements for Hospitals

Eligible hospitals under the EHR incentive program include those acute care inpatient hospitals that are paid under the hospital inpatient prospective payment system (IPPS) and are located in one of the 50 states or the District of Columbia and/or hospitals that are affiliated with qualifying Medicare Advantage (MA) organizations.[27] **Figure 24–2** illustrates these requirements.

Different Eligibility Requirements for EPs Under the Two Programs

Program eligibility for EPs differs between the Medicare HITECH incentive program and the Medicaid HITECH incentive program. The Medicare program recognizes doctors of medicine or osteopathy, dental surgery or dental medicine, podiatry, and optometry, along with chiropractors. The Medicaid program, on the other hand, recognizes physicians (primarily doctors of medicine and doctors of osteopathy), plus nurse practitioners, certified nurse–midwives, dentists, and certain physician assistants.[28] These different requirements are illustrated in **Figure 24–3**.

Eligible Hospitals Under the EHR Incentive Program include:	
Acute care inpatient hospitals* that are paid under the hospital inpatient prospective payment system (IPPS) and are located in one of the 50 states or the District of Columbia	
Hospitals that are affiliated with qualifying Medicare Advantage (MA) organizations	

*Defined as subsection (d) hospitals in section 1886 (d)(1)(B) of The American Recovery and Reinvestment Act (Recovery Act) of 2009.

Figure 24–2 Eligible Hospitals Under the EHR Incentive Program.
Reproduced from the Centers for Medicare and Medicaid Services. CMS Medicare Learning Network ICN #904626 (November 2010).

Eligible Professionals Under the Medicare EHR Incentive Program Include:	**Eligible Professionals Under the Medicaid EHR Incentive Program Include:**
Doctor of medicine or osteopathy	Physicians (primarily doctors of medicine and doctors of osteopathy)
Doctor of dental surgery or dental medicine	Nurse practitioner
Doctor of podiatry	Certified nurse–midwife
Doctor of optometry	Dentist
Chiropractor	Physician assistant who furnishes services in a Federally Qualified Health Center or Rural Health Clinic that is led by a physician assistant

Figure 24–3 Eligible Professionals: Medicare Versus Medicaid EHR Incentive Programs.
Reproduced from the Centers for Medicare and Medicaid Service. "EHR Incentive Programs: Who Is Eligible To Participate? - Eligibility Requirements for Professionals" (February 2013).

"MEANINGFUL USE" WITHIN THE HITECH PROGRAM

This section includes program definitions along with the benefits of meaningful use. Certified EHR technology is defined first because it is part of the meaningful use definition.

CERTIFIED EHR TECHNOLOGY DEFINED

"Certified EHR Technology" means an EHR that has been especially certified for the EHR Incentive Programs. For example, you may have an EHR system that has been qualified, or certified, for another CMS incentive program. But this does not mean your system is automatically certified for the HITECH program. The technology must be specifically certified for use in this particular program.[29]

Meaningful Use Defined

For this program, providers have to use their certified EHR technology in a meaningful manner in order to receive incentive payments. The technology must properly provide for the electronic exchange of health information. To show "meaningful use" also means successfully meeting, and reporting, the criteria for three different elements: core objectives, menu objectives, and quality control measures.[30]

Meaningful Use Benefits

The overall goal of meaningful use is as follows: "...to promote the spread of electronic health records to improve health care in the United States."[31]

It is true that electronic health records are able to provide many benefits for both providers and their patients. But it is also true that the benefits of electronic health records depend on the manner in which they are used.[32]

Meaningful use benefits include:

- Complete and more accurate information—providers will have more information to use in a more efficient manner
- Better access to this information—providers can share the information for better coordination of care
- Empowerment of the patient—patients can receive electronic information to encourage a more active role in their own health[33]

HITECH MEDICARE AND MEDICAID EHR INCENTIVE PROGRAMS AND RELATED MANAGEMENT DECISION POINTS

This section describes certain management decisions required for various elements of the initiative.

FURTHER CHOICES BETWEEN TWO HITECH PROGRAMS ARE REQUIRED

Management must choose the program and must also choose what year to enter that program, as further discussed below.

Choose the Program

Eligible hospitals can choose to participate in either the Medicare or the Medicaid EHR incentive program, or the hospital can choose to be "dual eligible." A dual eligible hospital would be able to participate in both the Medicare and Medicaid programs. This is not the case, however, for eligible professionals (EPs). They must choose either the Medicare or the Medicaid program, and they are only allowed to change programs once. Furthermore, that change can only occur before 2015.[34] The choices just described are illustrated in **Figure 24–4**.

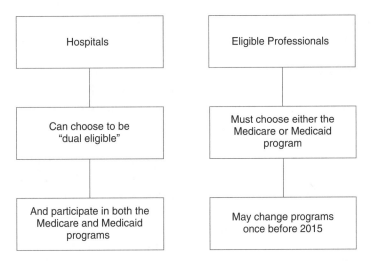

Figure 24–4 EHR Incentive Program Choices for Hospitals and Eligible Professionals.
Courtesy of J.J. Baker and R.W. Baker, Dallas, Texas.

Medicare EHR Incentive Program	Medicaid EHR Incentive Program
Run by CMS.	Run by your state Medicaid agency.
Maximum incentive amount is $44,000.	Maximum incentive amount is $63,750.
Payments over 5 consecutive years.	Payments over 6 years, does not have to be consecutive.
Payment adjustments will begin in 2015 for providers who are eligible but decide not to participate.	No Medicaid payment adjustments.
Providers must demonstrate meaningful use every year to receive incentive payments.	In the first year providers can receive an incentive payment for adopting, implementing, or upgrading EHR technology. Providers must demonstrate meaningful use in the remaining years to receive incentive payments.

Figure 24–5 Choosing an EHR Incentive Program: Medicare Versus Medicaid for Eligible Professionals.
Reproduced from the Centers for Medicare and Medicaid Services. "EHR Incentive Programs: Choosing a Program: Medicare or Medicaid?" (February 2013).

Further details about the eligible professionals program choices are illustrated in **Figure 24–5**. The first thing you will notice on Figure 24–5 is that the Medicare program is run by CMS, while the Medicaid program is run by your state Medicaid Agency. It is important to note that not every state in the United States will opt to provide a Medicaid EHR Incentive Program. The Medicaid incentive programs are administered by the individual states, and each state is free to participate or not. That means the EPs who practice in a state that is not participating will, of course, not have the advantage of a choice.

If the EP has a choice, however, the maximum incentive amount that could be earned is $44,000 for Medicare with payments over five consecutive years, versus $63,750 for Medicaid with payment over six years that do not have to be consecutive. The Medicare program imposes a penalty, called a "payment adjustment," that begins in 2015 for eligible EPs who decide not to participate.

At the time of this writing the Medicaid program does not impose a payment adjustment. Finally, in the Medicare program EPs must demonstrate meaningful use every year to receive the incentive payments. There is a somewhat different situation in the Medicaid program, because in the first year the EP can receive the incentive payment for adopting, implementing, or upgrading EHR technology. The EP must then demonstrate meaningful use in the remaining years to receive the payments.[35]

Many factors will enter into management's decision about which EP program to choose. A variety of elements must be considered, and each situation will be different. The choice is not a decision to be taken lightly.

Choose the Timing: What Year to Enter the Program

The Medicare EHR incentive program and the Medicaid EHR incentive program have different rules for each of the following:

- Number of payment years available
- Last year for which incentives may be received
- Last payment year for initiating the program[36]

Timing for the Medicare Program

Medicare program timeline dates include the following:

- 2014: Last year to begin participation in the program
- 2015: Payment adjustments (penalties) begin if not a meaningful user
- 2016: Last year to receive an incentive payment[37]

Timing for the Medicaid Program

Medicaid program timeline dates include the following:

- 2016: Last year to begin participation in the program
- 2012: Last year to receive an incentive payment[38]

Both programs' timelines are illustrated in **Figure 24–6**.

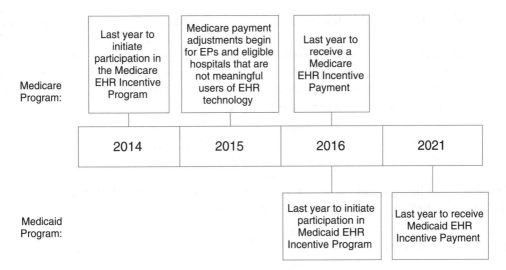

Figure 24–6 Milestone Timeline for EHR Incentive Programs.
Adapted from the Centers for Medicare and Medicaid Services (2010). EHR Incentive Programs, Milestone Timeline.
www.cms.gov/EHRIncentivePrograms.

CONSIDER PROGRAM BENEFITS AND COSTS

Program benefits and costs are discussed in this section.

Program Benefits

Medicare and Medicaid EHR Incentive Program Benefits
   "…we believe there are substantial benefits that can be obtained by eligible hospital and eligible professionals (EPs), including:

- Reductions in medical recordkeeping costs
- Reductions in repeat tests
- Decreases in length of stay
- Increased patient safety
- Reduced medical errors"[39]

Program Technology Costs

Healthcare organizations affected by these adoption requirements must adopt certified electronic health record technology. In order to do so, the organizations will have to update or acquire health information systems that provide the certified EHR technology. There must be cost incurred, and that cost may be substantial.

CMS has made it clear that the program's incentive payments are not for purchasing or replacing an EHR program. Instead the payments are for achieving meaningful use while using certified EHR technology.[40] Thus there will almost surely be a net cost over and above the program incentives received and the reductions in costs associated with certain benefits just described. How much these net costs incurred will be will vary substantially between and among the affected healthcare organizations.

MAKING STRATEGIC MANAGEMENT DECISIONS ABOUT MULTIPLE INITIATIVE CHOICES IS ALSO REQUIRED

Managers must be aware of the organizational environment in which they are operating. It is important to think strategically about the following items.

Multiple Current Initiatives Are in Place

Multiple initiatives are in place, with different requirements and often with different timelines. For example, CMS has pointed out three quality improvement programs that are in place for eligible professionals as follows: the Medicare EHR Incentive Program, the Physician Quality Reporting System (PQRS), and the Medicare Improvements for Patients and Providers Act (MIPPA) e-Prescribing Incentive Program.[41] It is important to note the fact of multiple initiatives, even though a further discussion of the PQRS and the MIPPA program is beyond the scope of this chapter.

Multiple Demands on Resources

Most, if not all, organizations have a finite limit of available resources such as cash, staffing, systems, space, and so on. Because many elements within the organization are competing for these resources, a project to adopt EHR is not operating in a vacuum. Managers must be aware that they may have to compete for resources that the project requires.

Potential Time Lag in Cash Flow Should Be Recognized

It is to be expected that adoption requirements of the EHR initiative will result in cash expenditures. It is also to be expected that successful participation in the program should result in cash received from incentive payments. However, a time lag in the cash flow (cash out versus expected cash in) is almost inevitable. Consequently managers should recognize this potential for a time lag and plan accordingly. It is important to also note that the incentive payments should not be expected to cover the full cost of EHR adoption.

THE PRIVATE SECTOR'S MANAGEMENT ALSO CONTRIBUTES TO EHR SYSTEM ADVANCES

Certain private sector healthcare organizations have also contributed to changes in healthcare information management. They have sometimes led the way in demonstrating how electronic health records can successfully be conceived and implemented.

"Private Sector" Means Nongovernmental

By "private sector" we mean those organizations that are not part of the government. These entities are part of the healthcare industry and may be either proprietary or nonprofit. However, as members of the private sector they all share one characteristic: they are not part of a government entity.

Kaiser Permanente Personal Health Record Statistics

Kaiser Permanente's business structure provides health plans and delivers managed health care across the continuum, including the hospital, medical group professionals, the laboratory, and the pharmacy. The Kaiser Permanente Information Technology group is also part of the organization.[42]

Kaiser Permanente (KP) is believed to have the largest private sector electronic health record system in the world and has received multiple awards for leadership in electronic health record implementation.[43] KP has implemented "My Health Manager," an electronic personal health record application that presently contains five elements as follows:

- My Medical Record (connected to the individual's electronic medical record)
- My Message Center (exchange secure email with the doctor's office)
- Appointment Center (book visits and/or consult the interactive symptom checker)
- Pharmacy Center (manage prescriptions and/or consult the drug encyclopedia feature)
- Manage My Plan and Coverage (obtain facts about the individual's plan and benefits and download forms)[44]

KP has nearly nine million members, so heavy usage of the electronic personal health record can be expected. In the first half of 2011, for example, KP reported that members "...have securely viewed 34.8 million laboratory results, exchanged 6.2 million emails with their KP caregivers and refilled 4.6 million prescriptions online."[45] Furthermore, at the time of this writing KP has released a mobile-optimized website and app. In the first month after the new application was released, KP reported that it was used more than a million times by members and patients.[46]

Unified EHR Adoption at Duke University Health System

Duke University Health System (Duke) includes three hospitals along with physician practices and other services such as home care and hospice, all based in North Carolina.[47] In July 2012, Duke began a multi-year information systems project to unify electronic medical records across the health system. The project, titled "Maestro Care," has a "tag line" motto: "One Patient, One Record, One Health System." Duke expects to implement the new technology in three phases as follows:

- Phase 1 (2012): 33 primary care practices
- Phase 2 (2013): Duke University Hospital plus all ambulatory clinics
- Phase 3 (2014): The 2 remaining hospitals (Durham Regional and Duke Raleigh)[48]

A 2012 Project Overview authored by the Duke Medicine Chief Information Officer listed the following six goals and objectives for Maestro Care:

- Reduce current IT fragmentation
- Improve clinician satisfaction
- Provide context-specific decision support
- Achieve "meaningful use" with a certified electronic health record
- Support the health system as it converts to ICD-10
- Establish a robust data foundation for research[49]

Incidentally, the goal/objective of reducing current IT fragmentation is certainly appropriate, as it is reported that Duke had more than 135 different clinical technology applications in use prior to the implementation of Maestro Care.[50]

As the project commenced in the summer of 2012, it was widely reported that the information technology project represented a $500 million investment. At that time the Duke Chief Medical Information Officer discussed related financial issues in a newspaper interview. He explained that the $500 million figure represented total ownership costs over a seven-year period. This amount included, therefore, the cost to maintain and upgrade the system over seven years in addition to the initial costs to acquire and begin to use the technology. He also explained that the $500 million was the gross investment figure. If you add up all the costs to maintain and to support the 135 applications that are being replaced, and if you then subtract that cost from the $500 million, you wind up with a net new investment that is "a little bit more than $300 million."[51] Finally, he also pointed out that the project should be eligible to receive "tens of millions of dollars in federal funding" that would help to partially cover costs of the investment.[52] (The federal funding referred to would, of course, come from the financial incentives discussed in a preceding section of this chapter.)

CONCLUSION: MANAGEMENT DECISIONS AND LEADERSHIP

This section discusses the process of innovation, leadership and the future.

THE PROCESS OF INNOVATION AND LEADERSHIP DECISIONS

Change and process flow are discussed in the following sections.

Innovation Defined

Innovation may be defined as "...an idea, practice or object that is perceived as new."[53] The new uses of health information technology that are discussed would certainly qualify as innovations.

How do the leaders of an organization approach an innovative project? E.M. Rogers, a communication and innovation researcher, comments upon reaction to an innovation as follows:

"An innovation presents an individual or an organization with a new alternative or alternatives, with new means of solving problems. But the probabilities of the new alternatives being superior to previous practice are not exactly known by the individual problem solvers. Thus, they are motivated to seek further information about the innovation to cope with the uncertainty that it creates."[54]

We visualize this type of information-seeking approach as a sequential decision process, as discussed in the following section.

The Process of Leadership Decisions

Leadership decisions are often made in a series of stages. **Figure 24–7** illustrates three decision stages that may lead to adoption, for example, of a health information technology project.

The three-stage decision process includes the following:

- "Gathers Information"—this stage seeks enough information to attain knowledge.
- "Forms an Opinion"—this stage uses that knowledge gained to reach an understanding that leads in turn to forming an opinion.
- "Makes a Decision"—this stage uses the opinion that has been formed to make a decision.

The last stage—"Makes a Decision"—should result in one of two outcomes. The decision will either be positive ("Yes: will adopt and implement") or negative ("No: will not adopt").

(There could be a third possible outcome on that last stage. R.W. once briefly worked with a boss who would never say "yes" or "no"; instead his decision would be "Take no action either way.") We should also note that a negative decision might not always be final, as it might be reversed at a later date.

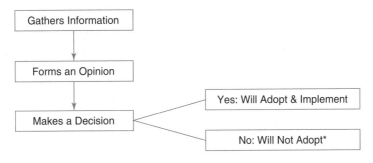

*Negative decisions may not be final.

Figure 24–7 Process Flow: Leadership Decision Stages.

Bringing About Innovation

How can a manager help to bring about an innovative concept such as the health information technology projects that are the subject of this chapter? He or she can help first to understand and then to diffuse.

Understanding the Required Framework

You as a manager can gather information and use it to understand the required framework. If requested, you can also actually assist in gathering information to provide to your upper-level management.

Diffusing the Information

You as a manager can also help to establish understanding about the innovative concept throughout your part of the organization. This could be by specific assignment, or through informal information sharing. In either case you would be assisting by helping to diffuse the information through individuals who need to know.

CHANGES IN LEADERSHIP MAY IMPACT THE STRATEGY AND PROGRESS OF HEALTHCARE INFORMATION MANAGEMENT

This section discusses management leadership and provides an impact-of-change example.

Management and the Impact of Leadership Changes

Firm, focused leadership is essential to guidance through the maze of health industry technology evolutions. Program compliance often extends over a period of years, and during those years leadership may change.

Leadership Change Within a Healthcare Organization

It seems obvious to say that leadership change within a healthcare organization may well result in a change in strategic direction. Still, this is often the case. Consequently certain resources and/or initiatives may now receive more support, while some other resources and/or initiatives may have their funds and staffing cut, or even eliminated. It is important for a manager to be aware of this possibility, and be ready to defend his/her projects with current well-organized information.

Leadership Change Within Legislative Bodies

Leadership change with legislative bodies can have a similar impact on projects in progress. An example follows.

When the Governor Changed, So Did the Project: An Example of Impact

A northeastern state's change-over of governors provides an instructive example of how leadership changes can affect the direction of a project.

The Project

Certain federal stimulus funding has been made available for states to create health information exchanges. (A health information exchange (HIE) in this context is defined as "... the electronic movement of health-related information among organizations according to nationally recognized standards."[55]) This type of information exchange typically requires a Health Information Organization, or HIO, to oversee it.[56] This state received around $17 million in funding to set up an HIE system that would be statewide.[57]

The Democratic Governor's Vision of the Project

The structure of the exchange entity can be quite centralized or quite decentralized. The Democratic governor that was in office at the beginning of the project envisioned a "one-stop repository" that would be built and then maintained by the state. In other words, his vision was a centralized project. He proceeded with this concept, reportedly to the point of receiving a contract proposal in the amount of over $31 million to build such a centralized exchange.[58]

The Newly-Elected Republican Governor Had a Different Vision

But election time came and went, and now the state had a new Republican governor. The new governor envisioned a decentralized "shared services" exchange system, whereby the state-run part of the system would be a much smaller operation that would be fed in turn by regional health information networks. This vision was very much a decentralized project.[59]

What Will Happen Next?

We do not know the end to this story. At the time of this writing the specifications for a "shared services" system were reportedly being written so a contract could go out for bids. Will the system be built? If so, will it be built along the lines of the decentralized version? Or, perhaps, will the process take so long that still another governor will come along and be able to change the direction of this project?

THE FUTURE

This section contains a brief look into the future.

Required Implementation Changes Still to Come

Future legislative and regulatory changes will certainly occur. Some are predictable at this time, while others are not. At the time of this writing, for example, we can reasonably predict that Stage 3 of the HITECH initiative will occur, and that it will be reasonably on schedule. We can also expect more stringent measures of meaningful use over time, but we cannot predict what shape they may take, nor what their ultimate future timing might be. Likewise, we cannot predict the outcome over the next few years of the current multiple challenges to other aspects of the healthcare law.

The "Glide Path"

In conclusion, we expect interpretations of the various health information technology strategic priorities, along with their supporting rules and regulations, to emerge over a considerable period of years. A formidable base of knowledge has been laid as a foundation for these directions. One official who must have had an aviation background was reported to have said we were now on the "glide path" to success in the area of health information technology, meaning that the sailing (or flying) would be smooth from now on. We hope he was correct.

TECHNOLOGY IN HEALTH CARE MINI-CASE STUDY

Even simple technological changes can improve workflow and increase efficiency. This fact is borne out by the Mini-Case Study entitled "Technology in Health Care: Automating Admissions Processes." Electronic records are powerful financial management tools that can bring about measurable results, as this case study proves.

APPENDIX 24-A: THE E-PRESCRIBING (eRx) INCENTIVE PROGRAM FOR PHYSICIANS AND OTHER ELIGIBLE PRESCRIBERS: A MATURED INITIATIVE

Appendix 24-A describes the Electronic Prescribing (eRx) Incentive Program for Physicians and Other Eligible Prescribers. The program was intended to encourage significant expansion of the use of e-prescribing, and it has done so through the use of payment incentives and financial penalties. This program is important because it laid much of the foundation for subsequent initiatives to build upon.

 INFORMATION CHECKPOINT

What is needed?	Some description of health information technology (HIT) as defined in the first part of this chapter. This could be a description of HIT within your place of work, or it could be advertising materials attempting to sell HIT hardware and/or software.
Where is it found?	Possibly in the information technology or administration offices at your place of work. There are many varied sources for HIT advertising materials.
How is it used?	The HIT description could be used to evaluate or assess current HIT status at your place of work, or such a description could be within a manual (but be careful about proprietary use if that is the case). The advertising materials, of course, are trying to sell the product.

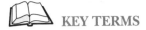 **KEY TERMS**

Certified EHR Technology
Electronic Health Record (EHR)
Electronic Prescribing (E-Prescribing)
Electronic Transaction Standards
Health Information Exchange
Health Information Technology (HIT)
Innovation
Meaningful Use
Private Sector
Version 5010 of Transaction Standards

 DISCUSSION QUESTIONS

1. Do you use electronic health records in your own work? If so, how do you use them?
2. Do you know of a healthcare organization that is either initially installing or upgrading its electronic health information technology? If so, can you describe how this organization is going about it?
3. Have you encountered materials either at your place of work or elsewhere that discuss the HITECH financial incentives for either hospitals or physicians? If so, do you think these materials did a good job of describing the incentives? Please explain.
4. Do you know of any private sector contributions to EHR such as those described in this chapter? If so, what are they? Please describe.

NOTES

1. By 1994 the Office of the Inspector General (OIG) had issued one of several reports about this issue. The OIG has three branches, one of which is the Office of Evaluation and Inspections (OEI). The OEI is responsible for short-term management and program evaluations such as these reports. At that time the Health Care Financing Administration (HCFA) was responsible for administering the Medicare and Medicaid programs, and the OIG report concerned HCFA's issues.
2. Office of Inspector General (OIG), Electronic Data Interchange and Paperless Processing: Issues and Challenges. OEI-12-93-00080 (March 1994) p. i.
3. American Medical Association (AMA), "HCFA becomes CMS: A name to live up to," *American Medical News* (July 23, 2001). www.ama-assn.org/amednews /2001/07/23/edsa0723.htm. In 2001 the Health Care Financing Administration (HCFA) name was changed to the Centers for Medicare and Medicaid Services, or CMS, as we know it today.

4. Electronic Data Interchange and Paperless Processing OEI-12-93-00080 p. 4.
5. ARRA Division B. Title IV Section 4101.
6. 73 Federal Register (FR) 69847 (November 29, 2008).
7. 74 Federal Register (FR) 3328 (January 16, 2009).
8. 77 Federal Register (FR) 54665 (September 5, 2012).
9. A. K. Jha et. al., "Use of Electronic Health Records in U.S. Hospitals," *New England Journal of Medicine* 360, no. 16 (2009), http://www.nejm.org/doi/full/10.1056/NEJMsa0900592.
10. Ibid.
11. ARRA Division A. Title XIII Section 3001. The Office of the National Coordinator for Health Information Technology is located within the Department of Health and Human Services.
12. CMS, "EHR Incentive Programs: Getting Started," http://www.cms.gov/Regulations-and-Guidance/Legislation/EHRIncentivePrograms/Getting_Started.html
13. Ibid.
14. Ibid.
15. ARRA Division A. Title XIII "Health Information Technology" (HITECH) and Division B. Title IV "Medicare and Medicaid Health Information Technology."
16. HealthIT.gov, "Policymaking, Regulation, & Strategy-Meaningful Use," www.healthit.gov/policy-researchers-implementers/meaningful-use (accessed January 23, 2013).
17. Ibid.
18. Ibid.
19. CMS, "EHR Incentive Programs: Getting Started," http://www.cms.gov/Regulations-and-Guidance/Legislation/EHRIncentivePrograms/Getting_Started.html
20. American Recovery and Reinvestment Act of 2009 (ARRA) Division A Title XIII Section 3000.
21. Ibid.
22. American Recovery and Reinvestment Act of 2009 (ARRA) Title IV Section 4101 (the HITECH Act).
23. ARRA Division B. Title IV Section 4102.
24. ARRA Division B. Title IV Section 4101.
25. Ibid.
26. Ibid.
27. CMS Medicare Learning Network ICN #904626 (November 2010) Figure 24–2.
28. www.cms.gov/EHRIncentivePrograms Figure 24–3.
29. CMS, "EHR Incentive Programs: Certified EHR Technology," http://www.cms.gov/Regulations-and-Guidance/Legislation/EHRIncentivePrograms/Certification.html
30. CMS, "EHR Incentive Programs: Meaningful Use," http://www.cms.gov/Regulations-and-Guidance/Legislation/EHRIncentivePrograms/Meaningful_Use.html and ARRA Division B Title IV Section 4102 (the HITECH Act).
31. HealthIT.gov, "Policymaking, Regulation, & Strategy-Meaningful Use." www.healthit.gov/policy-researchers-implementers/meaningful-use (accessed January 23, 2013).
32. Ibid.

33. Ibid.

34. CMS, "EHR Incentive Programs." http://www.cms.gov/Regulations-and-Guidance /Legislation/EHRIncentivePrograms/index.html.

35. Ibid.

36. 77 Federal Register (FR) 53974 (September 4, 2012) and 77 Federal Register (FR)13703 (March 7, 2012).

37. Ibid.

38. Ibid, Figure 24–6.

39. 77 Federal Register (FR) 53971 (September 4, 2012).

40. CMS, "EHR Incentive Programs," http://www.cms.gov/Regulations-and-Guidance /Legislation/EHRIncentivePrograms/index.html

41. CMS, "An Introduction to the Medicare EHR Incentive Program for Eligible Professionals", p.5.

42. Kaiser Permanente, "Kaiser Permanente Careers: Our Business Structure," www .kaiserpermanentejobs.org/our-business-structure.aspx (accessed January 21, 2013).

43. Kaiser Permanente, "Kaiser Permanente Receives Two Awards for Leadership in Electronic Health Records Implementation," http://xnet.kp.org/newscenter /pressreleases/nat/2012/022212stage7himssdavies.html (accessed January 21, 2013).

44. Kaiser Permanente, "My Health Manager: Get Wellness and Coverage Information," https://healthy.kaiserpermanente.org/health/care/consumer/my-health -manager (accessed January 21, 2013).

45. Kaiser Permanente, "Kaiser Foundation Hospitals and Health Plan Report Second Quarter 2011 Financial Results," http://xnet.kp.org/newscenter/pressreleases/nat /2011/080511q2financials.html (accessed July 25, 2012).

46. Kaiser Permanente, "Kaiser Permanente Receives Two Awards for Leadership in Electronic Health Records Implementation," http://xnet.kp.org/newscenter /pressreleases/nat/2012/022212stage7himssdavies.html (accessed December 24, 2012).

47. Duke, "Duke Human Resources: About Duke University Health System," www.hr.duke .edu/jobs/duke_durham/duhs.php (accessed January 21, 2013).

48. Duke, "Duke Starts to Transfer to Digital Electronic Health Record," www .dukehealth.org/duke-starts-transfer-to-digital-electronic-health-record (accessed January 21, 2013).

49. A. Glasgow, "Maestro Care: Duke University Health System Electronic Health Record Update," http://sites.duke.edu/techexpo/files/2012/01/2012_1_5_TechExpo _MAESTRO.pdf (accessed January 21, 2013). The motto mentioned in the preceding paragraph ("One Patient, One Record, One Health System") was also listed under the goals and objectives heading in the Overview.)

50. Duke, "Duke Starts to transfer to Digital Electronic Health Record," http://www .dukehealth.org/duke-starts-transfer-to-digital-electronic-health-record

51. D. Ranii, "Duke Kicks Off Digital Health Records Plan," www.newsobserver .com/2012/07/17/v-print/2204389/duke-kicks-off-digital-health.html (accessed January 21, 2013).

52. Ibid.

53. E.M. Rogers, Diffusion of Innovations, 4th ed. (New York: The Free Press, 1995).

54. Ibid., p.xvii.

55. Health Resources and Services Administration, "Health IT Toolbox: What is Health Information Exchange?" http://www.hrsa.gov/healthit/toolbox.html (accessed January 31, 2013).

56. American Health Information Management Association, "Resources: Health Information Exchange," http://www.ahima.org/resources/hie.aspx (accessed January 31, 2013).

57. B. Toland, "Pennsylvania Closes In On Health IT Network," *Pittsburgh Post-Gazette*, May 27, 2012.

58. Ibid.

59. Ibid.

The E-Prescribing (eRx) Incentive Program for Physicians and Other Eligible Prescribers: A Matured Initiative

This appendix describes and discusses the eRx incentive program.

INTRODUCTION

This initiative is an example of adoption requirement changes that have already largely occurred; thus we call it a "matured initiative." The E-Prescribing (eRx) Incentive Program for Physicians and Other Eligible Prescribers commenced January 1, 2009, and was intended to encourage "significant expansion" of the use of e-prescribing through the use of payment incentives and financial penalties.[1]

E-prescribing is, relatively speaking, a comparatively simple use of electronic technology. Its purpose and boundaries are understandable. Thus the eRx program serves as a workable first step and introduction to the current and more extensive use of electronic health technology such as that now required by the HITECH initiative.

eRx PROGRAM OVERVIEW

The E-Prescribing (eRx) Incentive Program was authorized by the Medicare Improvements for Patients and Providers Act (MIPPA), which was enacted on July 15, 2008. The incentive program is for eligible professionals who are successful electronic prescribers (e-prescribers) as defined by MIPPA. It is separate from, and is in addition to, the Physician Quality Reporting Initiative (PQRI).[2] Only services paid under the Medicare Physician Fee Schedule (MPFS) are included in the E-Prescribing Incentive Program.[3]

Note an important difference: the HITECH Medicare program incentives described earlier in this chapter are paid only to "physicians," as defined by law. The older E-Prescribing Incentive Program described in this Appendix pays "eligible professionals," which may include other eligible prescribers in addition to physicians, such as physician assistants, nurse practitioners, and certain therapists.[4]

Definitions

In the definitions that follow, be aware that over time the precise wording of such definitions may shift and/or expand for regulatory purposes.

- *E-prescribing* means "the transmission, using electronic media, of a prescription or prescription-related information, between a prescriber, dispenser, PBM, or health plan, either directly or through an intermediary, including an e-prescribing network."
- *Prescriber* means "a physician, dentist, or other person licensed, registered, or otherwise permitted by the U.S. or the jurisdiction in which he or she practices, to issue prescriptions for drugs for human use."
- *Dispenser* means "a person, or other legal entity, licensed, registered, or otherwise permitted by the jurisdiction in which the person practices or the entity is located, to provide drug products for human use on prescription in the course of professional practice."[5]

E-Prescribing Transactions

Generally speaking, transactions recognized as part of e-prescribing include the following:

- New prescription transaction
- Prescription refill request and response
- Prescription change request and response
- Cancel prescription request and response
- Ancillary messaging and administrative transactions[6]

As to the definition for "prescriber" above, CMS has commented elsewhere about other individuals who "are permitted to issue prescriptions for drugs for human use. These non-physician providers could include certified registered nurse anesthetists (CRNAs), nurse practitioners, and others."[7] (Naturally, these individuals would have to be properly licensed or registered in order to be a prescriber.)

Also note that this discussion is limited to the impact of e-prescribing on physicians and other eligible professionals who prescribe, because the technical aspects of other applications of e-prescribing (such as the impact on pharmacies as dispensers) are not within the scope of this book.

INCENTIVE PAYMENTS AND FINANCIAL PENALTIES FOR E-PRESCRIBERS

The eRx program encouraged significant expansion of the use of e-prescribing by providing incentive payments and imposing financial penalties.

Payments and Penalties

The eRx program provided these incentive payments through 2013. Beginning in 2012 and beyond there is then a penalty for noncompliance.[8]

Exhibit 24-A–1 E-Prescribing (eRx) Program for Physicians and Other Eligible Prescribers: Incentive Payments and Financial Penalties

INCENTIVE PAYMENTS FOR E-PRESCRIBERS	
Additional % of allowed charges paid	
2009	+2.0%
2010	+2.0%
2011	+1.0%
2012	+1.0%
2013	+1.0%
2014	–0–
Each subsequent year	–0–

FINANCIAL PENALTIES FOR NON-E-PRESCRIBERS	
% Reduction in fee schedule amount paid	
2009	–0–
2010	–0–
2011	–0–
2012	–1.0%
2013	–1.5%
2014	–2.0%
Each subsequent year*	–2.0%

*2.0% penalty continues for each subsequent year per 73 Federal Register 69847-8 (November 19, 2008).

Reproduced from the Centers for Medicare and Medicaid Services. MLN Matters Update #MM7879, p.5 (August 3, 2010).

Exhibit 24-A–1 illustrates the financial consequences of participation and nonparticipation in the program. Eligible e-prescribers could receive an additional percentage of allowed charges paid as follows: 2% in 2009 and 2010 and 1% in 2011, 2012, and 2013. On the other hand, non-e-prescribers are penalized by a percentage reduction in the fee schedule amount paid, as follows: 1% in 2012, 1.5% in 2013, and 2% in 2014. It is our understanding that the 2% reduction penalty for non-compliance continues for each subsequent year beyond 2014.[9]

Benefits

The benefits of e-prescribing can be administrative, financial and/or clinical. CMS has listed the following benefits as potentially improving quality and efficiency, and reducing costs:

- Speeds up the process of renewing medication
- Provides information about formulary-based drug coverage, including formulary alternatives and co pay information

- Actively promotes appropriate drug usage, such as following a medication regimen for a specific condition
- Prevents medication errors, in that each prescription can be electronically checked at the time of prescribing for dosage, interactions with other medications, and therapeutic duplication
- Provides instant connectivity among the healthcare provider, the pharmacy, health plans/pharmacy benefit managers (PBMs), and other entities, improving the speed and accuracy of prescription dispensing, pharmacy callbacks, renewal requests, eligibility checks, and medication history[10]

Costs

The cost of implementation to a practice may vary widely, based on practice size, location, and the degree of electronic adoption already under way within the office. However, three types of costs associated with e-prescribing can be identified as follows:

1. The initial purchase of hardware and software
2. Costs associated with daily use and maintenance, including online connectivity
3. Education and training[11]

Because of the wide variability, no official estimate of e-prescribing costs exists at the time of this writing. An older estimate of implementation costs has been published as follows. As background, in the past some health plans have offered to install an e-prescribing system for physicians that participate in their plan. In that regard, several years ago a health plan responded with comments to a CMS-proposed rule about e-prescribing. The health plan stated that:

> . . . it had spent three million dollars to equip 700 physicians with hardware and installation, software and training in their e-prescribing initiative (an average of almost $4,300 per physician). To boost participation, the health plan [was] piloting a program to grant honoraria (between $600 and $2,000) to physicians who write electronic prescriptions. The commenter believed that without the financial hardware/software and support incentives, the average physicians' practice would incur costs up to $2,500 per physician to adopt e-prescribing.[12]

In conclusion, adoption of e-prescribing by physicians was voluntary. Therefore each physician could make an individual decision about the costs and benefits of e-prescribing. Now that time has passed.

eRx PROGRAM IMPLEMENTATION

This section describes adoption rates and dates, implementation barriers, and successes of the E-Prescribing (eRx) Incentive Program.

Adoption Rates and Dates

Adoption rates and the final adoption date for this program are discussed as follows.

Adoption Rates for E-Prescribing Were Also Slow to Begin

Electronic prescribing among physicians and other professionals who prescribe has traditionally been low. A study published a few years ago estimated only 5 to 18% of providers used e-prescribing at that time.[13]

As to a real-life example of the low adoption rate, several years ago a Massachusetts collaborative project was partially funding the adoption of e-prescribing by physicians. While this project offered the technology to 21,000 physicians, it reported that only about 2,700, or 13%, of the targeted physicians had adopted the technology.[14]

E-Prescribing for Physicians: Final Adoption Date Without Penalty

As we have previously stated, those e-prescribers who have not yet complied with e-prescribing requirements are penalized by a percentage reduction in the fee schedule. The penalty commenced in 2012. It is thus our understanding that the last available adoption date without a penalty incurred is the calendar year (CY) 2011, as illustrated in **Figure 24-A–1**.[15]

Barriers

Barriers to physicians' implementation and increased usage of e-prescribing include the following:

- Costs of buying and installing a system
- Training
- Time and workflow impact
- Lack of knowledge about the benefits related to quality care
- Lack of reimbursement for costs and resources[16]

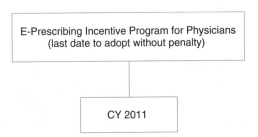

Figure 24-A–1 E-Prescribing Incentive Program for Physicians: Last Adoption Date Without Penalty. Reproduced from the Centers for Medicare and Medicaid Services. MLN Matters Update #MM7879, p.5 (August 3, 2010).

At least the "lack of reimbursement" barrier is lessening somewhat with the physician incentives that are now in place.

While the primary barrier to adoption of e-prescribing by physicians appears to be the cost of buying and installing the system, change is also a significant barrier, because implementation of a new system involves at least three types of change:

1. Changing the business practices of the physician's office
2. Changing record systems (from paper to electronic)
3. Training staff for change[17]

Another change-related barrier is resistance to actually using the electronic system, both by staff and by the physicians themselves.

Anecdotal Successes Within This Program

Certain physician practices that have provided anecdotal evidence of successful e-prescribing implementation to CMS are quoted as follows:

- A 53% reduction in calls to the pharmacy.
- Time savings of 1 hour per nurse and 30 minutes per file clerk per day by streamlining medication management processes.
- A large practice in Lexington, Kentucky, estimates that e-prescribing saves the group $48,000 a year in decreased time spent handling prescription renewal requests.
- Before implementation of e-prescribing, a large practice in Kokomo, Indiana, with 20 providers and 134,000 annual patient office visits was receiving 370 daily phone calls, 206 of which were related to prescriptions. Of the 206 prescription-related calls, 97 were prescription renewal requests. The remainder consisted of clarification calls from pharmacists or requests for new prescriptions. Staff time to process these calls included 28 hours per day of nurse time and 4 hours per day of physician time. Chart pulls were required in order to process half of the renewal requests. Implementation of an e-prescribing system produced dramatic time savings that permitted reallocation of nursing and chart room staff.[18]

Commentary

As a final note, we should point out that the Electronic Prescribing (eRx) Incentive Program is separate and apart from the Physician Quality Reporting System (previously known as the Physician Quality Reporting Initiative or PQRI). Confusion has arisen because both programs are voluntary, both involve electronic reporting, and both have been making incentive payments over the past few years. Even certain definitions such as "individual eligible professional" are identical for both programs. However, be aware they are two quite separate programs that serve different purposes.[19]

APPENDIX NOTES

1. 73 Federal Register (FR) 69847-8 (November 19, 2008) and CMS, "MLN Matters Update," #MM7879 p. 5 (Release Date August 3, 2010; Effective Date October 29, 2012). Technically speaking, individual eligible professionals who were successful electronic prescribers could enter the program on January 1, 2009, while eligible group practices could enter under the Group Practice Reporting Option (GPRO) beginning in 2010 (see p. 4 of MLN update).
2. CMS, Transmittal 459, CR 6394 (2009): C.
3. Medicare Learning Network, *MLN Matters* MM6394 (2009):9.
4. Ibid., 3.
5. 70 Federal Register (FR) 6265 (February 4, 2005).
6. Ibid.
7. 70 Federal Register (FR) 67572 (November 7, 2005).
8. 73 Federal Register (FR) 69847-8 (November 19, 2008) and CMS, "MLN Matters Update," #MM7879 p. 5 (Release Date August 3, 2010; Effective Date October 29, 2012).
9. CMS, "MLN Matters Update," #MM7879 p. 5 (Release Date August 3, 2010; Effective Date October 29, 2012).
10. 70 Federal Register (FR) 67569 (November 7, 2005).
11. Ibid., 67592.
12. Ibid., 67588.
13. (D.S. Bell & M.A. Friedman etc).
14. 70 Federal Register (FR) 67588 (November 7, 2005).
15. CMS, "MLN Matters Update," #MM7879 p. 5 (Release Date August 3, 2010; Effective Date October 29, 2012).
16. Adapted from 70 Federal Register (FR) 67569 (November 7, 2005).
17. 70 Federal Register (FR) 6370 (February 4, 2005).
18. 70 Federal Register (FR) 67589 (November 7, 2005).
19. CMS, "MLN Matters Update," #MM7879 p. 5 (Release Date August 3, 2010; Effective Date October 29, 2012).

Electronic Health Records Framework: Incentives, Standards, Measures, and Meaningful Use

WHY EXPLORE HOW THE HITECH EHR INITIATIVE WORKS?

This section introduces the background and framework of the HITECH EHR Initiative.

THE INITIATIVE: BACKGROUND

Recall policy and management issues involved in the HITECH "Medicare and Medicaid Electronic Health Record Incentive Programs" initiative. We can summarize this initiative as follows:

- Federal policymakers are working toward developing a health information technology (IT) infrastructure that allows for the electronic use and exchange of information and is nationwide.
- The Health Information Technology for Economic and Clinical Health Act, or HITECH, part of the American Recovery and Reinvestment Act of 2009 (ARRA), advances that goal by requiring programs to improve healthcare quality, safety, and efficiency through the use of the health IT infrastructure.
- The Act provides approximately $17 billion to establish HITECH Medicare and Medicaid EHR Incentive Programs that will provide payment incentives for hospitals and physicians.

WHY EXPLORE?

This chapter is dedicated to exploring how the HITECH EHR Initiative and its programs actually work. Why is this

After completing this chapter, you should be able to

1. Understand EHR program payments as incentives.
2. Define certified EHR Technology.
3. Define meaningful use.
4. Identify the three stages of meaningful use.
5. Understand core and menu sets of objectives.
6. Identify three types of measures for meaningful use.

important? Because managers can manage better if they truly understand the necessary components and computations, how the process works, and the reasoning behind it. This understanding gives you, the manager, the power to make appropriate decisions. You can better manage your part in the adoption and implementation process because you possess this underlying knowledge.

The HITECH initiative is also a good choice to explore because its implementation extends over such a long time period. Managers will be involved with the initiative's adoption and implementation for years to come. In this chapter we will discuss and describe the following:

- Program payments as incentives
- Standards and EHR
- Meaningful use and EHR
- Measures of meaningful use (and their objectives)
- Measurement methods (how the measures are computed)

We then provide two reporting examples—one for eligible professionals and one for hospitals—and work through their requirements and computations.

WHAT IS THE FRAMEWORK, OR STRUCTURE, OF THE HITECH EHR INITIATIVE?

The Initiative's Programs

The Centers for Medicare and Medicaid Services (CMS) describes these EHR Incentive Programs in a single sentence: "The Medicare and Medicaid EHR Incentive Programs provide incentive payments to eligible professionals, eligible hospitals and critical access hospitals (CAHs) as they adopt, implement, upgrade or demonstrate meaningful use of certified EHR technology."[1]

The Initiative's Framework

We consider the history and interpret the logic that led to this initiative. We can see a framework that holds the undertaking together. For simplicity's sake we can discuss that framework, or structure, in question-and-answer format about four elements, as follows.

Incentives

Question: How can we get providers to adopt EHR?
Answer: We will provide payments to get them to do so. The payments will be their incentive.

Standards

Question: How can the information be transmitted in a uniform manner?
Answer: We will require the use of uniform standards for health information technology (HIT) exchange.

Meaningful Use

Question: How can the providers show "meaningful use"?
Answer: We will require them to use certified EHR technology that is based upon the uniform standards, and we will require they meet certain objectives.

Measures (and Objectives)

Question: How can the provider meet the objectives?
Answer: By measuring predetermined sets of criteria, using performance measures.

INCENTIVES AND EHR

This section discusses program payments and program penalties.

Program Payments as Incentives

CMS has precedents for payments as an incentive for adoption. In fact, payments as an incentive to adopt electronic health records were actually recommended in the early 1990s, many years before this program was initiated.[2]

Incentive Payments to Eligible Professionals

The eligible professionals who may receive HITECH incentive payments represent those physicians who are defined by law as "meaningful EHR users." Note that this definition excludes hospital-based professionals from receiving payments.

Figure 25–1 presents a payment chart that is based on the first calendar year for which the eligible professional receives payment.

You will recall that the HITECH initiative contains two programs: one for Medicare and one for Medicaid. Both programs are shown, side by side, on the chart. The first year to receive payment is represented by the (horizontal) years across the top of the chart: calendar year (CY) 2011 to calendar year 2016. The year for which payment may be received is represented by the (vertical) years down the side of the chart: calendar year 2011 to calendar year 2021.[3]

The maximum amount an eligible professional can receive for the first year in the Medicare program decreases year by year. To see this effect, read the top line in each Medicare column across, as follows:

> Year 1 = $18,000 in 2011 or 2012
> Year 1 = $15,000 in 2013
> Year 1 = $12,000 in 2014

To further read the chart results, choose a first year of the program across the top and then read dollars by year down that vertical column.

If you follow the "Medicare" column down for each year and then refer to the "Total" on the last line, you find that the maximum incentive payments for the Medicare program range from a high of $44,000 for 2011 and 2012 to $39,000 for 2013 and $24,000 for 2014.

CY	CY 2011		CY 2012		CY 2013		CY 2014		CY 2015		CY 2016	
	Medicare	Medicaid	Medicare	Medicaid	Medicare	Medicaid	Medicare	Medicaid	Medicare	Medicaid	Medicare	Medicaid
2011	$18,000	$21,250										
2012	$12,000	$8,500	$18,000	$21,250								
2013	$8,000	$8,500	$12,000	$8,500	$15,000	$21,250						
2014	$4,000	$8,500	$8,000	$8,500	$12,000	$8,500	$12,000	$21,250				
2015	$2,000	$8,500	$4,000	$8,500	$8,000	$8,500	$8,000	$8,500		$21,250		
2016		$8,500	$2,000	$8,500	$4,000	$8,500	$4,000	$8,500		$8,500		$21,250
2017				$8,500		$8,500		$8,500		$8,500		$8,500
2018						$8,500		$8,500		$8,500		$8,500
2019								$8,500		$8,500		$8,500
2020										$8,500		$8,500
2021												$8,500
Total (if EP does not switch programs)	$44,000	$63,750	$44,000	$63,750	$39,000	$63,750	$24,000	$63,750	$0	$63,750	$0	$63,750

NOTE: Medicare Eligible Professionals may not receive EHR incentive payments under both Medicare and Medicaid.

NOTE: The amount of the annual EHR incentive payment limit for each payment year will be increased by 10 percent for EPs who predominantly furnish services in an area that is designated as a Health Professional Shortage Area.

Figure 25–1 Maximum EHR EP Incentive Payments.
Reproduced from the Centers for Medicare and Medicaid Services. CMS Medicare Learning Network ICN #905343, p. 2 (September 2010).

As you can see, there are no incentive payments for the Medicare program after calendar year 2014.

The chart also shows Medicaid program incentive payments. These payments all amount to a six-year total of $63,750, with Year 1 "front-loaded" in the amount of $21,250 and each remaining year amounting to $8,500. There are no incentive payments for the Medicaid program after the year 2016.

Incentive Payments to Eligible Hospitals

Hospital incentives are based upon inpatient hospital services, and the hospital must be a "meaningful electronic health records (EHR) user" to be eligible for payment. In general, under the Medicare program an eligible hospital can receive a two-part payment, as follows:

- An initial amount (the base amount)
- The "Medicare share" (a discharge-related formula that represents a percentage).

The hospital incentive payment computations are complex and details are beyond the scope of this text. However, at the time of this writing the following basic payment outline was in force. This outline is for illustration only; please refer to regulatory sources for additional information.

When computing incentive payments to eligible hospitals, this outline can be used:

- The initial or base amount equals $2,000,000.
- The discharge-related amount divides eligible hospitals into three classes of hospital based on the number of discharges during the applicable payment year.

- Thus the total possible amount to be received, including the $2,000,000 base amount is as follows for each class of hospital:

  - Class 1: Hospitals with 1,149 or fewer discharges during the payment year receive a zero discharge-related amount, so their total incentive payment is calculated on the $2,000,000 base amount only.
  - Class 2: Hospitals with at least 1,150 but no more than 23,000 discharges during the payment year receive a total incentive payment, including the base amount that ranges between $2,000,000 and $6,370,400 depending on the number of discharges.
  - Class 3: Hospitals with 23,001 or more discharges during the payment year receive an amount that is limited by law to $6,370,400, including the base amount.[4]

The hospital Medicare program incentive payments span a four-year period. For hospitals that first received incentive payments in fiscal years 2011, 2012, or 2013, the discharge-related payments are paid at 100% for year one; at 75% for year two; at 50% for year three; at 25% for year four; and nothing thereafter. For those first receiving payments in fiscal year 2014, the discharge-related payments are paid at 75% for year one; at 50% for year two; at 25% for year three; and nothing thereafter. Finally, for those first receiving payments in fiscal year 2015, the discharge-related payments are paid at 50% for year one; at 25% for year two; and nothing thereafter.[5]

Program Penalties as "Reluctant Incentives"

This section discusses program penalties.

Program "Payment Adjustments" Are Penalties

The HITECH Act assesses penalties if an eligible provider does not adopt by a certain date. Within the Act these penalties are called "Payment Adjustments." They work exactly as the term implies, in that the provider's payment is adjusted—downward.

We call this reduction in payment a "reluctant incentive" because some providers will reluctantly adopt (probably at the last minute) for only one reason: to avoid a reduction in revenue due to the payment adjustment penalty.

Payment Reductions for Eligible Providers

According to the Act, payment adjustments (reductions) may occur as follows:

- Eligible Professionals: If adoption has not occurred by calendar year 2015, the physician's fee schedule amount will be reduced by a percentage.[6]
- Hospitals: Eligible hospitals "…that are not meaningful users of certified EHR technology beginning in fiscal year 2015 will be subject to payment adjustments."[7]

Website Postings Are Another "Reluctant Incentive"

The HITECH Act also requires that the names of hospitals and physicians who are "meaningful EHR users" will be posted on the CMS website.[8] We consider this requirement to be another "reluctant incentive." It is not as strong a motivation as the payment adjustment penalty, but it can still be a factor, especially in deciding when to adopt. Management may believe that appearing on the website (and thus shown to the public to be a meaningful user) is a positive asset, and that not being present on the website is negative liability. (A number of factors such as area competition may influence this belief.)

The Payments Must Be Earned

The HITECH EHR initiative payments must be earned. In order to quality for payments, the provider must typically use certified EHR technology in a meaningful manner for the electronic interchange of health information and successfully report the results. These requirements are further described and discussed in the following sections of this chapter.

STANDARDS AND EHR

This section discusses electronic transmission standards and the certified EHR technology that utilizes these standards.

Electronic Transmission Standards

One of the first steps in establishing a nationwide health information technology (IT) infrastructure is to adopt uniform electronic transmission standards. Electronic transmission standards are standards that are adopted and used to facilitate the electronic transmission of healthcare information and related business transactions.

Accordingly, the Health Insurance Portability and Accountability Act of 1996 (HIPAA) Public Law 104-191 mandated adopting such standards for "electronically conducting certain health care administrative transactions between certain entities."[9] HIPPA requires these standards to be adopted and used to "facilitate the electronic transmission of certain health information and the conduct of certain business transactions."[10] The final section of this chapter briefly discusses the current version of these electronic transmission standards.

Certified EHR Technology

An electronic health record must both capture and share patient data in an efficient manner. In order to do so, the EHR needs to store data in a structured format.

Structured Data Defined

Structured data, according to CMS, "… allows patient information to be easily retrieved and transferred, and it allows the provider to use the EHR in ways that can aid patient care. CMS and the Office of the National Coordinator for Health Information Technology (ONC) have established standards and other criteria for structured data that EHRs must use in order to qualify for this incentive program."[11]

Certified EHR Technology Defined

"Certified EHR Technology" means an EHR that has been specially certified for the EHR Incentive Programs. According to CMS:

- "Certified EHR technology gives assurance to purchasers and other users that:
  - an EHR system or module offers the necessary technological capability, functionality and security
  - to help them meet the meaningful use criteria."[12]
- "Certification also helps providers and patients be confident that the electronic health IT products and systems they use:
  - are secure,
  - can maintain data confidentially, and
  - can work with other systems to share information."[13]

MEANINGFUL USE AND EHR

This section discusses how to establish meaningful use, its three stages, and its timelines.

HOW DO YOU ESTABLISH MEANINGFUL USE?

The overall goal of meaningful use is to improve health care in the United States by promoting the spread of electronic health records.[14]

The following definitions give more specific meaning to that goal.

"Meaningful Use" Defined

According to CMS, providers must show that they are "meaningfully using" their certified EHR technology by "... meeting thresholds for a number of objectives. CMS has established the objectives for "meaningful use" that eligible professionals, eligible hospitals, and critical access hospitals (CAHs) must meet in order to receive an incentive payment."[15]

By meeting "thresholds" CMS means meeting minimum levels. Note also that providers must successfully meet the criteria for three different elements (core objectives, menu objectives, and quality control measures) while using certified EHR technology. The differences among these elements is explained later in this chapter.

"Meaningful User" Defined

The HITECH Act legislation defined a meaningful electronic health records user as follows.
   "Meaningful electronic health records user" means the provider is:

- Using certified EHR in a meaningful manner
- Connected in a manner that provides for the electronic exchange of health information to improve the quality of health care, such as promoting care coordination
- Reporting on measures using EHR[16]

Establishing Meaningful Use

In order to establish meaningful use, we understand that four basic steps are required, as follows:

- Adopt and implement certified EHR technology
- Choose the appropriate incentive program
- Meet the criteria for your appropriate objectives
- Successfully report the required measures

Since the use of certified EHR technology is required for this initiative, the obvious first step is to adopt and implement a certified system. The second step concerns program choice. There are two programs under this initiative—one for Medicare and one for Medicaid. Hospitals can participate in either or both, but eligible professionals must choose between them. (This subject was more fully discussed in the previous chapter.)

The third step is to meet the criteria for your appropriate objectives. The properly certified EHR technology software that has been adopted for your hospital or physician practice should already have the programming for these criteria embedded in the system. User-friendly software will probably have drop-down menus and one-click entry options to make the process even more efficient. The fourth step is to successfully report the required measures, and the properly certified software should be able to also perform this function.

So why are we explaining how the computations work in this chapter if the software is supposed to automatically do the calculations? Because managers can be more effective if they really understand how the process works. You are, for example, much more able to recognize and catch something that is not functioning properly within your system.

MEANINGFUL USE PROGRESSES IN STAGES

This section discusses establishing meaningful use, its three stages, and its timelines for implementation.

The Reason for Stages

At the time of this writing, the HITECH initiative programs are supposed to advance in three sequential stages, and each stage requires a higher level of participation. The CMS regulations require completion of each stage before progressing to the next stage.[17]

What is the reason for the three levels, or stages, of participation? We can better understand the reason by labeling the stages as "Beginning," "Intermediate," and "Advanced."

Three Stages of Meaningful Use

The three stages of meaningful use, as illustrated in **Figure 25–2**, are summarized as follows:

- Stage 1 includes data capture and sharing
- Stage 2 includes advanced clinical processes
- Stage 3 includes improved outcomes

The criteria for each stage are described as follows.

Stage 1: "Beginning"

The Stage 1 criteria for meaningful use focus upon five items, as follows:

- Capture health information electronically in a standardized format
- Use that information in tracking key clinical conditions
- Communicate that information for processes of care coordination
- Begin to report clinical quality measures and public health information
- Use the information to engage patients and their families in their care[18]

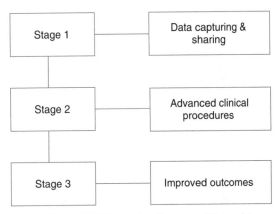

Figure 25–2 EHR Incentive Program: Three Stages of Meaningful Use.
Courtesy of J.J. Baker and R.W. Baker, Dallas, Texas.

Stage 2: "Intermediate"

The Stage 2 criteria for meaningful use focus upon four items, as follows:

- More rigorous health information exchange (HIE)
- Increased requirements for e-prescribing and incorporating lab results
- Electronic transmission of patient care summaries across multiple settings
- More patient-controlled data[19]

Stage 3: "Advanced"

The Stage 3 criteria for meaningful use focus upon five items, as follows:

- Improving quality, safety, and efficiency leading to improved health outcomes
- Decision support for national high-priority conditions
- Patient access to self-management tools
- Access to comprehensive patient data through patient-centered HIE
- Improving population health[20]

TIMELINES: ROLLING IMPLEMENTATION IN STAGES

This section discusses timelines as they relate to the three stages of meaningful use.

Stages of Meaningful Use by Year

The program is to be implemented in three stages as we have just discussed. A rolling implementation was visualized, with eligible providers having a choice as to what year they would enter the program. **Figure 25–3** illustrates this concept.

The vertical column labeled "1st Year" shows the applicable span of "first year" or "entry year" dates, ranging from 2011 to 2017. You can choose a first year date and read across to see when that provider must achieve Stages 1, 2, and 3. Note that a provider must meet two

1st Year	Stage of Meaningful Use By Year										
	2011	2012	2013	2014	2015	2016	2017	2018	2019	2020	2021
2011	1	1	1	2	2	3	3	TBD	TBD	TBD	TBD
2012		1	1	2	2	3	3	TBD	TBD	TBD	TBD
2013			1	1	2	2	3	3	TBD	TBD	TBD
2014				1	1	2	2	3	3	TBD	TBD
2015					1	1	2	2	3	3	TBD
2016						1	1	2	2	3	3
2017							1	1	2	2	3

Note that providers who were early demonstrators of meaningful use in 2011 will meet three consecutive years of meaningful use under the Stage 1 criteria before advancing to the Stage 2 criteria in 2014. All other providers would meet two years of meaningful use under the Stage 1 criteria before advancing to the Stage 2 criteria in their third year.

Figure 25–3 Stages of Meaningful Use by Year.
Reproduced from the Centers for Medicare and Medicaid Services. Stage 2 Overview Tipsheet. Updated August 2010.

years of meaningful use in Stage 1 before progressing to Stage 2. Then requirements for Stage 2 must be met before progressing to Stage 3.[21]

The horizontal headings begin with the year 2011 and end with the year 2021. For example, assume a first year entry in the year 2014. Select 2014 in the left-hand vertical column, then read across and find the matching "2014" column. On that line item you will then see that Stage 1 is required for the years 2014 and 2015, Stage 2 is required for the years 2016 and 2017, and Stage 3 is required for the years 2018 and 2019.

Reporting Periods Vary by Type of Provider

A typical reporting period covers 12 months. However, the beginning month and the ending month will vary between two types of providers as follows.

Reporting Periods for Eligible Professionals

The Eligible Professionals reporting period is a calendar year (CY). A calendar year runs like the calendar does, from January 1 to December 31.

Reporting Periods for Hospitals

The hospital reporting period, on the other hand, is a fiscal year (FY). Specifically, it is the federal fiscal year. This reporting period runs from October 1 of one year to September 30 of the following year.

MEASURES OF MEANINGFUL USE AND EHR

This section describes meaningful use objectives and the measures that support these objectives.

INTRODUCTION

The HITECH Act stipulated that under the initiative's Medicare program, "...the Medicare methods are segmented into Clinical Quality Measures (CQMs) and meaningful use objectives, both of which meaningful users must meet."[22]

We discuss core versus menu objectives and their supporting measures in the following sections. We also discuss how the clinical quality measures are treated.

MEANINGFUL USE OBJECTIVES: THE REASON FOR MEASURES

Meaningful use objectives support policy priorities in order to achieve the health outcomes. This program separates meaningful use objectives into two types. The two types (core versus menu) are described as follows. **Figure 25–4** further illustrates the concept.

Core Objectives

Core objectives are mandatory. That is, to achieve meaningful use, the provider must meet all the core objectives that pertain to the appropriate stage (Stage 1, 2, or 3).

Menu Objectives

Menu objectives, on the other hand, provide a choice. The provider is allowed to choose from a "menu" of objectives in order to achieve meaningful use. There are, however, a required number of these menu objectives that must be met in each stage.

STAGE 2 CORE AND MENU SETS OF OBJECTIVES

Stage 2 core and menu sets of objectives requirements to meet meaningful use at the time of this writing are as follows. Be aware that providers can claim an exclusion from an objective under certain circumstances, although the allowed methodology for such exclusions is extremely specific.

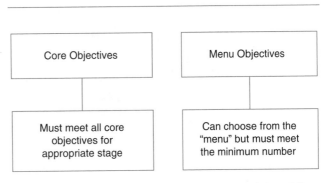

Figure 25–4 EHR Incentive Program: Characteristics of Core and Menu Objectives.
Courtesy of J.J. Baker and R.W. Baker, Dallas, Texas.

Hospitals

For eligible hospitals in Stage 2 there are a total of 16 core objectives and a total of 6 menu objectives. The hospital must meet the criteria (or show an exclusion) for all 16 core objectives. The hospital must also meet the criteria for 3 of the 6 menu objectives.[23]

Eligible Professionals

For eligible professionals (EPs) in Stage 2 there are a total of 17 core objectives and a total of 6 menu objectives. The EP must meet the criteria or report an exclusion for all 17 core objectives. The EP must also meet the criteria for 3 of the 6 menu objectives, "...unless an exclusion can be claimed for more than 3 of the menu objectives in which case the criteria for the remaining non-excluded objectives must be met."[24]

Clinical Quality Measures (CQMs) Were Originally Objectives

Clinical quality measures are a type of performance measure within this program. Generally speaking, clinical quality measures were originally designated as objectives within the program methodology. That methodology has now changed as follows. Beginning in 2014, clinical quality measure reporting will change for all providers. CQMs are to be reported electronically using EHR technology that is certified to the 2014 standards and that contains the new CQM criteria. Furthermore, both the CQM criteria and the certified standards may be adjusted annually in the years beyond 2014.[25]

Figure 25–5 illustrates the methodology requirements.

MEANINGFUL USE *includes*	HOSPITALS	ELIGIBLE PROFESSIONALS
STAGE 2 CORE OBJECTIVES*	16 Total *[Must meet all 16]*	17 Total *[Must meet all 17]*
STAGE 2 MENU OBJECTIVES*	6 Total *[Must report on 3 of the 6]*	6 Total *[Must report on 3 of the 6]*
CLINICAL QUALITY MEASURES	Beginning in 2014, CQM reporting will change for all providers. CQMs are to be reported electronically using EHR technology certified to the 2014 standards and that contains the new CQM criteria.**	

Source: *77 Federal Register 53980 (September 4, 2012)

**CMS: 2014 Clinical Quality Measures Tipsheet. Both CQM criteria and certified standards may be adjusted annually in years beyond 2014.

Figure 25–5 Stage 2 Core and Menu Meaningful Use Objectives for Hospitals and Eligible Professionals. Data from 77 Federal Register 53980 (September 4, 2012) and CMS: 2014 Clinical Quality Measures Tipsheet.

THE MEASURES THAT SUPPORT THE OBJECTIVES

This section discusses meaningful use measures, the relationship between measures and objectives, and establishing the measures.

Meaningful Use Measures

Meaningful use measures support the meaningful use objectives. How can you report that a certain objective has been met? That objective must be measured in some uniform manner for reporting purposes. In this program we have sets of criteria that are expressed as measures.

Relationship Between Measures and Objectives

The methodology works as follows. Every core measure is tied to its specific core objective. And likewise, every menu measure is tied to its specific menu objective.

Figure 25–6 illustrates this concept. It is important to also remember that certified EHR technology software should perform this function electronically.

Establishing the Measures

Measures will vary between types of providers and between stages, as discussed in the following sections.

Measures Differ Between Hospitals and Eligible Professionals

The operation of a hospital and the operation of an eligible professional's practice vary a great deal. It is logical, then, to recognize that this program's sets of criteria for measures must also vary in certain respects. Specific measures and their criteria have been created for hospitals. A different set of specific measures and their criteria have been created for eligible professionals. The certified EHR technology software in use will be electronically

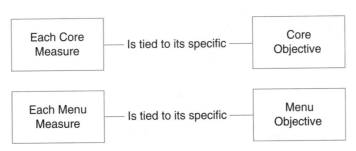

Figure 25–6 EHR Incentive Program: Relationship Between Meaningful Use Measures and Objectives. Courtesy of J.J. Baker and R.W. Baker, Dallas, Texas.

matched to one or the other of these sets of measures (that is, matched to either hospital or eligible professional objectives and measures).

Measures Differ Between Stage 1 and Stage 2

Stage 1 of meaningful use focuses upon data capturing and sharing while Stage 2 focuses upon advanced clinical procedures. The measures' criteria and their related objectives must vary between Stage 1 and Stage 2 in order to measure and report appropriately. Also note that sometimes the criteria for a stage can be modified midstream, so to speak. For example, some of the Stage 1 criteria were modified when the Stage 2 regulations were released.

STAGE 2 MEASUREMENT METHODS

This section describes measurement methods that are specific to Stage 2.

THREE TYPES OF MEANINGFUL USE MEASURES

At the time of this writing, the Stage 2 HITECH EHR program includes three types of meaningful use measures. Each is described below. (You will recall that "required threshold" means "required minimum." You may also recall that exclusions from a measure may be allowed under certain circumstances, although the methodology for such exclusions is extremely specific.)

System-Based Measures

System-based measures ask three questions, as follows:

- What function of our certified EHR technology system must be enabled?
- Do we meet the required threshold?
- Are we excluded from the measure?

Action-Based Measures

Action-based measures also ask three questions, as follows:

- What actions must we take?
- Do we meet the required threshold?
- Are we excluded from the measure?

Percentage-Based Measures

Percentage-based measures ask four questions, as follows:

- What makes up the denominator?
- What makes up the numerator?
- Do we meet the required threshold?
- Are we excluded from the measure?

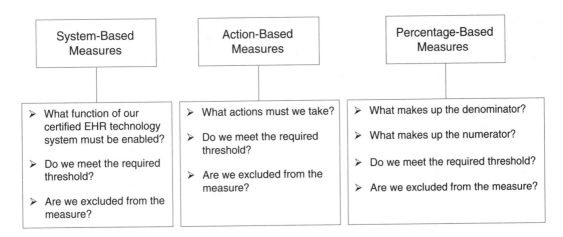

Figure 25–7 EHR Incentive Program: Types of Meaningful Use Measures.
Courtesy of J.J. Baker and R.W. Baker, Dallas, Texas.

Figure 25–7 further illustrates this concept.

PERCENTAGE-BASED MEASURES AS REPORTING REQUIREMENTS

The program's meaningful use objectives often use the percentage-based measures just described as reporting requirements. In fact, the regulations state that "...many of our meaningful use objectives use percentage-based measures wherever possible and if appropriate."[26] Thus we will explore the calculation of a percentage-based measure.

Computing a Percentage-Based Measurement

This section first discusses numerators and denominators and then provides a six-step computation method.

Numerators and Denominators

To compute a percentage you must first calculate a fraction, as illustrated in the six-step method that follows. A fraction has two parts—the numerator is the top number and the denominator is the bottom number. The line between the two parts signifies the division function. The denominator indicates the total number of parts available to be divided and the numerator indicates the number of parts of the denominator that are taken.

Why Is This Subject Important?

CMS has provided specifications for computing measures. Each specification for a percentage-based measure sets out what the composition of the denominator should be and what the composition of the numerator should be. Therefore it is important to understand the consequences of selecting a denominator and the consequences of what the numerator will be. We understand that electronic software will perform calculations, but managers should know how the method works in order to better understand the results produced for their organization. Therefore we provide two examples of the composition of denominators and numerators later in this chapter.

A Six-Step Computation Method

It works this way:

Step 1: Determine your denominator.
Step 2: Determine your numerator.
Step 3: Calculate the fraction (including the decimal).
Step 4: Convert the fraction to a percentage.
Step 5: Refer to the threshold percentage that is set for this particular measure.
Step 6: Compare your percentage to the threshold percentage; it must meet this threshold in order to count. (That is, it must meet a minimum level.)

For additional detail about the six steps, see the Supplemental Materials section entitled "The Mechanics of Percentage Computations."

Exceptions

Be aware that certain exceptions exist for particular measures. These exceptions don't have to be included in the numerator or denominator, so they won't count against you.

PERCENTAGE-BASED MEASURES FOR ELIGIBLE PROFESSIONALS

Percentage-based measures represent one of three types of reporting requirements for measures associated with Stage 2 meaningful use objectives. In this section we describe the Stage 2 denominators available for eligible professionals (EPs) along with certain related definitions.

STAGE 2 DENOMINATORS AVAILABLE FOR EPs

Only four denominators can be used by eligible professionals (EPs) in determining Stage 2 percentage-based measures.

The four denominators for EPs reporting in Stage 2 include the following:

- Unique patients seen by the EP during the EHR reporting period (stratified by age or previous office visit)
- Number of orders (medication, labs, radiology)
- Office visits
- Transitions of care/referrals[27]

DEFINITIONS FOR THE EP DENOMINATORS

"Office Visits" and "Number of Orders" are pretty much self-explanatory. However, the terms "Unique Patient" and "Transitions of Care" require definitions, as follows.

"Unique Patient" Defined

A "Unique Patient" for the EP denominator means if a patient is seen (or admitted) more than once during the EHR reporting period, that patient only counts once in the denominator for the office visit measure. This means, for example, if patient Susie Smith is seen three times within the reporting period, she can be counted only once in the denominator for this measure. Also note that a patient seen through telemedicine still counts as a patient that is seen by the eligible professional.[28]

"Transitions of Care" Defined

"Transitions of Care" for the EP denominator visualizes the movement of a patient from one setting of care to another. The care settings can be, for example, hospital, ambulatory primary care practice, ambulatory specialty care practice, long-term care, home health, or rehabilitation facility.[29]

For purposes of the EP denominator, transition of care/referrals can apply to either the EP that initiates the transition or referral, or the EP that receives the transition or referral:

- The initiating EP must include at a minimum those transitions and referrals that are ordered by the EP.
- On the other hand, the receiving EP must include at a minimum patient encounters whereby a summary of care record (regarding the transition/referral) is provided to him or her.[30]

ELIGIBLE PROFESSIONAL (EP) STAGE 2 REPORTING: AN EXAMPLE

This eligible professional reporting requirements example includes a discussion of the meaningful use objective, the measure, and computation of the measure's percentage. In order to meet this objective and its measure, an EP's electronic transmission must use specific capabilities and standards that have been adopted for EHR technology certification.[31] The Health Outcomes Policy Priority for this objective is as follows: "Engage patients and families in their health care."[32]

Objective, Measure, and Exclusion for the EP Stage 2 Example

This example is a "Core Set" objective. This measure is number 8 of 17 core measures.[33]

Objective

"Provide clinical summaries for patients for each office visit."

Measure

"Clinical summaries provided to patients or patient-authorized representatives within one business day for more than 50% of office visits."

Exclusion

"Any EP who has no office visits during the EHR reporting period."[34]

Definition of Terms

Two terms are defined as follows.

Office Visit Defined

Office visits "...include separate, billable encounters that result from evaluation and management services provided to the patient and include: (1) concurrent care or transfer of care visits, (2) consultant visits, or (3) prolong physician service without direct (face-to-face) patient contact (tele-health). A consultant visit occurs when a provider is asked to render an expert opinion/service for a specific condition or problem by a referring provider."[35]

Clinical Summary Defined

Clinical summary is "...an after-visit summary that provides a patient with relevant and actionable information and instructions."[36] Some 24 items are required to be included in the EP's clinical summary. These items are listed in **Exhibit 25–1**. (If any of this information is not available, that notation should be made instead.)[37]

Attestation Requirements: Calculating the Measure's Percentage

This measure's percentage represents the joint efforts of CMS and the Office of the National Coordinator for Health IT (ONC). Together they have defined the relevant denominator, the numerator, the threshold that must be met, and any exclusions as follows.

Denominator

Number of office visits conducted by the EP during the EHR reporting period.

Exhibit 25–1 Items Included in the After-Visit Clinical Summary

Patient name
Provider's name and office contact information
Date and location of the visit
Reason for the office visit
Current problem list
Current medication list
Current medication allergy list
Procedures performed during the visit
Immunizations or medications administered during the visit
Vital signs taken during the visit (or other recent vital signs)
Laboratory test results
List of diagnostic tests pending
Clinical instructions
Future appointments
Referrals to other providers
Future scheduled tests
Demographic information maintained within certified electronic health record technology (CEHRT) (sex, race, ethnicity, date of birth, preferred language)
Smoking status
Care plan field(s), including goals and instructions
Recommended patient decision aids (if applicable to the visit)

Reproduced from the Centers for Medicare and Medicaid Services. Stage 2 Eligible Professional Meaningful Use Core Measures. Measure 8 of 17 (October 2012).

Numerator

Number of office visits in the denominator where the patient or a patient-authorized person is provided a clinical summary of their visit within one business day.

Threshold

The resulting percentage must be more than 50% in order for an EP to meet this Stage 2 measure.

Exclusion

Any EP who has no office visits during the EHR reporting period.[38]

PERCENTAGE-BASED MEASURES FOR HOSPITALS

Percentage-based measures represent one of three types of reporting requirements for measures associated with Stage 2 meaningful use objectives. In this section we describe the Stage 2 denominators available for hospitals, along with certain related definitions.

STAGE 2 DENOMINATORS AVAILABLE FOR HOSPITALS

Only four denominators can be used by hospitals and critical access hospitals (CAHs) in determining Stage 2 percentage-based measures.

The four denominators for hospitals and CAHs reporting in Stage 2 are as follows:

- Unique patients admitted to the eligible hospital's or CAH's inpatient or emergency department during the EHR reporting period (stratified by age)
- Number of orders (medication, labs, radiology)
- Electronic lab orders received by the hospital from ambulatory providers
- Transitions of care[39]

DEFINITIONS FOR THE HOSPITAL DENOMINATOR

Two definitions follow.

"Electronic Lab Orders" Defined

The "electronic lab orders" measure matches a Stage 2 objective to "Provide structured electronic lab results to ambulatory providers." Also note that "electronic lab orders" means what it says; that is, to qualify the orders must be received using an electronic transmission method. This does not mean other methods such as an electronic fax, a paper document, or a telephone call.[40]

"Transitions of Care" Defined

For purposes of the hospital denominator, transition of care/referrals can apply to either the hospital that initiates the transition or referral, or the hospital that receives the transition or referral.

- When the initiating hospital is transitioning the patient, it must include all discharges from the inpatient department and after admission to the emergency department when follow-up care is ordered by an authorized provider of the hospital.
- On the other hand, the receiving hospital must include all admissions to both the inpatient and emergency departments that are related to such transition of care.[41]

HOSPITAL STAGE 2 REPORTING: AN EXAMPLE

This hospital reporting requirements example includes a discussion of the meaningful use objective, the measure, and computation of the measure's percentage. This objective and its measures actually include both hospitals and critical access hospitals (CAHs). Certain rural providers qualify as CAHs under the Medicare program. These CAHs are a separate provider type and are reimbursed under a separate payment method.[42] However, for purposes of ease in reading we have used the term "hospital" to include both types of providers.

In order to meet this objective and its measure, an eligible hospital's electronic transmission must use certified electronic technology capabilities and standards. The Health Outcomes Policy Priority for this objective is as follows: "Improving quality, safety, efficiency and reducing health disparities."[43]

Objective, Measure, and Exclusion for the Hospital Stage 2 Example

This example is a "Menu Set" objective. This measure is number one of six menu set measures.[44] The relevant elements are as follows.

Objective

"Record whether a patient 65 years old or older has an advance directive."

Measure

"More than 50 percent of all unique patients 65 years old or older admitted to the eligible hospital's or CAH's inpatient department (PO S21) during the EHR reporting period have an indication of an advance directive status recorded as structured data."

Exclusion

"An eligible hospital or CAH that admits no patients age 65 years old or older during the EHR reporting period."[45]

Definitions of Terms

Four terms are defined as follows.

Unique Patient Defined

If a patient is admitted to an eligible hospital's or CAH's inpatient department (POS 21) more than once during the EHR reporting period, then for purposes of measurement that patient is only counted once in the denominator for the measure.[46]

"Admitted to the Inpatient Department" Defined

There are two methods for calculating Emergency Department (ED) admissions for the denominators for these measures. CMS resources provide technical information regarding these calculation methods.[47]

Advance Directive Defined

Advance directives are legal documents in written form that allow the individual to convey his or her end-of-life decisions ahead of time. These legal documents are sometimes called by other names. For example, a living will is typically considered a type of advance directive.[48]

"Structured data" means data residing in an electronic health record system that stores the data in a structured format. (In this example, the system would be one that uses certified EHR technology.)[49]

Attestation Requirements: Calculating the Measure's Percentage

This measure's percentage represents the joint efforts of CMS and ONC. Together they have defined the relevant denominator, the numerator, the threshold that must be met, and any exclusions as follows.

Denominator

The number of unique patients age 65 or older admitted to an eligible hospital's inpatient department (Place of Service 21) during the EHR reporting period.

Numerator

The number of patients in the denominator who have an indication of an advance directive status entered using structured data.

Threshold

The resulting percentage must be more than 50% in order for an eligible hospital or CAH to meet this measure.

Exclusion

Any eligible hospital or CAH that admits no patients age 65 years old or older during the EHR reporting period.[50]

Commentary

As a matter of interest, note that "indication of an advance directive status" in the numerator doesn't mean the patient has to have an advance directive. Instead it means whether or not there is an advance directive should be noted.[51]

As another point of interest, this Stage 2 measure is limited only to the inpatient department of the hospital. Thus at the time of this writing, eligible professionals do not have to record information about advance directives.[52]

MORE ABOUT STANDARDS AND THEIR IMPACT

This section discusses version 5010 of electronic transmission standards and the impact of these standards on the healthcare industry.

Version 5010 of Electronic Transmission Standards

Earlier in this chapter under the heading "Standards and EHR" we described how standards were mandated by law to facilitate electronic transmission. This meant the healthcare industry had to use standard formats for electronic claims and claims-related transactions.[53] Version 5010 is the current version of these electronic transmission standards in force at the time of this writing.

Version 5010 was implemented as of January 1, 2012. This means any electronic transaction for which a standard was adopted had to be submitted using Version 5010 as of the first of the year in 2012. Electronic transactions not using Version 5010 were rejected, although there was an enforcement discretionary period through June 30, 2012, during which no enforcement action was taken.[54] (A further description of the rules and regulations surrounding standards is well beyond the scope of this text.)

Impact of Standards on the Healthcare Industry

Changes in electronic transaction standards directly impact providers, health plans, and others as illustrated in **Figure 25–8**. Providers affected include, at a minimum, hospitals, physicians, dentists, and pharmacies. Health plans affected include commercial health plans, the Blue Cross/Blue Shield plans, and all government plans such as Medicare and Medicaid. Other healthcare organizations that are affected include the electronic information clearinghouses and the vendors who provide hardware and software to the healthcare industry.

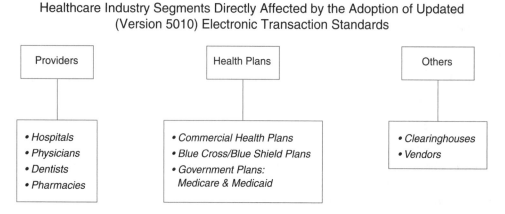

Healthcare Industry Segments Directly Affected by the Adoption of Updated (Version 5010) Electronic Transaction Standards

Figure 25–8 Healthcare Industry Segments Directly Affected by the Adoption of Updated (Version 5010) Electronic Transaction Standards.
Reproduced from 73 Federal Register 49761 (August 22, 2008).

SUMMARY

To summarize, the electronic transmission standards are coordinated with and are the beginning point for certified EHR technology. Providers must be able to obtain certified software that is updated with the latest version of such standards. Vendors must comply with updates. And finally, it is the responsibility of management to protect your electronic health records. Security and privacy are essential.

SUPPLEMENTARY MATERIALS: THE MECHANICS OF PERCENTAGE COMPUTATIONS

A brief description entitled "The Mechanics of Percentage Computations" appears in the "Supplementary Materials" section. This piece further describes the step-by-step mechanics of computing a percentage. We realize that electronic software generally performs this computation automatically. Nevertheless, every manager should be able do the calculation with paper and pencil. This knowledge is important to your understanding of the overall process described in this chapter.

 INFORMATION CHECKPOINT

What is needed?	Find a document that concerns the HITECH initiative reporting requirements as discussed in this chapter. (The document could be about meaningful use, percentage-based measures, CQMs, etc.)
Where is it found?	The subject affects many areas of responsibility, so it could be found within the IT department, with the individuals responsible for training, or in a finance, administrative, or clinical area.
How is it used?	Its use depends on the item that you find. It could be used for reference, for training, or for everyday look-up purposes.

 KEY TERMS

Certified EHR Technology
Core Objectives
Denominator
Electronic Transmission Standards
Meaningful Use
Meaningful User
Measures
Menu Objective

Numerator
Payment Adjustment
Structured Data
Threshold
Version 5010 Transmission Standards

 DISCUSSION QUESTIONS

1. Does your work involve dealing with "meaningful use" in some way? If so, will you describe how your work is involved?
2. Do you know of an organization that has progressed from Stage 1 to Stage 2 in the HITECH initiative? If so, can you describe this progression?
3. Do you think posting the names of the "meaningful health electronic record users" publicly on the CMS website is a good idea? If so, why? If not, why not?
4. Why do you think the federal policymakers decided to make the names public on a government website?

NOTES

1. CMS, "EHR Incentive Programs: Getting Started," http://www.cms.gov/Regulations-and-Guidance/Legislation/EHRIncentivePrograms/Getting_Started.html (August 27, 2012).
2. Office of Inspector General (OIG), "Electronic Data Interchange and Paperless Processing: Issues and Challenges," OEI-12-93-0080 (March 1994).
3. CMS, Medicare Learning Network ICN#905343, p.2 (September 2010).
4. CMS, Medicare Learning Network ICN #904626 Table 1. (November 2010). Note that this payment methodology is applicable to eligible hospitals that participate under both Medicare fee-for-service and MA incentive programs.
5. Ibid., Table 2.
6. ARRA Division B. Title IV Section 4101 (HITECH Act).
7. CMS, MLN ICN #904626, page 1.
8. ARRA Division B. Title IV Section 4102.
9. 73 Federal Register (FR) 49743 (August 22, 2008).
10. Ibid.
11. CMS, "EHR Incentive Programs: Certified EHR Technology," http://www.cms.gov/Regulations-and-Guidance/Legislation/EHRIncentivePrograms/Certification.html (August 21, 2012).
12. Ibid.
13. Ibid.
14. www.healthit.gov/policy-researchers-implementers/meaninful-use (accessed January 23, 2013).

15. CMS, "EHR Incentive Programs: 'Meaningful Use,'" http://www.cms.gov/Regulations-and-Guidance/Legislation/EHRIncentivePrograms/Meaningful_Use.html (September 20, 2012).

16. HITECH Act: ARRA Division B. Title IV Section. 4102. Note that the definition for hospital users originally said "…Submits information on clinical quality measures and other measures not yet determined." It is our understanding that CMS still retains the regulatory authority to require "other measures not yet determined."

17. CMS, "EHR Incentive Programs: 'Meaningful Use,'" http://www.cms.gov/Regulations-and-Guidance/Legislation/EHRIncentivePrograms/Meaningful_Use.html (September 20, 2012).

18. HealthIT.gov, "Policymaking, Regulation, & Strategy-Meaningful Use," www.healthit.gov/policy-researchers-implementers/meaningful-use (accessed January 23, 2013).

19. Ibid.

20. Ibid.

21. CMS, "Stage 2 Overview Tipsheet." (August 2012).

22. 77 Federal Register (FR) 54089 (September 4, 2012).

23. 77 Federal Register (FR) 53980 (September 4, 2012).

24. Ibid., FR p. 53980.

25. CMS, 2014 Clinical Quality Measures Tipsheet. (August 2012).

26. 77 Federal Register (FR) 13707 (March 7, 2012).

27. 77 Federal Register (FR) 53984 (September 4, 2012).

28. 77 Federal Register (FR) 53982-3 (September 4, 2012). And of course any patient seen or admitted only once during the EHR reporting period will also count once in the denominator.

29. 77 Federal Register (FR) 53983 (September 4, 2012).

30. 77 Federal Register (FR) 53984 (September 4, 2012).

31. 77 Federal Register (FR) 54001 (September 4, 2012).

32. 77 Federal Register (FR) 54046 (September 4, 2012).

33. CMS, "EHR Incentive Programs: Stage 2 Eligible Professional Meaningful Use Core Measures—Measure 8 of 17." (October 2012).

34. Ibid.

35. Ibid.

36. Ibid.

37. 77 Federal Register (FR) 54001 (September 4, 2012).

38. CMS, "EHR Incentive Programs: Stage 2 Eligible Professional Meaningful Use Core Measures—Measure 8 of 17." (October 2012).

39. 77 Federal Register (FR) 53984 (September 4, 2012) "Inpatient bed days" was initially proposed as a hospital Stage 2 measure but was not included in the final Stage 2 rule.

40. 77 Federal Register (FR) 53984 (September 4, 2012).

41. 77 Federal Register (FR) 53983-4 (September 4, 2012).

42. CMS, "Critical Access Hospitals," Medicare Learning Network Fact Sheet #ICN 006400 (January 2012).

43. 77 Federal Register (FR) 54048 (September 4, 2012).

44. CMS, "EHR Incentive Programs: Stage 2 Eligible Hospital and Critical Access Hospital Meaningful Use Menu Set Measures—Measure 1 of 6." (October 2012).

45. Ibid.

46. Ibid.

47. Ibid.

48. MedlinePlus, "Advance Directives," http://www.nlm.nih.gov/medlineplus /advancedirectives.html (accessed April 30, 2013).

49. CMS, "An Introduction to the Medicare EHR Incentive Program for Eligible Professionals," p.9. (January 2012).

50. CMS, "EHR Incentive Programs: Stage 2 Eligible Hospital and Critical Access Hospital Meaningful Use Menu Set Measures—Measure 1 of 6." (October 2012).

51. 77 Federal Register (FR) 54040-1 (September 4, 2012).

52. Ibid.

53. CMS, "New Health Care Electronic Transactions Standards Versions 5010, D.0, and 3.0," Medicare Learning Network Fact Sheet ICN #903192 (January 2010).

54. CMS, "Version 5010 Industry Resources," www.cms.gov/Regulations-and-Guidance /HIPAA-Administrative-Simplification/Versions5010andD0/Version_5010-Industry -Resources.html (accessed February 3, 2013).

New Information Systems: ICD-10 Implementation and the Manager's Viewpoint

ICD-10 E-RECORDS OVERVIEW AND IMPACT

This chapter provides an ICD-10 overview and describes the ICD-10 electronic records impact.

OVERVIEW OF THE ICD-10 CODING SYSTEM

The International Classification of Diseases, 10th Revision (ICD-10) is designed to "promote international comparability in the processing classification and presentation of mortality statistics."[1] The ICD is the international standard diagnostic classification for all general epidemiological issues, many health management purposes, and clinical use.[2]

This classification system has been developed by collaboration among the World Health Organization (WHO) and 10 international centers. Other countries that have already adopted ICD-10 include Australia, Canada, France, Germany, and the United Kingdom.[3]

ICD-10-CM AND ICD-10-PCS CODES

The National Center for Health Statistics (NCHS) is 1 of the 10 international centers collaborating with the WHO in the development and revisions of the ICD. The NCHS is an agency within the Centers for Disease Control and Prevention (CDC). As such, NCHS is the federal agency that is responsible for use of the ICD-10 in the United States.

Progress Notes

After completing this chapter, you should be able to

1. Understand the six benefits of transitioning to ICD-10.
2. Understand why the change to ICD-10 codes is a technology problem.
3. Identify the three types of ICD-10 implementation costs.
4. Understand why situational analysis is particularly appropriate for electronic records implementation such as ICD-10.
5. Identify the four components of a SWOT analysis.
6. Understand the five phases of project management.

WHO owns the ICD-10 copyright and has "authorized the development of an adaptation of ICD-10 for use in the United States for U.S. government purposes."[4] The NCHS, under the CDC, has developed a clinical modification of the ICD-10, termed "ICD-10-CM." The ICD-10-CM replaces the ICD-9-CM. The ICD-10-CM diagnosis classification system has been developed for use in all types of healthcare treatment settings in the United States.[5]

Meanwhile, the Centers for Medicare and Medicaid Services (CMS) has developed a procedure classification system, termed the "ICD-10-PCS." The ICD-10-PCS is for use in in-patient hospital settings only within the United States.[6] (Note this difference: ICD-10-CM is for use in all types of healthcare treatment settings, while ICD-10-PCS is for use in inpatient hospital settings only.)

Final Revised ICD-10 Compliance Date

CMS has extended the deadline for ICD-10 compliance by one year. Thus the compliance date for ICD-10-CM and ICD-10-PCS is now October 1, 2014, instead of October 1, 2013, as reflected in **Figure 26–1**. CMS officials believe this extension "...will give covered entities the additional time needed to synchronize system and business process preparation and changeover to the updated medical data code sets."[7]

Providers and Suppliers Impacted by the ICD-10 Transition

The change from ICD-9 to ICD-10 has a ripple effect that impacts nearly every corner of the healthcare industry in the United States. The companies and organizations impacted by the ICD-10 transition include inpatient providers, outpatient providers, and an array of other support services and suppliers.

Figure 26–2 illustrates the entities that are affected by the ICD-10 transition. Inpatient providers impacted include both hospitals and nursing facilities. Outpatient providers include, at a minimum, physician offices, outpatient care centers, medical diagnostic and imaging services, home health services, other ambulatory care services, and durable medical equipment providers. Support services and suppliers include health insurance carriers and third-party administrators, along with the vendors who provide computer system design and related services.[8] Note that pharmacies (both chain and independent pharmacies) are substantially impacted by the required electronic transaction standards updates for pharmacies, while ICD-10 adoption is generally more of a peripheral issue for pharmacies.

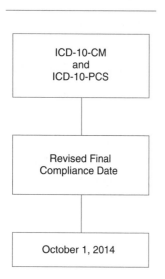

Figure 26–1 ICD-10 Revised Final Compliance Date.
Note: Date may be moved forward

E-RECORD STANDARDS AND THE ICD-10 TRANSITION

This section discusses Version 5010 of electronic record standards and provides an example of standards use.

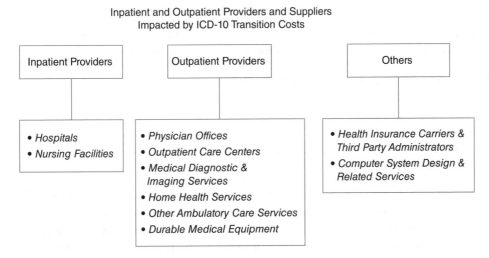

Figure 26–2 Inpatient and Outpatient Providers and Suppliers Impacted by the ICD-10 Transition. Reproduced from 74 Federal Register 3357 (January 16, 2009).

Version 5010 of Standards and the ICD-10 Transition

Version 5010 of electronic transmission standards includes infrastructure changes that were necessary in order to prepare for the adoption of ICD-10 codes. A whole array of sequential rules and regulations has evolved over the last two decades to create these electronic transaction standards and to require their adoption—a full description of such rules and regulations is well beyond the scope of this text.[9]

Example of Standards Use

However, two particular items are of interest to us in the context of the ICD-10 transition:

1. It was necessary to update many electronic transaction standards in order to accommodate the new ICD-10 codes. The groups, or sets, of codes (termed "standard medical data code sets")[10] to be used in those electronic transactions also had to be updated. (Note that at the time of this writing, the current standard to be adopted is Version 5010, although new versions will inevitably be introduced in the near future.)[11]
2. When the Centers for Medicare and Medicaid Services (CMS) staff compute transition costs, they divide some of these costs between the updating of transaction standards such as Version 5010 (which they argue would have to occur anyway) versus the cost of adopting and implementing the ICD-10 codes. We will be referring to this cost-splitting in a later discussion of implementation costs.

ICD-10 BENEFITS AND COSTS

The ICD-10 transition process will require management decisions that take both costs and benefits into account. A brief summary follows.

Benefits

Management will need to account for what their own organization will realize in conversion savings as benefits. CMS identified six benefits of transitioning to ICD-10:

- More accurate payments for new procedures
- Fewer rejected claims
- Fewer improper claims
- Improved disease management
- Better understanding of health conditions and healthcare outcomes
- Harmonization of disease monitoring and reporting worldwide[12]

In regard to recognition of other benefits, see our comment about cost-splitting in a previous paragraph, as the same concept applies to splitting benefits. Thus, the systems conversion to Version 5010 also recognizes three types of benefits, including operational savings (better standards), cost savings (increase in electronic claims transactions), and operational savings (increase in use of auxiliary transactions).[13]

Managers should also decide what potential governmental financial assistance might be available to their own organization. The ARRA legislation described in previous chapters provides financial incentives for the timely adoption of electronic health records. The ICD-10 conversion is, of course, part (but not all) of this adoption process. It is therefore logical for management to consider part of the financial incentives offered as relating to this system conversion when analyzing benefits.

Costs

Management must make decisions about major costs incurred in the ICD-10 transition, including direct adoption costs and cash flow disruption costs. Some costs will be one-time costs, while other costs will become recurring costs, and this factor must also be considered in the decision-making process.[14]

Three Types of ICD-10 Adoption Costs

CMS acknowledges that transition costs from ICD-9-CM to ICD-10 code sets are unavoidable and are incurred in addition to the Version 5010 standards conversion costs.[15] Three recognized types of ICD-10 adoption costs include the following:

1. System changes
2. Training costs
3. Productivity losses

CMS believes that large providers and institutions will most likely need to make system changes and software upgrades. However, CMS also believes small providers may only need software upgrades.[16] This belief is based upon findings that the majority of small providers have simplistic systems.[17]

Details about training costs and productivity losses are addressed within this chapter. As a final note, also see our comment about cost-splitting in a prior paragraph. Thus, systems conversion to Version 5010 recognizes two similar types of cost: system implementation costs and transition costs.[18]

Cash Flow Disruption Costs

Code set transition has a learning curve for all users. Thus, it is to be expected that a greater proportion of claims will be rejected during this learning curve. Rejected claims lead to cash flow disruption, and should be taken into account when decisions are made about implementation costs and benefits.

If certain contracts contain stipulations as to ICD-9 codes, these contracts may have to be renegotiated. The much greater specificity of the ICD-10 codes may make such renegotiation necessary in certain cases, and cash flow from contracts may be disrupted in the interim.

ICD-10 IMPLEMENTATION: SYSTEMS AFFECTED AND TECHNOLOGY ISSUES

ICD-10 implementation affects numerous computerized systems and creates complex technology issues, as discussed in the following sections.

SYSTEMS AND APPLICATIONS AFFECTED BY THE ICD-10 CHANGE

The ICD-10 technology changes that we will discuss in the following section impact a broad variety of systems and applications. It is important for the manager to fully understand the breadth and depth of change that is required by the technological transition from ICD-9 to ICD-10. **Figure 26–3** illustrates the types of systems and applications that must change.

Necessary Revisions to Vendor Software and Systems for Transition from ICD-9 to ICD-10 include:

Ambulatory systems
Billing systems
Patient accounting systems
Physician office systems
Practice management systems
Quality measurement systems

Emergency department software
Contract management programs
Reimbursement modeling programs

Financial functions such as:
    Code assignment
    Medical records abstraction
    Claims submission
    Other financial functions

Systems used to model or calculate are also impacted by the use of ICD-10 code sets:

Acuity systems
Decision support systems and content
Patient care systems
Patient risk systems
Staffing needs systems
Selection criteria within electronic medical
    records
Presentation of clinical content for support of
    plans of care

Specifications that will need to be revised for ICD-10 use include specifications for:

Data file extracts
Reporting programs and external interfaces
Analytic software that performs business analysis
Analytic software that provides decision support
    analytics for financial and clinical management
Business rules guided by patient condition or
    procedure

Figure 26–3 Systems and Applications Affected by the ICD-10 Change.
Reproduced from 74 Federal Register 3348-9 (January 16, 2009).

Twenty-five different examples of various systems and applications are contained in Figure 26–3, divided into three categories as follows:

1. Necessary revisions to vendor software and systems
2. Systems used to model or calculate that are impacted
3. Specifications that will need to be revised[19]

UNDERSTAND TECHNOLOGY ISSUES AND PROBLEMS

Examining the details of ICD-10 code set changes will help you more fully understand the technological problems that management will face in this transition. The scope of change is illustrated in the next three exhibits.

Comparison of ICD-9-CM and ICD-10-CM Diagnosis Codes

There were approximately 13,000 ICD-9-CM diagnosis codes; now ICD-10-CM has approximately 68,000 diagnosis codes, more than a 500% increase. ICD-9-CM diagnosis codes had three to five characters in length, while ICD-10-CM's characters are three to seven characters in length. This generally means input fields have to be lengthened in order to accommodate seven characters. In addition, ICD-9-CM's first digit may be alpha (E or V) or numeric, and digits two to five are numeric, while ICD-10-CM's first digit is alpha, digits two and three are numeric, and digits four to seven are either alpha or numeric. This change means reprogramming will be required for many applications. **Exhibit 26–1** sets out a comparison of ICD-9-CM versus ICD-10-CM diagnosis codes. The exhibit includes six benefits of the new code set in addition to the three differentials previously discussed in this paragraph.[20]

Comparison of ICD-9-CM and ICD-10-CM Procedure Codes

There were approximately 3,000 ICD-9-CM procedure codes; now ICD-10-CM has approximately 87,000 available procedure codes, or 29 times as many available codes. ICD-9-CM procedure codes had three to four numbers in length, while ICD-10-CM's characters are alpha-numeric and seven characters in length. This generally means input fields have to be lengthened in order to accommodate seven characters and possibly reprogrammed to accept alpha characters. **Exhibit 26–2** sets out a comparison of ICD-9-CM versus ICD-10-CM procedure codes. The exhibit includes seven benefits of the new code set in addition to the two differentials previously discussed in this paragraph.[21]

AN EXAMPLE: COMPARISON OF OLD AND NEW ANGIOPLASTY CODES

Exhibit 26–3 sets out one example of the proliferation of codes. In the ICD-9-CM, angioplasty had one code (39.50). In the ICD-10-PCS, angioplasty has 1,170 codes.[22] *The Wall Street Journal* even used this example in a headline: "Why We Need 1,170 Angioplasty Codes."[23]

ICD-10 IMPLEMENTATION: TRAINING AND LOST PRODUCTIVITY COSTS

This section describes training and lost productivity costs for the ICD-10 transition. Also see this chapter's Appendix, entitled "ICD-10 Conversion Costs for a Midwestern Community Hospital."

Exhibit 26–1 Comparison of ICD-9-CM and ICD-10-CM Diagnosis Codes

ICD-9-CM Diagnosis Codes	ICD-10-CM Diagnosis Codes
3–5 characters in length	3–7 characters in length
Approximately 13,000 codes	Approximately 68,000 available codes
First digit may be alpha (E or V) or numeric; digits 2–5 are numeric	Digit 1 is alpha; digits 2 and 3 are numeric; digits 4–7 are alpha or numeric
Limited space for adding new codes	Flexible for adding new codes
Lacks detail	Very specific
Lacks laterality	Has laterality
Difficult to analyze data due to nonspecific codes	Specificity improves coding accuracy and richness of data for analysis
Codes are nonspecific and do not adequately define diagnoses needed for medical research	Detail improves the accuracy of data used for medical research
Does not support interoperability because it is not used by other countries	Supports interoperability and the exchange of health data between other countries and the United States

Reproduced from 73 Federal Register 49803 (August 22, 2008).

WHO GETS TRAINED ON ICD-10?

CMS identified three types of individuals who would require varying levels of training on ICD-10. These included coders, code users, and physicians.

Coders

It is vital that coders receive adequate training on the ICD-10 coding changes. CMS, therefore, estimated training costs for both full-time and part-time coders. In producing cost estimates, CMS assumed that full-time coders were primarily dedicated to hospital inpatient coding and that part-time coders worked in outpatient ambulatory settings. The difference is based on the job setting for a reason. CMS further assumed that all coders will need to learn ICD-10-CM, while the coders who work in the hospital inpatient job setting will also need to learn ICD-10-PCS.[24]

Code Users

CMS refers to the American Health Information Management Association (AHIMA) definition of code users as "anyone who needs to have some level of understanding of the

Exhibit 26–2 Comparison of ICD-9-CM and ICD-10-CM Procedure Codes

ICD-9-CM Procedure Codes	ICD-10-CM Procedure Codes
3–4 numbers in length	7 alpha-numeric characters in length
Approximately 3,000 codes	Approximately 87,000 available codes
Based upon outdated technology	Reflects current usage of medical terminology and devices
Limited space for adding new codes	Flexible for adding new codes
Lacks detail	Very specific
Lacks laterality	Has laterality
Generic terms for body parts	Detailed descriptions for body parts
Lacks description of methodology and approach for procedures	Provides detailed descriptions of methodology and approach for procedures
Limits DRG assignment	Allows DRG definitions to better recognize new technologies and devices
Lacks precision to adequately define procedures	Precisely defines procedures with detail regarding body part, approach, any device used, and qualifying information

Reproduced from 73 Federal Register 49803 (August 22, 2008).

coding system, because they review coded data, rely on reports that contain coded data, etc., but are not people who actually assign codes."[25] These users can be people who are outside of healthcare facilities: individuals such as researchers, consultants, or auditors, for example. Or these users might actually be inside the healthcare facility but are not coders. Such facility users might include upper-level management, business office and accounting personnel, clinicians and clinical departments, or corporate compliance personnel.[26]

Physicians

CMS believed that the majority of physicians did not work with codes and thus would not need training. The initial assumption was that only 1 in 10 physicians would require such knowledge. (CMS also believed that physicians would probably obtain the needed training through continuing professional education courses that they would attend anyway.)[27]

COSTS OF TRAINING

ICD-10 training costs were estimated for each category described above: coders, code users, and physicians.

Exhibit 26–3 Comparison of Old and New Angioplasty Codes

Old Code:
ICD-9-CM
Angioplasty
1 code (39.50)

New Code:
ICD-10-PCS
Angioplasty Codes
1,170 codes

Specifying body part, approach, and device, including:

047K04Z	Dilation of right femoral artery with drug-eluting intraluminal device, open approach
047KODZ	Dilation of right femoral artery with intraluminal device, open approach
047KOZZ	Dilation of right femoral artery, open approach
047K24Z	Dilation of right femoral artery with drug-eluting intraluminal device, open endoscopic approach
047K2DZ	Dilation of right femoral artery with intraluminal device, open endoscopic approach

Reproduced from the Centers for Medicare and Medicaid Services. "ICD-10 Clinical Modification/Procedure Coding System." ICN #901044 (October 2008).

Coder Training Costs

CMS initially assumed the following:

1. There were 50,000 full-time hospital coders that would need 40 hours of training apiece on both ICD-10-CM and ICD-10-PCS. The 40 hours of training was estimated to cost $2,750 apiece, including lost work time of $2,200, plus $550 for the expenses of training, for a total of $2,750 per coder.
2. Training of full-time coders would start the year before ICD-10 implementation. It was further assumed that 15% of training costs would be expended in this initial year, 75% would be expended in the year of implementation, and the remaining 15% would be expended in the year after implementation.
3. There were approximately 179,000 part-time coders who would require training only on ICD-10-CM (and not on ICD-10-PCS). The part-time coders' training expense would amount to $110 for the expenses of training, plus $440 for lost work time, for a total of $550.[28]

Code Users Training Costs

CMS estimated there were approximately 250,000 code users, of which 150,000 would work directly with codes. Each code user was estimated to need eight hours of training at $31.50 per hour or approximately $250 apiece.[29]

Physician Training Costs

CMS estimated there were approximately 1.5 million physicians in the United States, of which 1 in 10 would require training. Each physician was estimated to need four hours of training at $137 per hour or approximately $548 apiece.[30]

COSTS OF LOST PRODUCTIVITY

CMS used a productivity loss definition as follows: "The cost resulting from a slow-down in coding bills and claims because of the need to learn the new coding systems."[31] Thus, the productivity loss slowdown reflects the extra staff hours that are needed to code the same number of claims per hour as prior to the ICD-10 conversion. (For instance, Jane normally codes x claims per hour; during the first month learning the new system, she slows down to xx claims per hour.)

CMS estimated that inpatient coders would incur productivity losses for the first six months after ICD-10 implementation; they further estimated that productivity would increase (and losses thus decrease) month by month over the initial six-month period until by the end of six months, productivity has returned to its former level. It was estimated that inpatient coders would take an extra 1.7 minutes per inpatient claim in the first month. At $50 per hour, 1.7 minutes equates to $1.41 per claim.[32] ($50.00 per hour divided by 60 minutes equals $0.8333 per minute times 1.7 minutes equals $1.41 per claim.)

CMS assumed the same six-month productivity loss period for outpatient coders. CMS further assumed that outpatient claims require much less time to code. In fact, the initial assumption was that outpatient claims would take one-hundredth of the time for a hospital inpatient claim. Thus, one-hundredth of the inpatient 1.7 minute productivity loss equals 0.017 minutes. At the same $50 per hour, one-hundredth of the $1.41 inpatient loss equals 0.014 per claim, or about 1.5 cents.[33] (To compute one-hundredth of $1.41, move the decimal to the left two places. Thus $1.41 becomes $0.014.) The reasoning for this small amount of coding time per claim is that physician offices "may use preprinted forms or touch-screens that require virtually no time to code."[34]

ICD-10 IMPLEMENTATION: SITUATIONAL ANALYSIS

System implementation on this scale requires multiple planning cycles. Recommendations for implementation planning that include situational analysis are described as follows.

IMPLEMENTATION PLANNING RECOMMENDATIONS

CMS recommends that healthcare organizations plan for implementation of ICD-10-CM/PCS by developing a three-step organizational plan that includes the following:

- Step 1: Situational Analysis
- Step 2: Strategic Implementation/Organizing
- Step 3: Planning for Strategic Control[35]

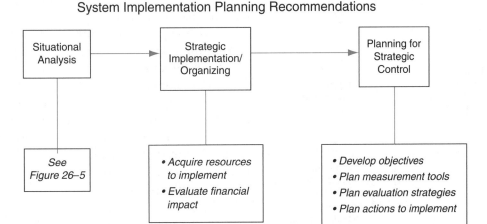

Figure 26–4 System Implementation Planning Recommendations.
Adapted from the Centers for Medicare and Medicaid Services. "ICD-10 Clinical Modification/Procedure Coding System." ICN #901044 (October 2008).

Figure 26–4 illustrates these steps. We believe that development of a timeline and a map of individual responsibilities should also be an important part of this planning process, as follows:

1. Situational Analysis: Situational analysis is defined and discussed in the following section.
2. Strategic Implementation and Organizing: The strategic implementation and organizing planning step includes acquiring the resources to implement the plan and evaluating the financial impact of the plan. In actual fact, these two steps should be reversed, as the scope of the financial impact should be considered before resources are acquired.
3. Planning for Strategic Control: Developing objectives should, of course, be the first step in planning for strategic control. The remaining planning recommendations are action steps. They include planning measurement tools, evaluation strategies, and actions to implement.[36]

SITUATIONAL ANALYSIS RECOMMENDATIONS

This section provides background plus recommendations for an ICD-10 situational analysis.

Background

You will recall that situational analysis does two things. It reviews the organization's internal operations for strengths and weaknesses and it explores the organization's

Situational Analysis Recommendations

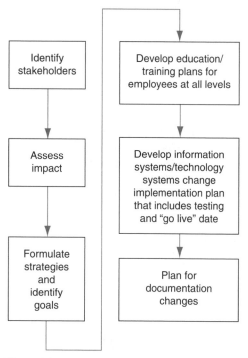

Figure 26–5 Situational Analysis
Recommendations.
Adapted from the Centers for Medicare and Medicaid
Services. "ICD-10 Clinical Modification/Procedure
Coding System." ICN #901044 (October 2008).

external environment for opportunities
and threats. Thus it is called "SWOT," for
strengths-weaknesses-opportunities-threats.

Situational analysis is particularly appropriate for the analysis of electronic records
systems implementation such as ICD-10 because such implementation requires the collaboration of multiple knowledge areas. A
meeting of the minds can better occur with
the discipline that a situational analysis can
impose. As we have previously said, it is a powerful tool when properly applied.

CMS Recommendations for ICD-10 Adoption

CMS recommends six steps for an ICD-10 adoption situational analysis. We believe the six steps
should be divided into two parts. The first part
contains strategic steps that must be addressed
at the beginning of the project. The second
part of the analysis contains developmental
steps that we believe can only be properly accomplished after the strategic steps have been
completed. (That said, however, we must also
acknowledge that sometimes immovable deadlines and/or lack of sufficient planning resources do not allow the ideal two-part process.)
Figure 26–5 illustrates the CMS situational analysis recommendations for ICD-10 adoption.

Strategic Steps

The strategic steps that CMS recommends include three steps, as follows:

1. Stakeholders: Step 1 is to identify stakeholders. This traditional first step is an important
   beginning point for the analysis. The array of stakeholders will vary depending upon
   the size and nature of the healthcare organization. Payers should always be one of the
   stakeholders. Regulatory agencies may also be recognized as stakeholders.
2. Impacts: Step 2 involves assessing the impact of the ICD-10 transition. Impacts on
   all aspects of the organization should be recognized. As with stakeholders, the
   transition's impact will also vary significantly depending upon the size and type of
   healthcare organization.
3. Strategies and Goals: Step 3 involves formulating strategies and identifying goals. The
   larger the organization the more likely there will be competing strategies and goals.
   Compromises may have to be negotiated. Tight deadlines and/or lack of planning
   resources may work to shortchange this component of the situational analysis.[37]

Developmental Steps

The developmental steps that CMS recommends also include three steps, discussed as follows. Note that different knowledge areas are required for these different steps.

1. Training Plans: Training plans must be developed for employees at all levels. The cost of training for ICD-10-CM/PCS implementation is discussed and illustrated in the following chapter.
2. Systems Change Implementation Plan: Information systems and/or technology systems "change implementation plans" must be developed. These plans must include timelines and individual responsibilities. The timelines should leave sufficient time for testing. (Insufficient testing time is a common pitfall.) A "go live" date is another important part of this plan. If hardware and/or software vendors are involved in a facility's implementation plan, all timelines and the final "go live" date must also be coordinated closely with the vendor.
3. Documentation Change Plan: The documentation change plan will hopefully cover all areas of the organization where documents exist that will reflect ICD-10-CM/PCS changes. A document inventory is the ideal beginning point for a documentation change plan. The inventory allows for a full and complete change plan, but lack of resources often means completing the full document inventory is not possible.[38]

COMMENCING AN INFORMATION TECHNOLOGY SWOT MATRIX FOR ICD-10

This section discusses building a situational analysis matrix. The example used involves ICD-10 adoption as the project under consideration and information technology as the division or department involved in the project.

Background

Building a SWOT matrix can be an important strategic process. Each of the four components of a SWOT (strengths, weaknesses, opportunities, and threats) was discussed in a previous chapter about strategic planning. The SWOT analysis matrix containing all four components was also presented in that chapter. You will recall that the "Strengths" and "Weaknesses" sectors of the matrix were labeled "Internal," while the "Opportunities" and "Threats" sectors were labeled "External." We will use this format in the following section.

Building the Matrix

As to the internal components, the SWOT team or task force needs to evaluate resources and thus identify those that should belong in the strengths and weaknesses sectors of the SWOT matrix. For example, for an Information Technology (IT) analysis such as the ICD-10 adoption issue, the team might enter "Financial Resources" as a main heading and "Capital Resources Available" as one of the Financial Resources subheadings in the strengths and weaknesses categories.

The team might also enter "Information Technology" as a main heading. Because this is an IT project, some of the subheadings in the strengths and weaknesses categories might include the following:

- IT Hardware Resources
- IT Software Resources
- IT Storage Capacity
- IT Staffing Capacity
- IT Staffing Knowledge Levels

Understand that the SWOT matrix is built as these resources are evaluated. As to the external components, the SWOT team or task force would likewise evaluate the external opportunities and threats as a parallel exercise. In an IT analysis such as the ICD-10 adoption issue, the team might logically enter the government's incentive payment as an external opportunity (potential dollars received) and an external threat (compliance requirements to be met).

The basic SWOT matrix in its present stage is illustrated in **Figure 26–6**. For further information about building a situational analysis, see the SWOT Worksheets and related Question Guides that appear as an Appendix to the Strategic Planning chapter.

Summary

The four-part SWOT matrix is built as the key internal resources, both strengths and weaknesses, are evaluated, and the key external opportunities and threats are identified and evaluated. We can tie the CMS recommendations in the preceding section to the process of building a SWOT matrix as follows. Identifying stakeholders and commencing to assess impacts of the ICD-10 adoption are considered part of building the SWOT matrix. Formulating strategies and identifying goals would most likely come after building the initial matrix, because these actions would be influenced and should naturally carry forward from the evaluations performed as part of the SWOT matrix-building process. Finally, the remaining three developmental steps, each of which involves creating a plan, should all come as final steps in the situational analysis process.

As we have previously mentioned, there are a variety of approaches to performing a situational analysis, and this brief discussion features only the single approach as recommended by CMS. The important point is this: no matter what approach is utilized, a situational analysis is an important planning tool.

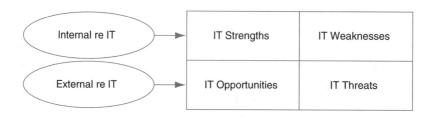

Figure 26–6 Basic Information Technology SWOT Analysis Format.

PROJECT MANAGEMENT FROM THE MANAGER'S VIEWPOINT

This section addresses the manager's challenge, presents a project management format for ICD-10 transition, and closes with comments about the manager's role.

THE MANAGER'S CHALLENGE

Information systems are both a challenge and an opportunity for the manager. Consider the recent and ongoing healthcare changes. This chapter discusses the technical aspects of the ICD-10 transition and what you need to know about implementing the necessary changes.

The overall system changes are expected to transition over a period of years due to a variety of compliance date deadlines. During this transition period, a manager who understands the underlying technology issues can develop and/or strengthen needed skills. Then, he or she is in a position to support the implementation plan and work to assist change within the organization.

PROJECT MANAGEMENT BY PHASES

We have divided the essential activities for an ICD-10 transition project into five sequential phases as follows. Certain activities as described may be switched or time-frames may be shortened in the case of smaller organizations with fewer personnel. **Figure 26–7** summarizes the management phases. The five phases are further described as follows.

Phase 1

Phase 1 sets up the project. The choices made for these first steps may well determine success of the overall transition project.

Create a Project Team

The ICD-10 transition affects virtually all areas of the organization's operations. For that reason the ICD-10 project team should be multidisciplinary. Suggested team members include the following:

- Senior management
- Health information management
- Finance
- Coding
- Billing
- Revenue cycle management
- Information systems and technology[39]

In a smaller organization it is possible that a single individual may fulfill more than one of the roles listed above.

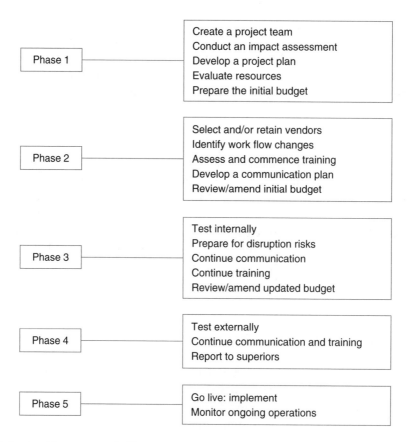

Figure 26–7 Project Management in Phases.
Courtesy of J.J. Baker and R.W. Baker, Dallas, Texas.

The team should first identify initial tasks and a project manager. Team priorities as the project commences should include the following:

- Create a project budget
- Identify stakeholders
- Develop a project timeline
- Establish a schedule of team meetings[40]

The project budget should include relevant costs such as software and training. This budget should be both comprehensive and realistic. Both internal and external stakeholders should be identified and their involvement assured. The project timeline should be realistic, well-defined, and suited to your organization.[41]

Conduct an Impact Assessment

The impact assessment issue has been discussed in a previous section of this chapter. It is important to allow adequate time to prepare and review an effective assessment.

Develop a Project Plan

The project plan should contain, as a minimum, the following:

- Identify and document project tasks
- Incorporate results of impact assessment
- Create an initial timeline
- Develop project milestones[42]

Each task involved in the project should be identified within the project plan. The deadline and the responsible person must also be identified. All of this information about tasks should then be documented in a structured format. A timeline should be developed to commence the project, with the knowledge that an initial timeline will unavoidably change as the project moves forward. The milestones that are developed for accountability will also have to move when the timeline is amended.

Evaluate Resources

Several types of resources should be evaluated at this point, including the following:

- The ICD-10 impact assessment
- Internal financial and staffing resources
- External information resources

The impact assessment will provide invaluable resource information if it has been properly prepared. The assessment should then guide an evaluation of internal financial and staffing resources. The external information resources are typically gathered from sources such as reliable trade organizations. The information resources should include data about best practices for this project.

Prepare the Initial Budget

The project budget should be first estimated. The budget's funding should then be secured. Budget items for this project would typically include the following:

- Updates to information technology systems specifically for ICD-10
- Updates to management systems that will also refer to ICD-10
- New coding guides and other related materials
- Staff training[43]

The budget's funding requirements should match the project timeline, but this ideal state of affairs does not always happen. The project manager is responsible for coordinating the availability of necessary funds.

Phase 2

Phase 2 commences the actual transition. In this phase the manager must fully understand the entire scope of the project, and his or her role in it, including timelines and accountability.

Select and/or Retain Vendors

Vendors may include software and/or systems salesmen, clearinghouses, and billing services. Review each contract and/or proposal. Ask potential vendors about required system changes (or a new system) and costs, guarantees, and system support. Ask about their testing schedules, including a start date and an end date for the transition project. Also ask to what degree your organization's own staff may be involved.[44]

Identify Work Flow Changes

The organization's work flow and processes will necessarily undergo changes due to ICD-10 implementation within items such as the following:

- Clinical documentation
- Internal reporting forms
- Quality measures reporting
- Public health reporting[45]

It is advisable to document the existing work flow and then specify the changes that will have to occur.

Assess and Commence Training

First, perform a needs assessment to determine who will need training within the organization. Then develop a training plan that indicates how much training each individual will require, at basic, intermediate, or advanced levels.

Gather information about available training resources. CMS and industry organizations such as the American Hospital Association and the American Medical Association are all good sources for training modules. Finally, commence training in accordance with a planned timeline.

Develop a Communication Plan

CMS has described the purpose of a communication and awareness plan, saying that it "ensures that all your employees and other internal departments as well as external business partners understand their roles and responsibilities for ICD-10 implementation. Think of this communication plan as a formal roadmap for communicating about ICD-10 throughout the transition."[46] Include both payers and vendors as external business partners in the communication plan. Ask them for scheduled updates, and incorporate these updates as milestones within your plan.[47]

Review/Amend Initial Budget

Review and amend your initial budget as needed. As time goes on, the project progresses and circumstances change. The project's budget needs to be reviewed and updated to reflect these changes.

Phase 3

At Phase 3 the organization should be well into transition mode. In this phase the manager must keep his or her part of the project on track. Cooperation among team members is essential.

Test Internally

The internal transaction testing should be performed along with related payer communication. Specifically, payers should be asked the following:

- Will you be able to meet the ICD-10 deadline and where are you currently in your transition process?
- Will you accept test transactions from my organization? If so, when? What are your specifications?
- Will there be any policy changes due to the ICD-10 transition? Do you anticipate any payment delays?[48]

Prepare for Disruption Risks

The transition from ICD-9 to ICD-10 may cause problems with billing. Disruption in billing means delay in receiving payment for services rendered, and sometimes these delays can be for a significant time period. If so, normal cash flow can be severely diminished or even cut off for a time. It is good planning to secure a line of credit as a precaution. Another plan to cushion the risk of disruption is to arrange for the potential backup services of a billing company.[49]

Continue Communication

Continue communication with internal team members, internal and external stakeholders and your vendors, payers, clearinghouses, and billing companies. Continue to share any revised implementation plans and timelines so that transition activities are coordinated.[50]

Continue Training

Basic training modules and most intermediate training modules should be completed by Phase 3. At this stage it may be helpful to use the actual internal testing results at the advanced training level.

Review/Amend Updated Budget

Review the project's progress and current needs. Then review the project's budget to see if it is still realistic and amend as needed. It is not always easy to increase the project budget at this point, but success of the transition may depend upon having the financial resources that are necessary for success.

Phase 4

Phase 4 is the final phase before actually going live. In this phase the manager should find and correct any weak spots in the systems.

Test Externally

Allow for plenty of time while testing multiple types of transactions, especially claims.[51] As in any well-run transition plan, it is desirable to run parallel for awhile before abandoning the old existing system. Therefore the timeframe must accommodate this run-parallel testing phase as well.

Continue Communication and Training

Continue communication and training as appropriate. It is especially important to plan structured and uniform training courses for new staff members who may be hired after the transition is completed. Also plan to share lessons learned from prior phases of the project.

Report to Superiors

Now is the time to prepare a progress report on the transition project. The report should contain mention of team members, timelines, milestones achieved, and adherence to the project budget.

Phase 5

Phase 5 represents completion of the transition project. Now it is time to actually implement the ICD-10 system.

Go Live: Implement

"Going live" means fully implementing the new ICD-10 system. At this stage it is up and running and should be fully operational. Some problems will still arise, but they should be handled with more or less routine troubleshooting.

Monitor Ongoing Operations

The responsibility and accountability for this project should be handed over to operations personnel at the close of the transition project. However, ongoing operations should continue to be monitored in a structured reporting format by the operations staff.

THE MANAGER'S ROLE

You the manager need to identify tasks required during the transition period and perform them. These tasks could involve aspects of planning, creating, evaluating, testing, or even all of the above. In other words, you as an observant manager can work to support aspects of the implementation plan that fall within your areas of responsibility, whether it involves, for example, information technology or the training plans. Understanding the scope, depth, and importance of the ICD-10 transition project will help you be a successful manager.

APPENDIX 26-A: ICD-10 CONVERSION COSTS FOR A MIDWESTERN COMMUNITY HOSPITAL

Appendix 26-A describes ICD-10 conversion costs for a midwestern community hospital.

INFORMATION CHECKPOINT

What is needed?	An ICD-10 newsletter or course announcement or an ICD-10 training manual.
Where is it found?	Within your place of work or posted on the website of an industry trade organization.
How is it used?	It is used for the purpose of ICD-10 training.

 KEY TERMS

Code Users
ICD-10 Codes
Project Management Phases
Situational Analysis
SWOT Analysis
Version 5010 of Standards

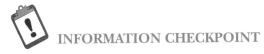 DISCUSSION QUESTIONS

1. Do you believe your place of work (the organization) has been affected by the ICD-10 transition? If so, how has your organization been affected? If not, why not?
2. Has your own area of work been involved in the transition to ICD-10? If so, are you aware of how project management progressed? If you had to ability to do so, how would you have changed management of the project?
3. Do you believe it was a good idea to extend the deadline for ICD-10 implementation? If so, why? If not, why not?

NOTES

1. National Center for Health Statistics, International Classification of Diseases, Tenth Revision (ICD-10). www.cdc.gov/nchs/about/major/dvs/icd10des.htm
2. World Health Organization, Classifications. www.who.int/classifications/icd/en/
3. CMS, ICD-10 Clinical Modification/Procedure Coding System Fact Sheet. www.cms.hhs.gov/MLNProducts/downloads/ICD-10factsheet2008.pdf
4. National Center for Health Statistics (NCHS), About the International Classification of Diseases, Tenth Revision, Clinical Modification (ICD-10-CM). www.cdc.gov/nchs/icd/icd10cm.htm

5. CMS, ICD-10-CM-PCS Fact Sheet.

6. Ibid.

7. 77 Federal Register (FR) 54665 (September 5, 2012).

8. 74 Federal Register (FR) 3357 (January 16, 2009).

9. CMS, "New Health Care Electronic Transactions Standards Versions 5010, D.0, and 3.0," Medicare Learning Network Fact Sheet ICN #903192 (January 2010).

10. 74 Federal Register (FR) 3328 (January 16, 2009).

11. 73 Federal Register (FR) 49745 (August 22, 2008).

12. 73 Federal Register (FR) 49821 (August 22, 2008).

13. Ibid., 49769.

14. Ibid., 49811.

15. Ibid., 49813.

16. Ibid., 49818.

17. Ibid., 49829.

18. Ibid., 49769.

19. 74 Federal Register (FR) 3348-9 (January 16, 2009).

20. 73 Federal Register (FR) 49803 (August 22, 2008).

21. Ibid.

22. CMS, ICD-10-CM-PCS Fact Sheet.

23. J. Zhang, "Why We Need 1,170 Angioplasty Codes," *Wall Street Journal*, November 11, 2008.

24. 73 Federal Register (FR) 49814-5 (August 22, 2008).

25. Ibid., 49815-6.

26. Ibid., 49815.

27. Ibid., 49816.

28. Ibid., 49815.

29. Ibid., 49816 and 74 Federal Register (FR) 3346-7 (January 16, 2009).

30. Ibid., 49816.

31. M. Libicki and I. Brahmakulam, The Costs and Benefits of Moving to the ICD-10 Code Sets (Santa Monica, CA: RAND Corporation, 2004), 10. http://www.rand .org/pubs/technical_reports/2004/RAND_TR132.pdf

32. 73 Federal Register (FR) 49816 (August 22, 2008) and 74 Federal Register (FR) 3346-7 (January 16, 2009).

33. 73 Federal Register (FR) 49817 (August 22, 2008).

34. Ibid., 49816-7.

35. CMS, ICD-10-CM-PCS Fact Sheet.

36. Ibid.

37. Ibid.

38. Ibid.

39. CMS, ICD-10 News Updates (January 10, 2013) and (August 1, 2012).

40. Ibid.

41. Ibid.

42. CMS, ICD-10 News Updates (January 10, 2013).

43. Ibid.

44. CMS, ICD-10 News Updates (January 10, 2013) and (August 1, 2012).
45. CMS, ICD-10 Basics for Medical Practices Fact Sheet (September 2012).
46. CMS, ICD-10 News Updates (August 16, 2012).
47. Ibid. (January 10, 2013).
48. Ibid. (November 7, 2012).
49. Ibid. (January 3, 2013).
50. Ibid. (October 3, 2012).
51. Ibid. (January 3, 2013).

ICD-10 Conversion Costs for a Midwestern Community Hospital

AUTHORS' NOTE

This CMS example illustrates the computation of hospital training costs and productivity loss costs and estimates a cost for system changes and upgrades in order to arrive at a total hospital ICD-10 conversion cost. We have numbered the paragraphs for easy reference. (And FYI, when the scenario below says "we" it means CMS, not the authors.)

Introduction

To further illustrate the computation of hospital ICD-10 conversion costs, CMS staff developed a scenario for a typical community hospital in the Midwest. The material presented in the appendix was published in the proposed rule as an example of costs that might be incurred by a hospital. The data were drawn from the American Hospital Directory, available at www.AHD.com. While based on an actual hospital in a midwestern state, the data have been altered to make calculations simpler.

The Scenario

1. The hospital has 100 beds, 4,000 discharges annually, and gross revenues of $200 million. Using the factors presented in the impact analysis, we estimated training costs (including the cost of the actual training as well as lost time away from the job), productivity loss for the first six months resulting from becoming familiar with the diagnostic and procedure codes, and the cost of system changes.
2. For our scenario, we assumed that the hospital employs three full-time coders who will require eight hours of training at $500 per coder for $1,500 ($500 times 3). While they are in training, the hospital will have to substitute other staff, either by hiring temporary coders if possible, or by shifting staff. The estimated cost at $50 per hour is $1,200 (8 hours times 3 staff times $50 per hour).
3. In estimating the productivity loss, we are only looking at the initial six months after implementation. Therefore, we divided the annual number of discharges of 4,000 by 2 to equal 2,000. We assume that three-quarters of the discharges are surgical, giving us 1,500 discharges requiring use of PCS codes. Dividing this by six months yields an average monthly discharge rate of 250.

4. We performed a similar calculation for outpatient claims. Of the 13,000 outpatient claims, the monthly average is 1,083 (we do not distinguish between medical and surgical outpatient claims).

5. Applying the 1.7 extra minutes per discharge, we estimated it would take an extra 425 minutes (1.7 times 250) to code the discharges in the first month. At $50 per hour, the cost per minute is $0.83 ($50 divided by 60 minutes) and the cost per claim is $1.41 ($0.83 times 1.7). For the first month, the productivity loss for inpatient coding is $353 ($1.41 times 250). Assuming for simplicity's sake that the resumption of productivity over the six-month period would increase in a straight line, we divide the $353 by six to come up with $59. We reduce the productivity loss by this amount each month through the sixth month. The total loss for the six-month period is $1,233.

6. We apply the same method to determine the outpatient productivity loss. Based on our assumption that outpatient claims will require one-hundredth of the time for hospital inpatient claims, when applying the 0.17 extra minutes per claim, we estimate it would take an extra 18.41 minutes (0.017 times 1,083) to code the discharges in the first month. At $50 per hour, the cost per minute is $0.83 ($50 divided by 60 minutes) and the cost per claim is $0.14 ($0.83 times 0.017). For the first month, the productivity loss for outpatient coding is $15.28 ($0.014 times 1,083). Assuming for simplicity sake that the resumption of productivity over the six-month period would increase in a straight line, we divide the $15.28 by six, coming up with $2.55. We reduce the productivity loss by this amount each month through the sixth month. Thus the total loss for the first six months will equal $53.

7. In estimating the cost of system changes and software upgrades, we deliberately chose a value that we think overstates the cost. We assumed that the hospital will have to spend $300,000 on its data infrastructure to accommodate the new codes. Summing the training costs, productivity losses, and system upgrades, we estimate the total cost to the hospital will equal approximately $303,990. Finally, in order to determine the percentage of the hospital's revenue that would be diverted to funding the conversion to the ICD-10, we compared the estimated cost associated with the conversion to ICD-10 to the total hospital revenue of $200 million. The costs amount to 0.15% of the hospital's annual revenues.

8. We note that although the impact in our scenario of 0.15% is significantly larger than the estimated impact of 0.03% for inpatient facilities (set out in the rule), it is still significantly below the threshold the Department considers a significant economic impact. We are of the opinion that, for most providers and suppliers, payers, and computer firms involved in facilitating the transition, the costs will be relatively small.

Source: 73 Federal Register 49830 (August 22, 2008).

Case Studies

Case Study: Strategic Financial Planning in Long-Term Care

## 27

Neil R. Dworkin, PhD

BACKGROUND

John Maxwell, CEO of Seabury Nursing Center, a not-for-profit long-term care organization located in suburban Connecticut, had just emerged from a board of directors meeting. He was contemplating the instructions he had received from the board's executive committee to assess the financial feasibility of adding a home care program to the Center's array of services.

Seabury's current services consist of two levels of inpatient care, chronic care, and subacute units, and a senior citizens' apartment complex financed in part by the Federal Department of Housing and Urban Development. In keeping with its mission, Seabury has a reputation of providing personalized, high-quality, and compassionate care across all levels of its continuum.

The CEO and his executive team agreed to meet the following week to plan the next steps.

FRAMEWORK OF THE BOARD'S MANDATE

At its last retreat, the board made clear that, reimbursement and payment systems notwithstanding, Seabury must establish realistic and achievable financial plans that are consistent with their strategic plans. Accordingly, three points relative to integrating strategic planning and financial planning should hold sway:

1. Both are the primary responsibility of the board
2. Strategic planning should precede financial planning
3. The board should play an active role in the financial planning process

Ultimately, every important investment decision involves three general principles:

1. Does it make sense financially?
2. Does it make sense operationally?
3. Does it make sense politically?

The board's interest in a possible home initiative was guided by these stipulations, particularly as they relate to Seabury's growth rate in assets and profitability objectives. As a result of the financial downturn, the organization is experiencing declining inpatient volumes, a deteriorating payer mix, and a higher cost of capital, all of which have the potential to weaken its liquidity position.

Taking the strategic service line path to a home care program would be less capital intensive and should appeal broadly to the significant baby boomer population residing in its service area, whose preference would undoubtedly be to be treated in their homes.

INDUSTRY PROFILE

When John Maxwell convened his executive team the following week, he had already decided to present an overview of the home health industry as gleaned by Seabury's Planning Department. He prefaced his comments by drawing on recent research by the federal Agency for Healthcare Research and Quality that detailed why home health care in the 21st century is different from that which has existed in the past. He cited four reasons:

1. We're living longer and more of us want to "age in place" with dignity.
2. We have more chronic, complex conditions.
3. We're leaving the hospital earlier and thus need more intensive care.
4. Sophisticated medical technology has moved into our homes. Devices that were used only in medical offices are now in our living rooms and bedrooms. For example, home caregivers regularly manage dialysis treatments, infuse strong medications via central lines, and use computer-based equipment to monitor the health of loved ones.[1]

The CEO presented a profile of national home care data as compiled by the National Association for Home Care and Hospice as follows:

- Approximately 12 million people in the United States require some form of home health care.
- More than 33,000 home healthcare providers exist today.
- Almost two-thirds (63.8%) of home healthcare recipients are women.
- More than two-thirds (69.1%) of home healthcare recipients are over age 65.
- Conditions requiring home health care most frequently include diabetes, heart failure, chronic ulcer of the skin, osteoarthritis, and hypertension.
- Medicare is the largest single payer of home care services. In 2009, Medicare spending was approximately 41% of the total home healthcare and hospice expenditure.[2]

According to the U.S. Census Bureau, he continued, in 2010 Connecticut's population was 3,574,097 of which 14.4% were age 65 or older.[3] A Visiting Nurse Association (VNA) analysis of revenue by payer source in the state indicated that 60% of revenue was derived from Medicare.[4]

FEASIBILITY DETERMINATION

The CEO went on to explain that the feasibility determination would be based on initially setting the home care program's capacity at 50 clients because that was the minimum required for Certificate-of-Need (CON) approval in Connecticut. He distributed a model developed by healthcare finance expert William O. Cleverly (**Figure 27–1**), which presents the *logic* behind the integration of strategic and financial planning.

In essence, he said, financial planning is influenced by the definition of programs and services in consort with the mission and goals. The next step entails financial feasibility of the proposed homecare program. Among the components that should be considered in determining financial feasibility are the following:

- The configuration and cost of staff
- The prevailing Medicare and Medicaid reimbursement rates

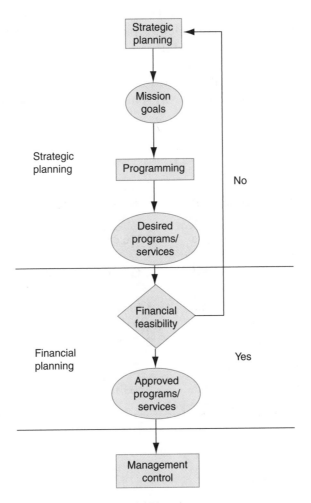

Figure 27–1 Integration of Strategic and Financial Planning.
Reproduced from W.O. Cleverley, *Essentials of Health Care Finance,* 7th ed. (Sudbury, MA: Jones & Bartlett), 289.

- A projection of visit frequency by provider category based on the most prevalent clinical conditions
- The physical location of the program and its attendant costs (e.g., rent, new construction)
- A projection of cash flows

Direct care staff associated with the home care program includes:

- Medical Social Worker (MSW)
- Physical Therapist (PT)
- Home Health Aide (HHA)
- Registered Nurse (RN)
- Registered Dietitian (RD)

Maxwell indicated that it would be useful to create a scenario depicting a home health visit abstract incorporating prevailing Medicare and Medicaid reimbursement rates for a 70-year-old male with heart failure and no comorbidities in order to gain traction and project potential cash flow. As previously noted, heart failure is a condition frequently requiring home healthcare services. Productivity in the home is typically based on the average number of visits per day by provider category. The visit scenario is depicted in **Table 27–1**.

Table 27–1 A Home Health Visit Scenario

Services	Visit Frequency	Payer	Rate	Rate x 4.2*	Medicare Cost	Medicaid Cost
Nursing (RN)	2x/month, every other week	Mc	$ 166.83	$ 700.69	$ 700.69	
Medical Social Worker (MSW)	Visits wkly for 4 wks	MA	$ 119.51	$ 501.94		$ 501.94
Physical Therapist (PT)	3x wkly for 2 wks	Mc	$ 103.22	$ 433.52	$ 433.52	
Home Health Aide (HHA)	Visits 4hrs MWF wkly for 60 days	Mc	$ 25.00	$ 1,260.00	$ 1,260.00	
Registered Dietitian (RD)	3x wkly for 1 wk	MA	$ 103.16			$ 309.48

Mc = Medicare

MA = Medicaid

*4.2 = The state's formula for the #wks/ per month

Total monthly Medicaid budget = $826.95

Total monthly Medicare budget = $2,394.21

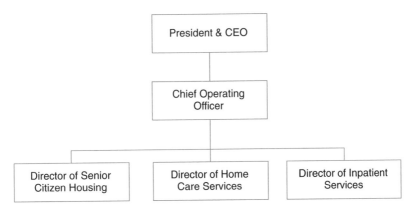

Figure 27–2 Seabury Nursing Center's Home Healthcare-Related Organization Chart.

Once the board decides to move ahead with the home care program and it is approved by the state, implementation and ongoing operations becomes a management control issue (see the Cleverly model in Figure 27–1). The CEO refers to a proposed table of organization as illustrated in **Figure 27–2**.

Given the paucity of other home care programs in its service area, Maxwell knows that Seabury is likely to be accorded a green light.

As he and his team reflect on this, the looming question will be where will the clients come from? He knows that likely referral sources will include Seabury's subacute inpatient population and residents from its senior citizens' apartment complex who are "aging in place." Other likely sources will be recently discharged patients from the region's two community hospitals, both bereft of home care programs. A premium will be placed on effective case management, and direct marketing to the community will also be necessary.

NOTES

1. U.S. Department of Health and Human Services, "Human Factors Challenges in Home Health Care," *Research Activities,* no. 376 (December 2011).
2. National Association for Home Care and Hospice, *Basic Statistics about Home Care* (Updated 2010).
3. Department of Commerce, U.S. Census Bureau, *2010 Demographic Profile.*
4. Visiting Nurse Association, *VNA Healthcare Annual Report* (Hartford, CT: Hartford Healthcare, 2012).

Case Study: Metropolis Health System

## 28

BACKGROUND

1. The Hospital System

Metropolis Health System (MHS) offers comprehensive healthcare services. It is a midsize taxing district hospital. Although MHS has the power to raise revenues through taxes, it has not done so for the past seven years.

2. The Area

MHS is located in the town of Metropolis, which has a population of 50,000. The town has a small college and a modest number of environmentally clean industries.

3. MHS Services

MHS has taken significant steps to reduce hospital stays. It has developed a comprehensive array of services that are accessible, cost-effective, and responsive to the community's needs. These services are wellness oriented in that they strive for prevention rather than treatment. As a result of these steps, inpatient visits have increased overall by only 1,000 per year since 2008, whereas outpatient/same-day surgery visits have had an increase of over 50,000 per year.

A number of programmatic, service, and facility enhancements support this major transition in the community's institutional health care. They are geared to provide the quality, convenience, affordability, and personal care that best suit the health needs of the people whom MHS serves.

- Rehabilitation and Wellness Center—for outpatient physical therapy and return-to-work services, plus cardiac and pulmonary rehabilitation, to get people back to a normal way of living.
- Home Health Services—bringing skilled care, therapy, and medical social services into the home; a comfortable and affordable alternative in longer-term care.
- Same-Day Surgery (SDS)—eliminating the need for an overnight stay. Since 1998, same-day surgery procedures have doubled at MHS.
- Skilled Nursing Facility—inpatient service to assist patients in returning more fully to an independent lifestyle.

- Community Health and Wellness—community health outreach programs that provide educational seminars on a variety of health issues, a diabetes education center, support services for patients with cancer, health awareness events, and a women's health resource center.
- Occupational Health Services—helping to reduce workplace injury costs at over 100 area businesses through consultation on injury avoidance and work-specific rehabilitation services.
- Recovery Services—offering mental health services, including substance abuse programs and support groups, along with individual and family counseling.

4. MHS's Plant

The central building for the hospital is in the center of a two-square-block area. A physicians' office building is to the west. Two administrative offices, converted from former residences, are on one corner. The new ambulatory center, completed two years ago, has an L shape and sits on one corner of the western block. A laundry and maintenance building sits on the extreme back of the property. A four-story parking garage is located on the eastern back corner. An employee parking lot sits beside the laundry and maintenance building. Visitor parking lots fill the front eastern portion of the property. A helipad is on the extreme western edge of the property behind the physicians' office building.

5. MHS Board of Trustees

Eight local community leaders who bring diverse skills to the board govern MHS. The trustees generously volunteer their time to plan the strategic direction of MHS, thus ensuring the system's ability to provide quality comprehensive health care to the community.

6. MHS Management

A chief executive officer manages MHS. Seven senior vice presidents report to the CEO. MHS is organized into 23 major responsibility centers.

7. MHS Employees

All 500 team members employed by MHS are integral to achieving the high standards for which the system strives. The quality improvement program, reviewed and reestablished in 2010, is aimed at meeting client needs sooner, better, and more cost-effectively. Participants in the program are from all areas of the system.

8. MHS Physicians

The MHS medical staff is a key part of MHS's ability to provide excellence in health care. Over 75 physicians cover more than 30 medical specialties. The high quality of their training and their commitment to the practice of medicine are great assets to the health of the community.

The physicians are very much a part of MHS's drive for continual improvement on the quality of healthcare services offered in the community. MHS brings in medical experts from around the country to provide training in new techniques, made possible by MHS's technologic advancements. MHS also ensures that physicians are offered seminars, symposiums, and continuing education programs that permit them to remain current with changes in the medical field.

The medical staff's quality improvement program has begun a care path initiative to track effective means for diagnosis, treatment, and follow-up. This initiative will help avoid unnecessary or duplicate use of expensive medications or technologies.

9. MHS Foundation

Metropolis Health Foundation is presently being created to serve as the philanthropic arm of MHS. It will operate in a separate corporation governed by a board of 12 community leaders and supported by a 15-member special events board. The mission of the foundation will be to secure financial and nonfinancial support for realizing the MHS vision of providing comprehensive health care for the community.

Funds donated by individuals, businesses, foundations, and organizations will be designated for a variety of purposes at MHS, including the operation of specific departments, community outreach programs, continuing education for employees, endowment, equipment, and capital improvements.

10. MHS Volunteer Auxiliary

There are 500 volunteers who provide over 60,000 hours of service to MHS each year. These men and women assist in virtually every part of the system's operations. They also conduct community programs on behalf of MHS.

The auxiliary funds its programs and makes financial contributions to MHS through money it raises on renting televisions and vending gifts and other items at the hospital. In the past, its donations to MHS have generally been designated for medical equipment purchases. The auxiliary has given $250,000 over the last five years.

11. Planning the Future for MHS

The MHS has identified five areas of desired service and programmatic enhancement in its five-year strategic plan:
I.   Ambulatory Services
II.   Physical Medicine and Rehabilitative Services
III.   Cardiovascular Services
IV.   Oncology Services
V.   Community Health Services

MHS has set out to answer the most critical health needs that are specific to its community. Over the next five years, the MHS strategic plan will continue a tradition of quality, community-oriented health care to meet future demands.

12. Financing the Future

MHS has established a corporate depreciation fund. The fund's purpose is to ease the financial burden of replacing fixed assets. Presently, it has almost $2 million for needed equipment and renovations.

MHS CASE STUDY

Financial Statements

- Balance Sheet (**Exhibit 28–1**)
- Statement of Revenue and Expense (**Exhibit 28–2**)

Exhibit 28–1 Balance Sheet

Metropolis Health System
Balance Sheet
March 31, 2____

Assets		Liabilities and Fund Balance	
Current Assets		Current Liabilities	
Cash and Cash Equivalents	$1,150,000	Current Maturities of Long-Term	
Assets Whose Use Is Limited	825,000	Debt	$525,000
Patient Accounts Receivable	7,400,000	Accounts Payable and Accrued	
(Net of $1,300,000 Allowance		Expenses	4,900,000
for Bad Debts)		Bond Interest Payable	300,000
Other Receivables	150,000	Reimbursement Settlement	
		Payable	100,000
Inventories	900,000		
Prepaid Expenses	200,000	Total Current Liabilities	5,825,000
Total Current Assets	10,625,000	Long-Term Debt	6,000,000
		Less Current Portion of	
Assets Whose Use Is Limited		Long-Term Debt	(525,000)
Corporate Funded		Net Long-Term Debt	5,475,000
Depreciation	1,950,000		
		Total Liabilities	11,300,000
Held by Trustee Under Bond			
Indenture Agreement	1,425,000	Fund Balances	
		General Fund	21,500,000
Total Assets Whose Use Is			
Limited	3,375,000	Total Fund Balances	21,500,000
Less Current Portion	(825,000)	Total Liabilities and Fund	
		Balances	$32,800,000
Net Assets Whose Use Is			
Limited	2,550,000		
Property, Plant, and			
Equipment, Net	19,300,000		
Other Assets	325,000		
Total Assets	$32,800,000		

Exhibit 28–2 Statement of Revenue and Expense

Metropolis Health System
Statement of Revenue and Expense
for the Year Ended March 31, 2___

Revenue		
Net patient service revenue	$34,000,000	
Other revenue	1,100,000	
Total Operating Revenue		$35,100,000
Expenses		
Nursing services	$5,025,000	
Other professional services	13,100,000	
General services	3,200,000	
Support services	8,300,000	
Depreciation	1,900,000	
Amortization	50,000	
Interest	325,000	
Provision for doubtful accounts	1,500,000	
Total Expenses		33,400,000
Income from Operations		$1,700,000
Nonoperating Gains (Losses)		
Unrestricted gifts and memorials	$20,000	
Interest income	80,000	
Nonoperating Gains, Net		100,000
Revenue and Gains in Excess of Expenses and Losses		$1,800,000

- Statement of Cash Flows (**Exhibit 28–3**)
- Statement of Changes in Fund Balance (**Exhibit 28–4**)
- Schedule of Property, Plant, and Equipment (**Exhibit 28–5**)
- Schedule of Patient Revenue (**Exhibit 28–6**)
- Schedule of Operating Expenses (**Exhibit 28–7**)

Statistics and Organizational Structure

- Hospital Statistical Data (**Exhibit 28–8**)
- MHS Nursing Practice and Administration Organization Chart (**Figure 28–1**)
- MHS Executive-Level Organization Chart (**Figure 28–2**)

Exhibit 28–3 Statement of Cash Flows

Metropolis Health System
Statement of Cash Flows
for the Year Ended March 31, 2___

Statement of Cash Flows

Operating Activities	
Income from operations	$1,700,000
Adjustments to reconcile income from operations	
to net cash flows from operating activities	
Depreciation and amortization	1,950,000
Changes in asset and liability accounts	
Patient accounts receivable	250,000
Other receivables	(50,000)
Inventories	(50,000)
Prepaid expenses and other assets	(50,000)
Accounts payable and accrued expenses	(400,000)
Reduction of bond interest payable	(25,000)
Estimated third-party payer settlements	(75,000)
Interest income received	80,000
Unrestricted gifts and memorials received	20,000
Net cash flow from operating activities	$3,350,000
Cash Flows from Capital and Related Financing Activities	
Repayment of long-term obligations	(500,000)
Cash Flows from Investing Activities	
Purchase of assets whose use is limited	(100,000)
Equipment purchases and building improvements	(2,000,000)
Net Increase (Decrease) in Cash and Cash Equivalents	$750,000
Cash and Cash Equivalents, Beginning of Year	400,000
Cash and Cash Equivalents, End of Year	$1,150,000

Exhibit 28–4 Statement of Changes in Fund Balance

Metropolis Health System Statement of Changes in Fund Balance for the Year Ended March 31, 2___	
General Fund Balance April 1, 2____	$19,700,000
Revenue and Gains in Excess of Expenses and Losses	1,800,000
General Fund Balance March 31, 2____	$21,500,000

Exhibit 28–5 Schedule of Property, Plant, and Equipment

Metropolis Health System Schedule of Property, Plant, and Equipment for the Year Ended March 31, 2___	
Buildings and Improvements	$14,700,000
Land Improvements	1,100,000
Equipment	28,900,000
Total	$44,700,000
Less Accumulated Depreciation	(26,100,000)
Net Depreciable Assets	$18,600,000
Land	480,000
Construction in Progress	220,000
Net Property, Plant, and Equipment	$19,300,000

Exhibit 28–6 Schedule of Patient Revenue

Metropolis Health System
Schedule of Patient Revenue
for the Year Ended March 31, 2___

Patient Services Revenue	
Routine revenue	$9,850,000
Laboratory	7,375,000
Radiology and CT scanner	5,825,000
OB–nursery	450,000
Pharmacy	3,175,000
Emergency service	2,200,000
Medical and surgical supply and IV	5,050,000
Operating rooms	5,250,000
Anesthesiology	1,600,000
Respiratory therapy	900,000
Physical therapy	1,475,000
EKG and EEG	1,050,000
Ambulance service	900,000
Oxygen	575,000
Home health and hospice	1,675,000
Substance abuse	375,000
Other	775,000
Subtotal	$48,500,000
Less allowances and charity care	(14,500,000)
Net Patient Service Revenue	$34,000,000

Exhibit 28–7 Schedule of Operating Expenses

Metropolis Health System
Schedule of Operating Expenses
for the Year Ended March 31, 2____

Nursing Services		General Services	
Routine Medical/Surgical	$3,880,000	Dietary	$1,055,000
Operating Room	300,000	Maintenance	1,000,000
Intensive Care Units	395,000	Laundry	295,000
OB–Nursery	150,000	Housekeeping	470,000
Other	300,000	Security	50,000
Total	$5,025,000	Medical Records	330,000
		Total	$3,200,000
Other Professional Services			
Laboratory	$2,375,000	Support Services	
Radiology and CT Scanner	1,700,000	General	$4,600,000
Pharmacy	1,375,000	Insurance	240,000
Emergency Service	950,000	Payroll Taxes	1,130,000
Medical and Surgical Supply	1,800,000	Employee Welfare	1,900,000
Operating Rooms and		Other	430,000
Anesthesia	1,525,000	Total	$8,300,000
Respiratory Therapy	525,000		
Physical Therapy	700,000	Depreciation	1,900,000
EKG and EEG	185,000	Amortization	50,000
Ambulance Service	80,000		
Substance Abuse	460,000	Interest Expense	325,000
Home Health and Hospice	1,295,000		
Other	130,000	Provision for Doubtful	
Total	$13,100,000	Accounts	1,500,000
		Total Operating Expenses	$33,400,000

Exhibit 28–8 Hospital Statistical Data

Metropolis Health System
Schedule of Hospital Statistics
for the Year Ended March 31, 2____

Inpatient Indicators:		Departmental Volume Indicators:	
Patient Days			
Medical and surgical	13,650	Respiratory therapy treatments	51,480
Obstetrics	1,080	Physical therapy treatments	34,050
Skilled nursing unit	4,500	Laboratory workload units	
		(in thousands)	2,750
Admissions		EKGs	8,900
Adult acute care	3,610	CT scans	2,780
Newborn	315	MRI scans	910
Skilled nursing unit	440	Emergency room visits	11,820
		Ambulance trips	2,320
Discharges		Home health visits	14,950
Adult acute care	3,580		
Newborn	315	Approximate number of employees	
Skilled nursing unit	445	(FTE)	510
Average Length of Stay (in days)	4.1		

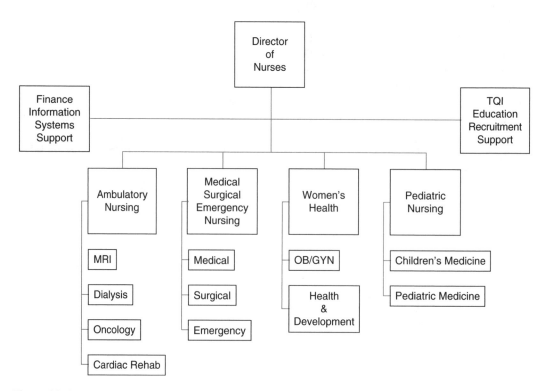

Figure 28–1 MHS Nursing Practice and Administration Organization Chart.
Courtesy of Resource Group, Ltd., Dallas, Texas.

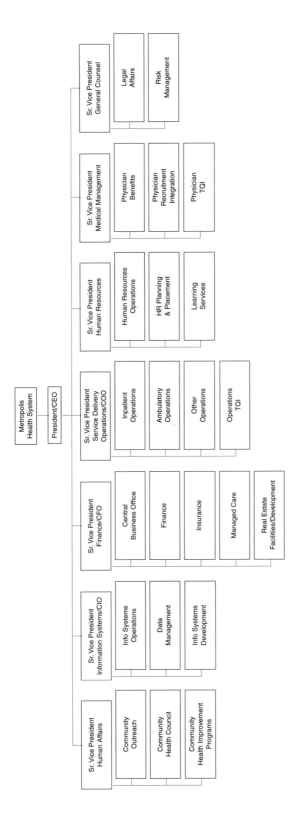

Figure 28–2 MHS Executive-Level Organization Chart.
Courtesy of Resource Group, Ltd., Dallas, Texas.

Metropolis Health System's Financial Statements and Excerpts from Notes

Metropolis Health System
Balance Sheet
March 31, 20X3 and 20X2

Assets

Current Assets		
Cash and cash equivalents	$1,150,000	$400,000
Assets whose use is limited	825,000	825,000
Patient accounts receivable	8,700,000	8,950,000
Less allowance for bad debts	(1,300,000)	(1,300,000)
Other receivables	150,000	100,000
Inventories of supplies	900,000	850,000
Prepaid expenses	200,000	150,000
Total Current Assets	10,625,000	9,975,000
Assets Whose Use Is Limited		
Corporate funded depreciation	1,950,000	1,800,000
Under bond indenture agreements— held by trustee	1,425,000	1,475,000
Total Assets Whose Use Is Limited	3,375,000	3,275,000
Less Current Portion	(825,000)	(825,000)
Net Assets Whose Use Is Limited	2,550,000	2,450,000
Property, Plant, and Equipment, Net	19,300,000	19,200,000
Other Assets	325,000	375,000
Total Assets	$32,800,000	$32,000,000

Metropolis Health System
Balance Sheet
March 31, 20X3 and 20X2

Liabilities and Fund Balance

Current Liabilities

Current maturities of long-term debt	$525,000	$500,000
Accounts payable and accrued expenses	4,900,000	5,300,000
Bond interest payable	300,000	325,000
Reimbursement settlement payable	100,000	175,000
Total Current Liabilities	5,825,000	6,300,000
Long-Term Debt	6,000,000	6,500,000
Less Current Portion of Long-Term Debt	(525,000)	(500,000)
Net Long-Term Debt	5,475,000	6,000,000
Total Liabilities	11,300,000	12,300,000

Fund Balances

General Fund	21,500,000	19,700,000
Total Fund Balances	21,500,000	19,700,000
Total Liabilities and Fund Balances	$32,800,000	$32,000,000

Metropolis Health System
Statement of Revenue and Expenses
for the Years Ended March 31, 20X3 and 20X2

Revenue

Net patient service revenue	$34,000,000		$33,600,000
Other revenue	1,100,000		1,000,000
Total Operating Revenue		35,100,000		34,600,000

Expenses

Nursing services	5,025,000		5,450,000
Other professional services	13,100,000		12,950,000
General services	3,200,000		3,220,000
Support services	8,300,000		8,340,000
Depreciation	1,900,000		1,800,000
Amortization	50,000		50,000
Interest	325,000		350,000
Provision for doubtful accounts	1,500,000		1,600,000
Total Expenses		33,400,000		33,760,000
Income from Operations		1,700,000		840,000

Nonoperating Gains (Losses)

Unrestricted gifts and memorials	20,000		70,000
Interest income	80,000		40,000
Nonoperating Gains, Net		100,000		110,000

Revenue and Gains in Excess of
Expenses and Losses $1,800,000 $950,000

Metropolis Health System
Statement of Changes in Fund Balance
for the Years Ended March 31, 20X3 and 20X2

General Fund Balance April 1st	$19,700,000	$18,750,000
Revenue and Gains in Excess of Expenses and Losses	1,800,000	950,000
General Fund Balance March 31st	$21,500,000	$19,700,000

Metropolis Health System
Schedule of Property, Plant, and Equipment
for the Years Ended March 31, 20X3 and 20X2

Buildings and Improvements	$14,700,000	$14,000,000
Land Improvements	1,100,000	1,100,000
Equipment	28,900,000	27,600,000
Total	44,700,000	42,700,000
Less Accumulated Depreciation	(26,100,000)	(24,200,000)
Net Depreciable Assets	18,600,000	18,500,000
Land	480,000	480,000
Construction in Progress	220,000	220,000
Net Property, Plant, and Equipment	$19,300,000	$19,200,000

Metropolis Health System
Schedule of Patient Revenue
for the Years Ended March 31, 20X3 and 20X2

Patient Services Revenue

	20X3	20X2
Routine revenue	$9,850,000	$9,750,000
Laboratory	7,375,000	7,300,000
Radiology and CT scanner	5,825,000	5,760,000
OB–nursery	450,000	445,000
Pharmacy	3,175,000	3,140,000
Emergency service	2,200,000	2,180,000
Medical and surgical supply and IV	5,050,000	5,000,000
Operating rooms	5,250,000	5,200,000
Anesthesiology	1,600,000	1,580,000
Respiratory therapy	900,000	890,000
Physical therapy	1,475,000	1,460,000
EKG and EEG	1,050,000	1,040,000
Ambulance services	900,000	890,000
Oxygen	575,000	570,000
Home health and hospice	1,675,000	1,660,000
Substance abuse	375,000	370,000
Other	775,000	765,000
Subtotal	48,500,000	48,000,000
Less Allowances and Charity Care	14,500,000	14,400,000
Net Patient Service Revenue	$34,000,000	$33,600,000

Metropolis Health System
Schedule of Operating Expenses
for the Years Ended March 31, 20X3 and 20X2

Nursing Services		
Routine Medical/Surgical	$3,880,000	$4,200,000
Operating Room	300,000	325,000
Intensive Care Units	395,000	430,000
OB–Nursery	150,000	165,000
Other	300,000	330,000
Total	$5,025,000	$5,450,000
Other Professional Services		
Laboratory	$2,375,000	$2,350,000
Radiology and CT Scanner	1,700,000	1,680,000
Pharmacy	1,375,000	1,360,000
Emergency Service	950,000	930,000
Medical and Surgical Supply	1,800,000	1,780,000
Operating Rooms and Anesthesia	1,525,000	1,515,000
Respiratory Therapy	525,000	530,000
Physical Therapy	700,000	695,000
EKG and EEG	185,000	180,000
Ambulance Services	80,000	80,000
Substance Abuse	460,000	450,000
Home Health and Hospice	1,295,000	1,280,000
Other	130,000	120,000
Total	$13,100,000	$12,950,000
General Services		
Dietary	$1,055,000	$1,060,000
Maintenance	1,000,000	1,010,000
Laundry	295,000	300,000
Housekeeping	470,000	475,000
Security	50,000	50,000
Medical Records	330,000	325,000
Total	$3,200,000	$3,220,000
Support Services		
General	$4,600,000	$4,540,000
Insurance	240,000	235,000
Payroll Taxes	1,130,000	1,180,000
Employee Welfare	1,900,000	1,950,000
Other	430,000	435,000
Total	$8,300,000	$8,340,000
Depreciation	$1,900,000	$1,800,000

Amortization	50,000	50,000
Interest Expense	325,000	350,000
Provision for Doubtful Accounts	1,500,000	1,600,000
Total Operating Expenses	$33,400,000	$33,760,000

EXCERPTS FROM METROPOLIS HEALTH SYSTEM NOTES TO FINANCIAL STATEMENTS

Note 1—Nature of Operations and Summary of Significant Accounting Policies

General

Metropolis Hospital System (Hospital) currently operates as a general acute care hospital. The hospital is a municipal corporation and body politic created under the hospital district laws of the state.

Cash and Cash Equivalents

For purposes of reporting cash flows, the hospital considers all liquid investments with an original maturity of three months or less to be cash equivalents.

Inventory

Inventory consists of supplies used for patients and is stated as the lower of cost or market. Cost is determined on the basis of most recent purchase price.

Investments

Investments, consisting primarily of debt securities, are carried at market value. Realized and unrealized gains and losses are reflected in the statement of revenue and expenses. Investment income from general fund investments is reported as nonoperating gains.

Income Taxes

As a municipal corporation of the state, the hospital is exempt from federal and state income taxes under Section 115 of the Internal Revenue Code.

Property, Plant, and Equipment

Expenditures for property, plant, and equipment, and items that substantially increase the useful lives of existing assets are capitalized at cost. The hospital provides for depreciation on the straight-line method at rates designed to depreciate the costs of assets over estimated useful lives as follows:

	Years
Equipment	5 to 20
Land Improvements	20 to 25
Buildings and Improvements	40

Funded Depreciation

The hospital's Board of Directors has adopted the policy of designating certain funds that are to be used to fund depreciation for the purpose of improvement, replacement, or expansion of plant assets.

Unamortized Debt Issue Costs

Revenue bond issue costs have been deferred and are being amortized.

Revenue and Gains in Excess of Expenses and Losses

The statement of revenue and expenses includes revenue and gains in excess of expenses and losses. Changes in unrestricted net assets that are excluded from excess of revenue over expenses, consistent with industry practice, would include such items as contributions of long-lived assets (including assets acquired using contributions that by donor restriction were to be used for the purposes of acquiring such assets) and extraordinary gains and losses. Such items are not present on the current financial statements.

Net Patient Service Revenue

Net patient service revenue is reported as the estimated net realizable amounts from patients, third-party payers, and others for services rendered, including estimated retroactive adjustments under reimbursement agreements with third-party payers. Retroactive adjustments are accrued on an estimated basis in the period the related services are rendered and adjusted in future periods as final settlements are determined.

Contractual Agreements with Third-Party Payers

The hospital has contractual agreements with third-party payers, primarily the Medicare and Medicaid programs. The Medicare program reimburses the hospital for inpatient services under the Prospective Payment System, which provides for payment at predetermined amounts based on the discharge diagnosis. The contractual agreement with the Medicaid program provides for reimbursement based upon rates established by the state, subject to state appropriations. The difference between established customary charge rates and reimbursement is accounted for as a contractual allowance.

Gifts and Bequests

Unrestricted gifts and bequests are recorded on the accrual basis as nonoperating gains.

Donated Services

No amounts have been reflected in the financial statements for donated services. The hospital pays for most services requiring specific expertise. However, many individuals volunteer their time and perform a variety of tasks that help the hospital with specific assistance programs and various committee assignments.

Note 2—Cash and Investments

Statutes require that all deposits of the hospital be secured by federal depository insurance or be fully collateralized by the banking institution in authorized investments. Authorized investments include those guaranteed by the full faith and credit of the United States of America as to principal and interest; or in bonds, notes, debentures, or other similar obligations of the United States of America or its agencies; in interest-bearing savings accounts or interest-bearing certificates of deposit; or in certain money market mutual funds.

At March 31, 20X3, the carrying amount and bank balance of the hospital's deposits with financial institutions were $190,000 and $227,000, respectively. The difference between the carrying amount and the bank balance primarily represents checks outstanding at March 31, 20X3. All deposits are fully insured by the Federal Deposit Insurance Corporation or collateralized with securities held in the hospital's name by the hospital agent.

	Carrying Amount	
	20X3	20X2
U.S. Government Securities or		
U.S. Government Agency Securities	$4,325,000	$3,575,000
Total Investments	4,325,000	3,575,000
Petty Cash	3,000	3,000
Deposits	190,000	93,000
Accrued Interest	7,000	4,000
Total	4,525,000	3,675,000
Consisting of		
Cash and Cash Equivalents—General Fund	1,150,000	400,000
Assets Whose Use Is Limited		
Corporate Funded Depreciation	1,950,000	1,800,000
Held by Trustee Under Bond Indenture Agreements	1,425,000	1,475,000
Total	$4,525,000	$3,675,000

Note 3—Charity Care

The hospital voluntarily provides free care to patients who lack financial resources and are deemed to be medically indigent. Such care is in compliance with the hospital's mission. Because the hospital does not pursue collection of amounts determined to qualify as charity care, they are not reported as revenue.

The hospital maintains records to identify and monitor the level of charity care it provides. These records include the amount of charges forgone for services and supplies furnished under its charity care policy. During the years ended March 31, 20X3 and 20X2, such charges forgone totaled $395,000 and $375,000, respectively.

Note 4—Net Patient Service Revenue

The hospital provides healthcare services through its inpatient and outpatient care facilities. The mix of receivables from patients and third-party payers at March 31, 20X3 and 20X2, is as follows:

	20X3	20X2
Medicare	30.0%	28.5%
Medicaid	15.0	16.0
Patients	13.0	12.5
Other third-party payers	42.0	43.0
Total	100.0%	100.0%

The hospital has agreements with third-party payers that provide for payments to the hospital at amounts different from its established rates. Contractual adjustments under third-party reimbursement programs represent the difference between the hospital's established rates for services and amounts paid by third-party payers. A summary of the payment arrangements with major third-party payers follows.

Medicare

Inpatient acute care rendered to Medicare program beneficiaries is paid at prospectively determined rates-per-discharge. These rates vary according to a patient classification system that is based on clinical, diagnostic, and other factors. Inpatient nonacute care services and certain outpatient services are paid based upon either a cost reimbursement method, established fee screens, or a combination thereof. The hospital is reimbursed for cost reimbursable items at a tentative rate with final settlement determination after submission of annual cost reports by the hospital and audits by the Medicare fiscal intermediary. At the current year end, all Medicare settlements for the previous two years are subject to audit and retroactive adjustments.

Medicaid

Inpatient services rendered to Medicaid program beneficiaries are reimbursed at prospectively determined rates-per-day. Outpatient services rendered to Medicaid program beneficiaries are reimbursed at prospectively determined rates-per-visit.

Blue Cross

Inpatient services rendered to Blue Cross subscribers are reimbursed under a cost reimbursement methodology. The hospital is reimbursed at a tentative rate with final settlement determined after submission of annual cost reports by the hospital and audits by Blue Cross. The Blue Cross cost report for the prior year end is subject to audit and retroactive adjustment.

The hospital has also entered into payment agreements with certain commercial insurance carriers, health maintenance organizations, and preferred provider organizations. The bases for payment under these agreements include discounts from established charges and prospectively determined daily rates.

Gross patient service revenue for services rendered by the hospital under the Medicare, Medicaid, and Blue Cross payment agreements for the years ended March 31, 20X3 and 20X2, is approximately as follows:

	20X3		20X2	
	Amount	%	Amount	%
Medicare	$20,850,000	43.0	$19,900,000	42.0
Medicaid	10,190,000	21.0	10,200,000	21.5
All other payers	17,460,000	36.0	17,300,000	36.5
	$48,500,000	100.0	$47,400,000	100.0

Note 5—Property, Plant, and Equipment

The hospital's property, plant, and equipment at March 31, 20X3 and 20X2, are as follows:

	20X3	20X2
Buildings and improvements	$14,700,000	$14,000,000
Land improvements	1,100,000	1,100,000
Equipment	28,900,000	27,600,000
Total	$44,700,000	$42,700,000
Accumulated depreciation	(26,100,000)	(24,200,000)
Net Depreciable Assets	$18,600,000	$18,500,000
Land	480,000	480,000
Construction in progress	220,000	220,000
Net Property, Plant, Equipment	$19,300,000	$19,200,000

Construction in progress, which involves a renovation project, has not progressed in the last 12-month period because of a zoning dispute. The project will not require significant outlay to reach completion, as anticipated additional expenditures are currently estimated at $100,000.

Note 6—Long-Term Debt

Long-term debt consists of the following:

Hospital Facility Revenue Bonds (Series 1995) at varying interest rates from 4.5% to 5.5%, depending on date of maturity through 2020.	20X3	20X2
	$6,000,000	$6,500,000

The future maturities of long-term debt are as follows:

Years Ending March 31

20X2	$ 475,000
20X3	500,000
20X4	525,000
20X5	550,000
20X6	575,000
20X7	600,000
Thereafter	3,750,000

Under the terms of the trust indenture the following funds (held by the trustee) were established: an interest fund, a bond sinking fund, and a debt service reserve fund.

Interest Fund

The hospital deposits (monthly) into the interest fund an amount equal to one-sixth of the next semi-annual interest payment due on the bonds.

Bond Sinking Fund

The hospital deposits (monthly) into the bond sinking fund an amount equal to one-twelfth of the principal due on the next July 1.

Debt Service Reserve Fund

The debt service reserve fund must be maintained at an amount equal to 10% of the aggregate principal amount of all bonds then outstanding. It is to be used to make up any deficiencies in the interest fund and bond sinking fund.

Assets held by the trustee under the trust indenture at March 31, 20X3 and 20X2 are as follows:

	20X3	20X2
Interest Fund	$ 300,000	$ 325,000
Bond Sinking Fund	525,000	500,000
Debt Service Reserve	600,000	650,000
Total	$1,425,000	$1,475,000

Note 7—Commitments

At March 31, 20X3, the hospital had commitments outstanding for a renovation project at the hospital of approximately $100,000. Construction in progress on the renovation has not progressed in the last 12-month period because of a zoning dispute. Upon resolution of the dispute, remaining construction costs will be funded from corporate funded depreciation cash reserves.

Comparative Analysis Using Financial Ratios and Benchmarking Helps Turn Around a Hospital in the Metropolis Health System

28-B

Sample General Hospital is another facility within the Metropolis Health System. Sample General Hospital has recently been acquired by Metropolis. It is a 100-bed hospital that has been losing money steadily over the last several years. The new chief financial officer (CFO) has decided to use benchmarking as an aid to turn around Sample's financial situation. Benchmarking will illustrate where the hospital stands in relationship to its peer group.

The CFO orders two benchmarking reports: one for the hospitals that are 100 beds or less and one for all hospitals, no matter the size. The 100-beds-or-less report will allow direct comparability for Sample, while the all-hospital report will give a universal or overall view of Sample's standing. Both reports appear at the end of this case study. **Exhibit 28-B–1** is the benchmark data report for Sample General Hospital compared with hospitals less than 100 beds, whereas **Exhibit 28-B–2** is the benchmark data report for Sample General Hospital compared with all hospitals.

When the reports arrive, the CFO writes a description of how the data are arranged so that his managers will better understand the information presented. His description includes the following points:

1. The percentile rankings are intended to present the hospital's performance ranked against all other performers in the comparison group. Whether the hospital's actual performance is good or bad depends on the statistic being evaluated.
2. The first column, labeled "Annual Average Year 1," provides a historical trend of actual performance of the hospital in the previous year. It is provided for reference only so that the reader can see the trend over time.
3. The column labeled "Q1 Year 2" represents the first quarter of the current year. These are the most recent data that this service has been provided for Sample General Hospital and are the data used in the comparison columns that follow.
4. The column labeled "50th %ile" represents the 50th percentile of all of the hospitals in the comparison group that supplied data for the individual line item.
5. The "Variance" column compares the data from Q1 Year 2 of Sample General Hospital with the 50th percentile information from the entire comparison group.
6. The column labeled "%ile Range" indicates where Sample General Hospital's individual score fell within a percentile range.

Exhibit 28-B–1 Hospital Statistical Data

Benchmark Data Report
Sample General Hospital
Compared to Hospitals of Less Than 100 Beds

	Annual Average Year 1	Q 1 Year 2	Current Quarter Benchmark		
			50%ile	Variance	%ile Range
Severity/Length of Stay					
Average Length of Stay	3.80	3.91	4.06	−0.15	35–40
Case Mix Index (All Patients)	1.02	1.04	1.04	0.005	50–55
Case Mix Index (Medicare)	1.24	1.26	1.19	0.07	80–85
Productivity/Labor Utilization					
FTE per Adjusted Occupied Bed	5.11	4.68	4.44	0.24	60–65
Paid Hours per Adjusted Patient Day	29.12	26.67	25.3	1.37	60–65
Paid Hours per Adjusted Discharge	110.53	104.19	109.5	−5.32	35–40
Salary Cost per Adjusted Discharge	$2,638	$2,510	$2,510	$0	50–55
Costs & Charges					
Cost per Adjusted Patient Day	$1,704	$1,608	$1,448	$161	70–75
Cost per Adjusted Discharge	$6,467	$6,282	$5,909	$373	55–60
Cost per CMI (All Pat.) Adj. Discharge	$6,328	$6,041	$5,837	$204	50–55
Cost per CMI (All Pat.) Adjusted Patient Day	$1,667	$1,546	$1,408	$139	60–65
Supply Cost per Adjusted Discharge	$1,046	$968	$867	$101	60–65
Supply Cost per CMI (All Pat.) Adj. Discharge	$1,024	$931	$829	$102	60–65
Gross Charges per Adjusted Discharge	$12,987	$14,155	$12,536	$1,620	60–65
Deductions Percentage	0.40%	58.46%	51.04%	7.42%	60–65
Net Charges per Adjusted Discharge	$6,112	$5,880	$5,929	($49)	45–50
Net Charges per Adjusted Patient Day	$1,610	$1,505	$1,424	$82	60–65
Utilization					
Average Daily Census	43.15	46.36	37.69	8.67	65–70
Occupancy Percentage	41.09%	46.36%	57.66%	−11.30%	10–15
Outpatient Charges Percentage	53.15%	54.02%	50.14%	3.88%	55–60
Beds in Use	100	100	66	34	90–95
Adjusted Occupied Beds	92.2	100.82	72.05	28.76	75–80
Total Patient Days Excluding Newborns	3,936	4,172	3,392	780	65–70
Total Discharges Excluding Newborns	1,036	1,068	751	317	80–85
Newborn Days as a % of Total Patient Days	6.95%	5.40%	4.61%	0.79%	60–65

Exhibit 28-B–1 Hospital Statistical Data *(continued)*

	Annual Average Year 1	Q 1 Year 2	Current Quarter Benchmark		
			50%ile	Variance	%ile Range
Financial Performance—Profitability Ratios					
Operating Margin	–2.26	–3.18	1.95	–5.13	15–20
Profit Margin	–2.26	–3.18	2.06	–5.24	20–25
Return on Total Assets					
(Annualized) (%)	–2.37%	–3.58%	1.22%	–4.80%	20–25
Return on Equity (Annualized) (%)	–6.56%	–11.19%	4.61%	–15.80%	15–20
Financial Performance—Liquidity Ratios					
Current Ratio	1.28	1.19	1.9	–0.71	15–20
Quick Ratio	0.54	0.56	1.56	–0.99	15–20
Net Days in Patient AR (Days)	50.73	49	51.86	–2.86	40–45
Financial Performance—Leverage and Solvency Ratios					
Total Asset Turnover—Annualized	1.07	1.13	0.99	0.14	65–70
Current Asset Turnover—Annualized	3.21	3.65	3.57	0.08	50–55
Equity Financing	0.38	0.32	0.47	–0.15	25–30
Long-Term Debt to Equity	0.77	0.85	0.56	0.28	70–75

For example, review the average length of stay information for hospitals less than 100 beds in Exhibit 28-B–1. For the Q1 Year 2, Sample General Hospital has a length of stay of 3.91 versus a benchmark comparison number of 4.06, a favorable performance against the 50th percentile by 0.15 (the −0.15 indicates an amount under the 50th percentile that, in the case of average length of stay, would be favorable). This performance places the hospital's score in the 35th to 40th percentile of all respondents.

As the CFO already knows, Sample General Hospital is in trouble. In most cases, the facility is either at or below (worse than) the 50th percentile information. Most of the labor productivity measures are in the 60th to 65th percentile range, with the cost information in the same relative range. This indicates that Sample is spending more than the peer group for labor and supplies. The utilization statistics also present a dismal picture.

Each statistic has to be evaluated against what it means to the institution before a conclusion can be drawn. For example, the occupancy percentage for Sample is 46.36% versus the 50th percentile of 57.66%. This places Sample in the 10th to 15th percentile range for the comparison group of hospitals less than 100 beds. In terms of utilization, the CFO knows that a facility should be in the 80th to 85th percentile range to use all of its assets effectively.

What other statistics should the CFO review to assure that a higher occupancy percentage is beneficial to the hospital? The answer is average length of stay. Sample General Hospital has a length of stay of 3.91 (as discussed earlier), which is favorable compared with the peer group, but an occupancy rate that is 11.30% below the 50th percentile for the peer

Exhibit 28-B–2 Hospital Statistical Data

Benchmark Data Report
Sample General Hospital
Compared to All Hospitals

	Annual Average Year 1	Q 1 Year 2	Current Quarter Benchmark 50%ile	Variance	%ile Range
Severity/Length of Stay					
Average Length of Stay	3.80	3.91	4.81	−0.91	10–15
Case Mix Index (All Patients)	1.02	1.04	1.14	−0.103	25–30
Case Mix Index (Medicare)	1.24	1.26	1.38	−0.118	30–35
Productivity/Labor Utilization					
FTE per Adjusted Occupied Bed	5.11	4.68	4.87	−0.19	40–45
Paid Hours per Adjusted Patient Day	29.12	26.67	27.77	−1.1	40–45
Paid Hours per Adjusted Discharge	110.53	104.19	134.6	−30.41	10–15
Salary Cost per Adjusted Discharge	$2,638	$2,510	$2,927	($417)	25–30
Costs & Charges					
Cost per Adjusted Patient Day	$1,704	$1,608	$1,530	$78	60–65
Cost per Adjusted Discharge	$6,467	$6,282	$7,284	($1,001)	30–35
Cost per CMI (All Pat.) Adj. Discharge	$6,328	$6,041	$6,115	($74)	45–50
Cost per CMI (All Pat.) Adjusted Patient Day	$1,667	$1,546	$1,268	$278	80–85
Supply Cost per Adjusted Discharge	$1,046	$968	$1,250	($282)	25–30
Supply Cost per CMI (All Pat.) Adj. Discharge	$1,024	$931	$1,069	($138)	30–35
Gross Charges per Adjusted Discharge	$12,987	$14,155	$17,196	($3,041)	35–40
Deductions Percentage	0.40%	58.46%	56.31%	2.15%	55–60
Net Charges per Adjusted Discharge	$6,112	$5,880	$7,419	($1,539)	20–25
Net Charges per Adjusted Patient Day	$1,610	$1,505	$1,529	($24)	45–50
Utilization					
Average Daily Census	43.15	46.36	142.98	−96.62	15–20
Occupancy Percentage	41.09%	46.36%	69.38%	−23.02%	< 5
Outpatient Charges Percentage	53.15%	54.02%	39.64%	14.38%	85–90
Beds in Use	100	100	206	−106	20–25
Adjusted Occupied Beds	92.2	100.82	225.9	−125.09	15–20
Total Patient Days Excluding Newborns	3,936	4,172	12,868	−8,696	15–20
Total Discharges Excluding Newborns	1,036	1,068	2,506	−1,438	20–25
Newborn Days as a % of Total Patient Days	6.95%	5.40%	4.52%	0.87%	60–65

Exhibit 28-B–2 Hospital Statistical Data *(continued)*

	Annual Average Year 1	Q 1 Year 2	Current Quarter Benchmark 50%ile	Variance	%ile Range
Financial Performance—Profitability Ratios					
Operating Margin	–2.26	–3.18	4.45	–7.63	10–15
Profit Margin	–2.26	–3.18	4.66	–7.84	10–15
Return on Total Assets					
(Annualized) (%)	–2.37%	–3.58%	4.04%	–7.62%	10–15
Return on Equity (Annualized) (%)	–6.56%	–11.19%	8.46%	–19.65%	5–10
Financial Performance—Liquidity Ratios					
Current Ratio	1.28	1.19	2.2	–1	10–15
Quick Ratio	0.54	0.56	1.74	–1.18	5–10
Net Days in Patient AR (Days)	50.73	49	55.76	–6.77	25–30
Financial Performance—Leverage and Solvency Ratios					
Total Asset Turnover—Annualized	1.07	1.13	0.93	0.2	70–75
Current Asset Turnover—Annualized	3.21	3.65	3.48	0.18	50–55
Equity Financing	0.38	0.32	0.5	–0.18	20–25
Long-Term Debt to Equity	0.77	0.85	0.59	0.26	65–70

group of hospitals less than 100 beds. If these two statistics are observed in combination, one could say that Sample efficiently manages its patients, but just does not have enough of them.

Other statistics bear the same message. The hospital is not profitable, and much of the problem is because the cost of running the institution exceeds the availability of patients to pay the bills. In other words, all institutions have core staffing requirements, and within a certain range of volume, most costs are fixed. Sample has 100 beds in use while the 50th percentile for its peer group shows 66 beds in use. Sample's plant is too big for its patient volume. These circumstances can mean the hospital is heading for disaster.

So what happened to Sample General Hospital? As you can surmise from the data, the previous year (labeled "Year 1" on Exhibits 28-B–1 and 28-B–2) was not favorable. Three years previous, the institution was losing money at a rate of over $1 million per month. The next two years showed improvement (even though the data still show concern), and the improvement trend continued through the year labeled "Year 2" on Exhibits 28-B–1 and 28-B–2. By using benchmarking data (and a lot of other analysis), management was able to determine and address many issues that forced this facility to perform below market averages. By improving quality, managing costs, and controlling productivity, the hospital was able to stabilize its financial position. In addition, with creative management and attention to both clinical quality and customer service, the occupancy percentage rose to above the 50th percentile. Finally, the operating margin improved dramatically. In the first quarter of year 2, the margin was minus 3.18. By the end of year 3, results showed a positive margin of greater than 2.5%, a dramatic turnaround. Benchmarking assisted in this turnaround by showing management where the need for improvement was greatest.

Mini-Case
Studies

Mini-Case Study 1:

Proposal to Add a Retail Pharmacy to a Hospital in the Metropolis Health System

Sample General Hospital belongs to the Metropolis Health System. The new chief financial officer (CFO) at Sample Hospital has been attempting to find new sources of badly needed revenue for the facility. Consequently, the CFO is preparing a proposal to add a retail pharmacy within the hospital itself. If the proposal is accepted, this would generate a new revenue stream. The CFO has prepared four exhibits, all of which appear at the end of this case study. **Exhibit 29–1**, a three-year retail pharmacy profitability analysis, is the primary document. It is supported by **Exhibit 29–2**, the retail pharmacy proposal assumptions. The profitability analysis is further supported by **Exhibit 29–3**, a year 1 monthly income statement detail. Finally, **Exhibit 29–4** presents the supporting year 1 monthly cash flow detail and assumptions.

When the controller reviewed the exhibits, she asked how the working capital of $49,789 was derived. The CFO explained that it represents 3 months of departmental expense. He also explained that the cost of drugs purchased for the first 60 days was offset by these purchases' accounts payable cycle, so the net effect was 0. In essence, the vendors were financing the drug purchases. Thus, the working capital reconciled as follows:

Working Capital:	
Cost of drugs (2 months)	$303,400
Vendor financing (accounts payable)	($303,400)
Departmental expense (3 months)	$49,789
Total Working Capital Required	$49,789

The controller also noticed on Exhibit 29–4 that the cost of renovations to the building is estimated at $80,000 and equipment purchases are estimated at $50,000 for a total capital expenditure of $130,000. The building renovations are depreciated on a straight-line basis over a useful life of 15 years, whereas the equipment purchases are depreciated on a straight-line basis over a useful life of 5 years. The required capital is proposed to be obtained from hospital sources, and no borrowing would be necessary. In addition, the total capital expenditure is projected to be retrieved through operating cash flows before the end of year 1.

Exhibit 29–1 Sample General Hospital 3-Year Retail Pharmacy Profitability Analysis

	Year 1	Year 2	Year 3
Rx Sales	2,587,613	2,692,152	2,828,375
Cost of Goods Sold	2,047,950	2,088,909	2,151,576
Gross Margin	539,663	603,243	676,799
GM %	20.9%	22.4%	23.9%
EXPENSES			
Salaries and Wages	192,000	197,760	203,693
Benefits	38,400	39,552	40,739
Materials and Supplies	12,000	14,400	17,280
Contract Services and Fees	14,400	17,280	20,736
Depreciation and Amortization	15,333	15,333	15,333
Interest	—	—	—
Provision for Bad Debts	25,876	26,922	28,284
Misc. Exp.	3,600	4,320	5,184
Total Expense	301,609	315,567	331,248
Net Income	238,053	287,676	345,550
Operating Margin	9.2%	10.7%	12.2%

Cash Flow

	Year 1	Year 2	Year 3
Sources			
Net Income	238,053	287,676	345,550
Depreciation	15,333	15,333	15,333
Borrowing	—	—	—
Total Sources	253,386	303,010	360,884
Uses			
Capital Purchasing	130,000	—	—
Working Capital	49,789	—	—
Total Uses	179,789	—	—
Cash at Beginning of Period	—	73,597	376,607
Net Cash Activities	73,597	303,010	360,884
Cash at Ending of Period	73,597	376,607	737,490

Volume

	Year 1	Year 2	Year 3
Number of Prescriptions Sold	55,350	56,457	58,151

Courtesy of Resource Group, Ltd., Dallas, Texas.

Exhibit 29–2 Sample General Hospital Retail Pharmacy Proposal Assumptions

		Prescriptions	
		Per Day	Annual
1. Annual Prescription Estimates—Rate of Growth/Capture			
Year 1		225	55,350
Year 2	2.0%	230	56,457
Year 3	3.0%	236	58,151
2. Average Net Revenue per Prescription—Yearly Increases			
Year 1			$ 46.75
Year 2	2.0%		$ 47.69
Year 3	2.0%		$ 48.64
3. Bad Debt Percentage	1.0%		
4. Average Cost per Prescription—Yearly Increases			
Year 1			$ 37.00
Year 2	3.0%		$ 38.11
Year 3	3.0%		$ 39.25
5. Inflation Rates—Per Year			
Salary and Wages			3.0%
Other Than Prescriptions			2.0%
Benefits as a % of Salaries			20.0%
6. Initial Capital Requirements			
Building			80,000
Equipment			50,000
Working Capital			49,789
Total			179,789

	Year 1	Year 2	Year 3
Gross Margin	539,663	603,243	676,799
Net Income before Taxes	238,053	287,676	345,550

	Year 1	Year 2	Year 3
Beginning Cash Balance	—	73,597	376,607
Net Cash Activity	73,597	303,010	360,884
Ending Cash Balance	73,597	376,607	737,490

Courtesy of Resource Group, Ltd., Dallas, Texas.

Exhibit 29–3 Sample General Hospital Retail Pharmacy Proposal Year 1 Monthly Income Statement Detail

	Month 1	Month 2	Month 3	Month 4	Month 5	Month 6	Month 7	Month 8	Month 9	Month 10	Month 11	Month 12
Return on Investment Analysis												
Average Rx Sales Price	$47	$47	$47	$47	$47	$47	$47	$47	$47	$47	$47	$47
Average Rx Cost	$37	$37	$37	$37	$37	$37	$37	$37	$37	$37	$37	$37
Gross Margin	21%	21%	21%	21%	21%	21%	21%	21%	21%	21%	21%	21%
Scripts per Day	225	225	225	225	225	225	225	225	225	225	225	225
	7.4%	7.4%	7.4%	7.8%	7.8%	8.3%	8.3%	8.7%	9.1%	9.3%	9.3%	9.3%
Business Days in the Month	20.5	20.5	20.5	20.5	20.5	20.5	20.5	20.5	20.5	20.5	20.5	20.5
Monthly Scripts	4,100	4,100	4,100	4,305	4,305	4,612.5	4,612.5	4,817.5	5,022.5	5,125	5,125	5,125
Rx Sales	$191,675	$191,675	$191,675	$201,259	$201,259	$215,634	$215,634	$225,218	$234,802	$239,594	$239,594	$239,594
COG Sold	$151,700	$151,700	$151,700	$159,285	$159,285	$170,663	$170,663	$178,248	$185,833	$189,625	$189,625	$189,625
Gross Margin	$39,975	$39,975	$39,975	$41,974	$41,974	$44,972	$44,972	$46,971	$48,969	$49,969	$49,969	$49,969
GM %	21%	21%	21%	21%	21%	21%	21%	21%	21%	21%	21%	21%
EXPENSES												
Salaries and Wages	$16,000	$16,000	$16,000	$16,000	$16,000	$16,000	$16,000	$16,000	$16,000	$16,000	$16,000	$16,000
Benefits	$3,200	$3,200	$3,200	$3,200	$3,200	$3,200	$3,200	$3,200	$3,200	$3,200	$3,200	$3,200
Materials and Supplies	$1,000	$1,000	$1,000	$1,000	$1,000	$1,000	$1,000	$1,000	$1,000	$1,000	$1,000	$1,000
Contract Services and Fees	$1,200	$1,200	$1,200	$1,200	$1,200	$1,200	$1,200	$1,200	$1,200	$1,200	$1,200	$1,200
Depreciation and Amortization	$1,278	$1,278	$1,278	$1,278	$1,278	$1,278	$1,278	$1,278	$1,278	$1,278	$1,278	$1,278
Interest	$0	$0	$0	$0	$0	$0	$0	$0	$0	$0	$0	$0
Provision for Bad Debts	$1,917	$1,917	$1,917	$2,013	$2,013	$2,156	$2,156	$2,252	$2,348	$2,396	$2,396	$2,396
Misc. Exp.	$300	$300	$300	$300	$300	$300	$300	$300	$300	$300	$300	$300
Total Expenses	$24,895	$24,895	$24,895	$24,991	$24,991	$25,134	$25,134	$25,230	$25,326	$25,374	$25,374	$25,374
Net Income	$15,080	$15,080	$15,080	$16,983	$16,983	$19,838	$19,838	$21,740	$23,643	$24,595	$24,595	$24,595
Accumulated Profits	$15,080	$30,161	$45,241	$62,224	$79,207	$99,045	$118,882	$140,623	$164,266	$188,861	$213,456	$238,050

Courtesy of Resource Group, Ltd., Dallas, Texas.

Exhibit 29–4 Sample General Hospital Retail Pharmacy Proposal Year 1 Monthly Cash Flow Detail and Assumptions

	Years		Month 1	Month 2	Month 3	Month 4	Month 5	Month 6	Month 7	Month 8	Month 9	Month 10	Month 11	Month 12
Depreciation														
Renovations	15	80,000	444	444	444	444	444	444	444	444	444	444	444	444
Equipment	5	50,000	833	833	833	833	833	833	833	833	833	833	833	833
Total Depreciation		130,000	1,278	1,278	1,278	1,278	1,278	1,278	1,278	1,278	1,278	1,278	1,278	1,278
Cash Flow														
Beginning Balance			$0	($163,431)	($147,073)	($130,714)	($112,453)	($94,192)	($73,076)	($51,961)	($28,942)	($4,021)	$21,852	$47,725
Sources														
Net Income			$15,080	$15,080	$15,080	$16,983	$16,983	$19,838	$19,838	$21,741	$23,644	$24,595	$24,595	$24,595
Depreciation			1,278	1,278	1,278	1,278	1,278	1,278	1,278	1,278	1,278	1,278	1,278	1,278
Borrowing			0	0	0	0	0	0	0	0	0	0	0	0
Total Sources			$16,358	$16,358	$16,358	$18,261	$18,261	$21,116	$21,116	$23,018	$24,921	$25,873	$25,873	$25,873
Uses														
Capital Purchasing			130,000	0	0	0	0	0	0	0	0	0	0	0
Working Capital			49,789	0	0	0	0	0	0	0	0	0	0	0
Total Uses			179,789	0	0	0	0	0	0	0	0	0	0	0
Net Cash Activities			($163,431)	$16,358	$16,358	$18,261	$18,261	$21,116	$21,116	$23,018	$24,921	$25,873	$25,873	$25,873
Ending Balance			($163,431)	($147,073)	($130,714)	($112,453)	($94,192)	($73,076)	($51,961)	($28,942)	($4,021)	$21,852	$47,725	$73,597

Courtesy of Resource Group, Ltd., Dallas, Texas.

So how was the proposal received by the hospital's board of trustees? They first asked for a small market study to test the amount of prescription sales projected within the proposal. When the market study results came back positive, the board approved the project, and renovations are about to commence.

Mini-Case Study 2:

The Economic Significance of Resource Misallocation: Client Flow Through the Women, Infants, and Children Public Health Program*

Billie Ann Brotman, Mary Bumgarner,
and Penelope Prime

CONFRONTING THE OPERATIONAL PROBLEM

The Women, Infants, and Children (WIC) Program, a federal program managed by the county boards of health, provides a mandated health service under strict federal guidelines to women and young children. In this chapter, we analyze how a WIC clinic, located in the Atlanta metropolitan area, can serve its clientele more efficiently in an environment of constraints. We focus on achieving shorter waiting times for WIC clients through better management of the flow of clients through the clinic. We apply the peak-load framework from economics to this basic operations research problem.

THE ENVIRONMENT

The WIC program provides nutrition counseling, limited physical examinations, and food vouchers for low-income pregnant women and for children with nutritional deficiencies who are five years old or less. WIC represents just one part of the integrated services provided to women and children by the county clinic. Other services include inoculations, medical visits with the nurse, and a variety of social services. Providing more than one health service at the county clinic is advantageous because it reinforces good health practices, provides intervention where necessary, and is convenient for the clients. However, it also complicates the management of service provision and makes it more difficult to improve the delivery of WIC's services.

To participate in the WIC program, a certification of income and health status is required. The first step for a client is to schedule an appointment for certification with a clinic nurse. Once certified, the client is immediately eligible to receive food vouchers and can return to the clinic to pick up her vouchers for up to a year without revisiting a nurse. Vouchers may also be picked up when a client comes to the clinic for nutritional classes, which are required periodically.

From the providers' point of view, several activities directly related to the WIC program are managed simultaneously. They include the scheduling of appointments for

---

*B.A. Brotman, M. Bumgarner, and P. Prime, "Client Flow through the Women, Infants, and Children Public Health Program," *Journal of Health Care Finance* 25, no. 1 (1998): 72–77.

certification, meeting previously scheduled certification appointments by the nurses, accommodating unscheduled clients who walk in seeking certification, and distributing food vouchers to eligible clients. (Eligible clients include those certified by the county clinic as well as those who have been certified by Kennestone Hospital and Home Visits, and Child Health.)

In principle, the appointment system is designed to regulate these activities. In practice, several factors, none of which are within the control of the clinic staff, undermine it. First, because clients come to the clinic for other services as well, they often are delayed for their WIC appointments. Second, of those that make appointments, 40 to 50% of them do not keep them because they either arrive late or simply do not come. Understanding the obstacles many of the clients face when arranging work schedules, getting transportation to the clinic, and arranging for child care, the clinic's management has instituted a policy of waiting 20 minutes for a client to arrive before rescheduling the appointment. Third, walk-ins are common and, according to federal guidelines, must be accommodated. In addition, the clinic has difficulty retaining qualified staff, and its physical space is limited. The end result is that women and children are often in the clinic for hours, are uncomfortable, and are unable to adequately care for their children during this time.

THE PEAK-LOAD PROBLEM

The economic problem faced by the clinic is one of demand exceeding capacity, leading to excessive wait times for the clinic's patrons as well as inefficient use of clinic nurses and clerks. The problem arises because the clinic's services are beneficial to the health of expectant mothers and children, and are provided without fee to the patient. Without a price mechanism to ration demand, quantity demanded exceeds quantity supplied. This problem is not uncommon. It is encountered often in the public or quasi-public sector, when the price of the good or service does not adequately reflect the benefits of the good or service as perceived by the public.

In this case, the problem of disequilibrium between demand and supply is exacerbated by the fact that demand for the clinic's services is unpredictable. Clients often do not keep their appointments or arrive at unscheduled times. As a result, appointments may go unfilled, or two or more clients may seek the same appointment time.

On the supply side, capacity constraints, coupled with a persistent lack of sufficient numbers of experienced clerks and nurses, hamper the clinic's ability to respond to unexpected demand shifts. Moreover, due to employee turnover experienced by the clinic, few employees become sufficiently skilled to work as part-time clerks during periods of peak demand.

The economic significance of the problem is one of resource misallocation. In this case, too many resources are employed in the production of WIC services. The market solution is to increase the price of the service, thereby matching demand with capacity. But because that option is not available, efficiently managing demand and supply is necessary if the amount of resources used in providing WIC services is to be reduced.

Federal guidelines for the WIC program leave little maneuvering room to improve the delivery of services. For example, the clinic cannot refuse to see unscheduled walk-ins, all clients must see a nurse for certification, all clients must attend nutrition classes, and vouchers must be closely monitored. Based on the data and information provided by the clinic, we determined that the fundamental cause of the queuing problem was the time spent by clients waiting to see clerks and nurses. Our hypothesis is that the flow of traffic through the clinic can be managed more efficiently by changing the current policy of waiting 20 minutes before filling a broken appointment with a "walk-in," to a new policy of filling the appointment immediately.

METHOD

We began by collecting information on the average daily client volume, the pattern of client flow through various services, the waiting points and times, and services rendered to the clients.

The data were collected by clinic personnel, recorded in a chart throughout the day in periodic intervals, and included nine items:

1. Number of clerks available
2. Number of nurses available
3. Waiting time to see clerks for walk-ins and appointments
4. Waiting time to see nurses for walk-ins and appointments
5. Total time in the clinic for walk-ins and appointments
6. Waiting time to get vouchers
7. Number of nutrition classes
8. Number of appointments met
9. Number of appointments missed

The actual flow of traffic through the clinic is depicted in **Figure 30–1**.

Clients visit the clinic to keep an appointment with the nurse, attend a nutrition class, or as an unscheduled walk-in. All clients first see a clerk to arrange for their records to be pulled. They then check in and wait to be called to their class or appointment. At the completion of the appointment, they see a clerk to pick up vouchers. Vouchers are also distributed at the end of the nutrition classes.

The General Purpose Simulation System for personal computer model simulates the average flow of traffic through the clinic. Estimation of traffic flow through the clinic is initiated when the client signs in and continues as the client meets with the clerks and the nurses. The model estimates the average amount of time a client spends in the clinic as well as average waiting times at each station. Clerk and nurse utilization rates are also generated assuming a variety of staffing levels. For comparison purposes, each version of the model is run with a 20-minute time lag before a late appointment is filled and then run with a 1-minute lag.

Six versions of the model are estimated using different combinations of numbers of clerks and nurses. Model A assumes that the clinic is staffed with three nurses and three clerks, Model B with two clerks and three nurses, and Model C with two clerks and two nurses.

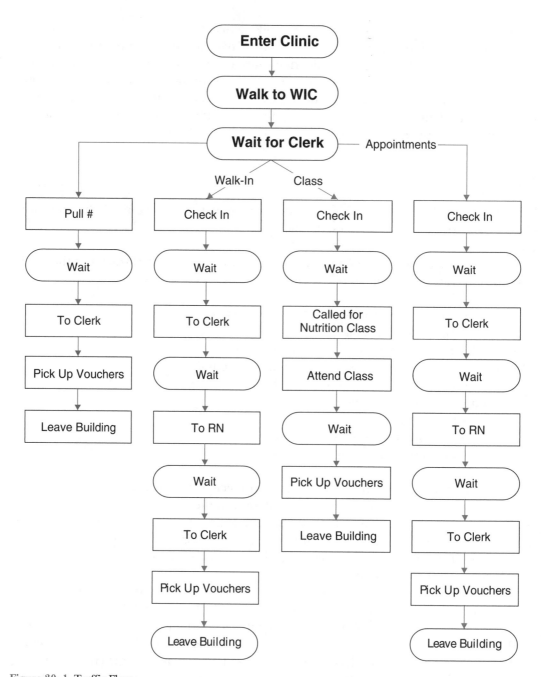

Figure 30–1 Traffic Flow.
Republished with permission of Wolters Kluwer Law & Business, from Brotman et al. Client Flow through the Women, Infants, and Children Public Health Program, *Journal of Health Care Finance* 25, no. 1 (1998): 72–77.

RESULTS

Models A, B, and C present the results of all the computer simulations.

Model A: Three Nurses and Three Clerks

A comparison of the results generated changing a 20-minute wait to a 1-minute wait show that reducing the time before an appointment is filled results in the following:

1. A decrease in the total time in the clinic for the client from 3 hours and 16 minutes to 1 hour and 11 minutes
2. A decrease in the time spent waiting for the clerk from 1 hour and 9 minutes to approximately 3 minutes
3. An increase in time spent waiting for a nurse from 3 minutes to 10 minutes
4. A decrease in the utilization of clerks from 91.6% to 53.2%
5. An increase in the utilization of nurses from 46.7% to 61.2%

Model B: Three Nurses and Two Clerks

1. A decrease in the total time in the clinic for the client from 3 hours and 13 minutes to 1 hour and 27 minutes
2. A decrease in the time spent waiting for the clerk from 1 hour and 19 minutes to approximately 1 minute
3. An increase in time spent waiting for a nurse from 8 minutes to 43 minutes
4. A decrease in the utilization of clerks from 91.6% to 46.8%
5. An increase in the utilization of nurses from 51.2% to 73.3%

Model C: Two Nurses and Two Clerks

1. A decrease in the total time in the clinic for the client from 1 hour and 50 minutes to 1 hour and 9 minutes
2. A decrease in the time spent waiting for the clerk from 19 minutes to less than 1 minute
3. A decrease in time spent waiting for a nurse from 18 minutes to 13 minutes
4. A decrease in the utilization of clerks from 76.6% to 30.3%
5. A decrease in the utilization of nurses from 64.6% to 53.7%

In all three versions of the model that were estimated, the results of the simulations reveal that reducing the time before a late appointment is filled significantly decreases the time spent in the clinic by the client, on average, for all clients. Furthermore, the time spent waiting for both clerks and nurses decreases, the utilization of the clerks decreases, and the utilization of the nurses increases in two of the three estimations.

Greater decreases in waiting time occur when the clinic is staffed with three nurses and either three or two clerks. Smaller decreases occur when only two nurses and two clerks are available. This suggests that the clinic has little to no scheduling flexibility on days when it is understaffed, and a policy of filling late appointments immediately should be particularly beneficial.

The utilization of clerks and the time spent waiting for a clerk decreases in all three models when appointments are filled within one minute, and in every case but one, the utilization rate of nurses increases when appointments are filled immediately. This suggests that the flow of clients through the clinic is improved by filling appointments quickly. Utilization rates of nurses decreases only when the clinic is staffed with three nurses and three clerks. One explanation for this result is that the clinic is overstaffed with this combination of nurses and clerks. A supporting piece of evidence for this conclusion is that the change in rates of utilization for both nurses and clerks is the smallest when three of each are employed.

Another implication of these results is that if the clinic does not implement the expedited scheduling policy, it makes little difference to time spent in the clinic whether it is staffed with two nurses and two clerks or three nurses and two clerks. Both scenarios result in clients spending approximately 3.25 hours in the clinic. With the 20-minute wait before rescheduling, the clinic must be staffed with three nurses and three clerks if the time spent in the clinic by the client is to fall below 2 hours.

In summary, our results suggest that following a policy of immediately rescheduling missed appointments reduces the misallocation of resources employed in the clinic and thus permits the clinic to respond to its clients' needs more efficiently. Although this approach cannot duplicate the increase in efficiency that could be realized through the use of a price mechanism, it does improve the overall welfare of the clinic's clients. Filling appointments immediately results in shorter wait times for all clients, so no client is made worse off by the new policy. Moreover, as the patients realize that timeliness is important, more will arrive on time, further increasing the clinic's ability to monitor demand and provide services for its clients.

Mini-Case Study 3:
Technology in Health Care: Automating Admissions Processes*

Eric Christ

Alexander Bain was a clever fellow. He invented the electric clock and the first electric printing telegraph. He also invented the fax machine, the device that many long-term care providers rely on for patient referral and admissions communications. That was in 1843.

That's right, the technology at the core of the referral and admissions process for many continuing care providers is more than 150 years old.

Needless to say, a lot has changed since then. Providers can benefit from these changes by looking at their patient intake processes and considering ways to use the Internet and other technological advances to automate and accelerate admissions and referral management.

ASSESS ADMISSIONS PROCESS

The first step for providers who are considering improved tools for patient intake is to assess current processes. Here are some good questions to start with:

- How many referrals are received per day or per month?
- How many sources (hospitals, physicians, liaisons, other long-term care providers) send referrals?
- How many pages of documents are associated with each referral?
- How are patient review and approval tasks assigned and tracked?
- How are referral and intake activities collected and reported?

Many providers do not realize what vast mountains of paper they manage. Results from a 2007 survey of about 400 skilled nursing facilities and home health agencies indicate the average provider receives 4 referrals per day, each with 22 pages of related documents. That's 1,460 referrals and 32,120 pages of documents per year—an 8-foot stack of paper for the average provider to process, review, and manage.

In a study conducted by a Canadian health policy organization, nursing facility admissions processes were found to involve 160 steps, including 69 handling steps, 36 forms to

---

*E. Christ, "Technology in Health Care: Automating Admissions Processes," *Provider Magazine* (Oct. 2008): 81–84. Reprinted with permission from *Provider Magazine*.

complete, 4 family trips to the facility that involved 53 steps and 5 staff members, and 9 forms.

AREAS TO AUTOMATE

Clearly, providers have many opportunities to streamline the admissions process. For example, there are typically four to five steps between an initial inquiry and a response to the referral source, after which insurance must be verified before a final decision to admit is made.

Once a provider has identified the steps in its admissions process, it can evaluate ways to apply messaging, management, and workflow technologies that can improve admissions in the following areas: fax and document management, communications, referral tracking and approval, and reporting.

FAX AND DOCUMENT MANAGEMENT

"Any solution that doesn't address the fax challenges will typically fall short," says Felicia Wilson, a licensed nursing facility administrator and director of the human services program at Shorter College in Rome, Georgia. "Experience has shown that providers must take steps to minimize receipt and management of faxed paper documents to make referral management more efficient."

Providers also may not realize how frequently fax errors occur that could delay or block inbound referrals. Typically, about 8% of outbound faxes do not reach their intended destination on the first try.

One option for providers is to convert faxed documents into an electronic format. Fax servers can provide this capability at a reasonable cost.

Providers may also benefit from software that helps organize and manage those electronic documents, which helps facilitate a smooth transition away from paper-filing processes.

It is important to note that providers should not let discussions about waiting for universal healthcare data standards for electronic medical records sidetrack attempts to automate. Just storing and managing documents in a common electronic document format, such as the ubiquitous PDF, is a huge incremental improvement over paper filing.

COMMUNICATION IS IMPORTANT

Both internal and external communications are critical to a responsive, efficient admissions team. In the May 2008 *Provider* cover story, Donna Shaw, administrator of Woodbine Rehabilitation Health Care in Alexandria, Virginia, summed up the critical need for responsive communications with referral sources: "Relationships with social workers and discharge planners at the hospitals are key," she said. "In an effort to move patients out quickly, hospitals are now expediting their placing process, which, in many cases, means a patient is referred to the facility that has the first available bed."

That urgency means providers cannot afford to miss calls or play phone tag with referral sources. Messaging and alerting systems can help providers know immediately when a referral comes in and send automated emails or faxes back to the referral source to update the status.

There are also emerging technologies to instantly confirm patient information, such as insurance verification—a step that typically requires multiple phone calls and can delay an admissions decision.

Some hospitals have adopted e-referral solutions that facilitate faster exchange of referral communications. These e-referrals still represent a small percentage of inbound referrals, however—about 6% according to the 2007 admissions survey. About 80% of new referral inquiries still arrive by fax or phone.

Providers should adopt tools and processes to effectively manage all inbound referrals, from all sources or methods, and communicate instantly with those referral sources.

REFERRAL TRACKING AND APPROVAL

Referral tracking and approval often remains a decidedly low-tech operation. A hospital or other source faxes in a referral request. The intake coordinator receives the fax, captures it in a handwritten log book or spreadsheet, makes copies of the paper documents, and distributes them to the appropriate clinical and management staff for review, with sticky notes affixed providing further instructions.

While this process may ultimately work, it is slow and inefficient. It also does not provide any mechanism for viewing the status of multiple active referral cases.

Some providers have adopted workflow automation software that can enable the admissions team to do several things:

- Notify staff when a new referral arrives
- Set review tasks for multiple staff members
- Capture and share notes related to the referrals
- Provide a quick update of referral status

"In an area where every second counts, workflow automation can make the difference between winning or losing a qualified patient referral," says Wilson.

ANALYZING REFERRAL ACTIVITY

Admissions staff often must report referral activity to management weekly or even daily. Much like the typical referral review process, this effort usually involves manually capturing information from multiple sources and compiling it into a written report or spreadsheet.

These manual processes make it extremely difficult to analyze referral activity, capacities, and win-loss data and create a particular challenge for multi-location providers that seek to view and analyze referral activity across all locations. They struggle to identify and deliver the services that are most in demand, prioritize and measure marketing programs, and keep admissions at peak levels.

One of the greatest advantages of automating admissions and referral processes is the enhanced ability to see and analyze referral activity. If a provider adopts a system that helps manage referral documents and workflows, by nature, that system will be capturing information that can help the provider make more informed decisions related to the admissions process.

There are several things a provider can expect to get a better view of with an automated system, including wins and losses; referral sources, types, and methods; reasons for decline; referral status and performance across locations; and acceptance rates.

Any provider considering solutions for automating admissions should evaluate up front what data it wants to report.

HOURS SAVED

One six-location skilled nursing provider implemented a web automation solution for centralized admissions and has seen the potential for tremendous gains in responsiveness and efficiency. An analysis that examined the time the provider spent on daily referral management processes revealed that the provider will save an estimated 1,175 hours, or 29.5 work weeks per year, by expediting referral review and communications processes.

This helps the provider meet goals to improve responsiveness to referral sources and maintain a competitive advantage in its marketplace.

The good news for providers seeking similar results is that many of the associated technologies are fairly simple, such as fax servers, e-mail messaging and alerting tools, and electronic document formats.

Providers may also benefit from web-based subscription solutions. Accessing a program through a web portal that is utilized as a monthly or annual subscription can eliminate upfront investments, such as software and hardware, as well as the need to install upgrades.

Providers simply need to assess their current admission processes and identify and apply the right mix to make admissions faster, smarter, and more effective.

Checklists

Checklist A-1 Reviewing a Budget

1. Is this budget static (not adjusted for volume) or flexible (adjusted for volume during the year)?

2. Are the figures designated as fixed or variable?

3. Is the budget for a defined unit of authority?

4. Are the line items within the budget all expenses (and revenues, if applicable) that are controllable by the manager?

5. Is the format of the budget comparable with that of previous periods so that several reports over time can be compared if so desired?

6. Are actual and budget for the same period?

7. Are the figures annualized?

8. Test one line-item calculation. Is the math for the dollar difference computed correctly? Is the percentage properly computed based on a percentage of the budget figure?

Checklist A-2   Building a Budget

1. What is the proposed volume for the new budget period?

2. What is the appropriate inflow (revenues) and outflow (cost of services delivered) relationship?

3. What will the appropriate dollar cost be?

    (Note: this question requires a series of assumptions about the nature of the operation for the new budget period.)

    3a. Forecast service-related workload.

    3b. Forecast non-service-related workload.

    3c. Forecast special project workload if applicable.

    3d. Coordinate assumptions for proportionate share of interdepartmental projects.

4. Will additional resources be available?

5. Will this budget accomplish the appropriate managerial objectives for the organization?

Checklist A-3   Balance Sheet Review

1. What is the date on the balance sheet?

2. Are there large discrepancies in balances between the prior year and the current year?

3. Did total assets increase over the prior year?

4. Did current assets increase, decrease, or stay about the same?

5. Did current liabilities increase, decrease, or stay about the same?

6. Did land, plant, and equipment increase or decrease significantly over the prior year?

7. Did long-term debt increase or decrease significantly over the prior year?

Courtesy of J.J. Baker and R.W. Baker, Dallas, Texas.

Checklist A-4   Review of the Statement of Revenue and Expense

1. What is the period reported on the statement of revenue and expense?

2. Is it one year or a shorter period? If it is a shorter period, why is that?

3. Are there large discrepancies in balances between the prior year operations and the current year operations?

4. Did total operating revenue increase over the prior year?

5. Did total operating expenses increase, decrease, or stay about the same? Is any particular line item unusually large or small?

6. Did income from operations increase, decrease, or stay about the same?

7. Are there unusual nonoperating gains or losses?

8. Did the current year result in an excess of revenue over expense? Is it as much as that of the prior year?

9. Did long-term debt increase or decrease significantly over the prior year?

Checklist A-5   Considerations for Forecasting Equipment Acquisition

- Only one location?
- Equipment—single purpose or multi-purpose?
- Technology—new, middle-aged, old (obsolete vs. untested)?
- Equipment compatibility
- Medical supply cost
- High or low capital investment?
- Buy new or used (refurbished)?
- Buy or lease?
- Lease for a number of years or lease on a pay-per-procedure deal?
- How much staff training is required?
- Certification required?
- Square footage required for equipment
- Is the required square footage available?
- Cleaning methods and equipment (and staff level required)
- Repairs and maintenance expense (high, medium, low?)

Web-Based and Software Learning Tools

HOMEPAGE FOR HEALTHCARE FINANCE

Health Care Finance: Basic Tools for Nonfinancial Managers, 4th edition, has its own page on the Jones & Bartlett Learning website. The homepage contains resources for both instructors and students. The site can be accessed using the following URL: http://www.jblearning.com/catalog/9781284029864/.

SOFTWARE TOOLS

Microsoft software and its web-based applications are universally available across the United States, and Microsoft Office Excel offers an array of computation tools. Relevant information is available at www.microsoft.com/office.

For example, click on "function reference/financial" for a listing of Excel's financial computations. And of course the formulas within Excel spreadsheets provide calculator capability for every-day addition, subtraction, multiplication, and division. The website also offers supporting resources such as online tutorials and a "help and how-to" feature, along with tips about using the various Excel features.

OTHER WEB-BASED TOOLS

A user who prefers to use a business analyst calculator (as opposed to computer spreadsheets) can search the Web for a calculator distributor who posts an operating guidebook.

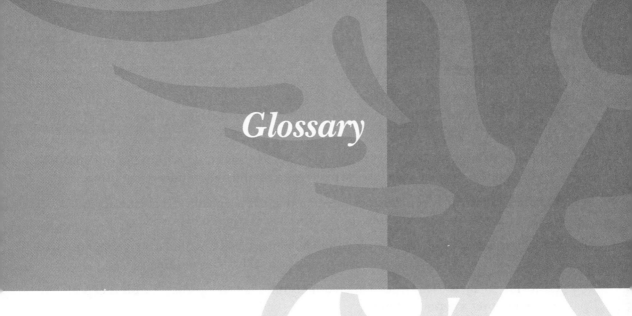

Glossary

Accounting Rate of Return: See Unadjusted Rate of Return.

Accounting System: Records the evidence that some event has occurred in the healthcare financial system.

Accrual Basis Accounting: Revenue is recorded when it is earned, not when payment is received. Expenses are recorded when they are incurred, not when they are paid. The opposite of accrual basis is cash basis accounting.

Action Plan: A detailed plan of operations that shows how one part of a particular objective will be accomplished.

Annualize: To convert data to an annual (12-month) period.

Assets: The net value of what an organization owns.

Balance Sheet: One of the four basic financial statements. Generally speaking, the balance sheet records what an organization owns, what it owes, and what it is worth at a particular point in time.

Benchmarking: The continuous process of measuring products, services, and activities against the best levels of performance. Best levels may be found inside or outside of the organization.

Book Value: The book value (also known as net book value) of a fixed asset is a balance sheet figure that represents the remaining undepreciated portion of the fixed asset cost.

Break-Even Point: The point when the contribution margin (i.e., net revenues less variable costs) equals the fixed costs.

Budget: The organization-wide instrument through which activities are quantified in financial terms.

Business Plan: A document that is typically prepared in order to obtain funding and/or financing.

Capital: Represents the financial resources of the organization. Generally considered to be a combination of debt and equity.

Capital Expenditure Budget: A budget usually intended to plan, monitor, and control long-term financial issues.

Capital Structure: Means the proportion of debt versus equity within the organization. The phrase "capital structure" actually refers to the debt–equity relationship.

Case Mix Adjusted: A performance measure that has been adjusted for the acuity level of the patient and, presumably, the resource level required to provide care.

Cash Basis Accounting: A transaction does not enter the books until cash is either received or paid out. The opposite of cash basis is accrual basis accounting.

Cash Flow Analysis: This type of analysis illustrates how the project's cash is expected to move over a period of time.

Certified EHR Technology: An electronic health record (EHR) that has been specially certified for use in the EHR Incentive Programs.

Chart of Accounts: Maps out account titles in a uniform manner through a method of numeric coding.

Code Users: Any individual who needs to have some level of understanding of the coding system, but does not actually assign codes.

Common Sizing: A process of converting dollar amounts to percentages to put information on the same relative basis. Also known as vertical analysis.

Common Stock: Stocks represent equity, or net worth, in a company. Common stock typically pays a proportionate share of net income out as a dividend to its investors.

Contribution Income Statement: Specifically identifies the contribution margin within the income statement format.

Contribution Margin: Called this because it contributes to fixed costs and to profits. Computed as net revenues less variable costs.

Controllable Expenses: Subject to a manager's own decision making and thus "controllable."

Controlling: Making sure that each area of the organization is following the plans that have been established.

Core Objectives: EHR Incentive Program criteria that is necessary to achieve meaningful use. Core objectives are mandatory; thus the provider must meet all applicable core objectives. See also Menu Objective.

Cost: The amount of cash expended (or property transferred, services performed, or liability incurred) in consideration of goods or services received or to be received.

Cost-Profit-Volume: A method of illustrating the break-even point, whereby the three elements of cost, profit, and volume are accounted for within the computation.

Cost Object: Any unit for which a separate cost measurement is desired.

Critical Access Hospitals (CAHs): Certain rural providers qualify as CAHs under the Medicare program. These eligible CAHs are a separate provider type and are reimbursed using a separate payment method.

Cumulative Cash Flow: The accumulated effect of cash inflows and cash outflows are added and/or subtracted to show the overall net accumulated result.

Current Ratio: A liquidity ratio considered to be a measure of short-term debt-paying ability. Computed by dividing current assets by current liabilities.

Days Cash on Hand Ratio: A liquidity ratio that indicates the number of days of operating expenses represented in the amount of unrestricted cash on hand. Computed by dividing unrestricted cash and cash equivalents by the cash operating expenses divided by number of days in the period.

Days Receivables Ratio: A liquidity ratio that represents the number of days in receivables. Computed by dividing net receivables by net credit revenues divided by number of days in the period.

Debentures: Bonds that are unsecured. Debentures are backed by revenues that the issuing organization can earn.

Debt Service Coverage Ratio: A solvency ratio universally used in credit analysis to measure ability to pay debt service. Computed by dividing change in unrestricted net assets (net income) plus interest, depreciation, and amortization by maximum annual debt service.

Decision Making: Making choices among available alternatives.

Deflation: A contraction in the volume of available money and credit that results in a general decline in prices.

Denominator: The bottom part of a fraction. The denominator indicates the total number of parts available to be divided. See also Numerator.

Depreciation: Depreciation expense spreads, or allocates, the cost of a fixed asset over the useful life of that asset.

Diagnoses: A common method of grouping healthcare expenses for purposes of planning and control. Such a grouping may be by major diagnostic categories or by diagnosis-related groups.

Direct Costs: These costs are incurred for the sole benefit of a particular operating unit. They can therefore be specifically associated with a particular unit or department or patient. Laboratory tests are an example of a direct cost.

Discounted Fee-for-Service: The provider of services is paid according to an agreed-upon contracted discount and after the service is delivered.

Dispenser: Either a person or other legal entity who provides drug products for human use on prescription in the course of professional practice, and who is licensed, registered, or otherwise permitted by the jurisdiction in which the person practices, or the entity is located, to do so.

Electronic Data Interchange: The electronic transfer of information such as electronic media claims. The transfer is made in a standard format between trading partners.

Electronic Health Record (EHR): A health-related electronic record of an individual that includes patient demographic and clinical information and that has the capacity to provide clinical decision support, support physician order entry, capture and query quality information, and exchange and integrate electronic health information.

Electronic Prescribing (E-Prescribing): Transmitting a prescription or prescription-related information using electronic media between a prescriber, dispenser, PBM, or health plan. The transmission may be either direct or through an intermediary, including an e-prescribing network.

Electronic Transaction Standards: Standards that are adopted and used to facilitate the electronic transmission of healthcare information and related business transactions.

Eligible Professional: In this context, physicians, practitioners, and therapists who are eligible for payment in the e-prescribing incentives program.

Equity: Claims held by the owners of the business because they have invested in the business; what the business is worth on paper, net of liabilities.

Estimates: A judgment that takes the place of actual measurement.

Expenses: Actual or expected cash outflows incurred in the course of doing business. Expenses are the costs that relate to the earning of revenue. An example is salary expense for labor performed.

Expired Costs: Costs that are used up in the current period and are matched against current revenues.

Fee-for-Service: The provider of services is paid according to the service performed and after the service is delivered.

FIFO: The First-In, First-Out (FIFO) inventory costing method recognizes the first costs placed into inventory as the first costs moved out into cost of goods sold when a sale occurs.

Financial Accounting: Is generally for outside, or third-party, use and thus emphasizes external reporting.

Financial Forecast: "Forecasted" prospective financial statements. Forecasts are based on assumptions that are expected to exist, and that reflect actions that are expected to occur.

Financial Lease: A formal agreement that may be called a lease but is actually a contract to purchase. This type of lease must meet certain criteria.

Financial Projection: "Projected" prospective financial statements that are often prepared to answer "what-if" questions. The statements "project" a view of future events, projects, or operations using a set of presumed, or hypothetical, assumptions.

Fixed Costs: Those costs that do not vary in total when activity levels or volume of operations change. Rent expense is an example of fixed cost.

Flexible Budget: A budget based on a range of activity or volume. The flexible budget is adjusted, or flexed (thus "flexible") to the actual level of output achieved or expected to be achieved during the budget period.

Forecasts: Information used for purposes of planning for the future. Forecasts can be short, intermediate, or long range.

For-Profit Organization: A proprietary organization that is generally subject to income tax.

Full-Time Equivalent: A measure to express the equivalent of an employee (annualized) or a position (staffed) for the full time required (thus, "full-time equivalent," or FTE).

Fund Balance: The difference between net assets and net liabilities; a term generally used by not-for-profit organizations.

General Ledger: A document in which all transactions for the period reside.

General Services Expenses: This type of expense provides services necessary to maintain the patient, but the service is not directly related to patient care. Examples of general services expenses are laundry and dietary.

Goal: A statement of aim or purpose that is part of a strategic plan.

Gross Domestic Product (GDP): A measure of the output of goods and services produced by labor and property located in the United States. The Bureau of Economic Analysis (BEA) is responsible for releasing quarterly estimates of the GDP.

Health Information Exchange (HIE): The electronic movement, or transmission, of health-related information between and among organizations using nationally recognized standards.

Health Information Technology (HIT): Technology that is designed for, or supports use by, healthcare entities or patients. Includes hardware, software, integrated technologies or related licenses, intellectual property, upgrades, or packaged solutions.

Horizontal Analysis: The process of comparing and analyzing figures over several time periods. Also known as trend analysis.

ICD-10 Codes: The International Classification of Diseases (ICD) is the international standard for diagnostic disease classifications. ICD-10 indicates the tenth revision.

Indirect Cost: These costs are incurred on behalf of the overall operation and therefore cannot be associated with the provision of specific health services. The finance office is an example of an indirect cost. Also known as joint costs.

Inflation: An increase in the volume of money and credit relative to available goods and services resulting in a continuing rise in the general price level.

Information System: Gathers the evidence that some event has occurred in the healthcare financial system.

Innovation: An idea, practice, or object that is perceived as new.

Internal Rate of Return: A return on investment method, defined as the rate of interest that discounts future net inflows (from the proposed investment) down to the amount invested.

Inventory: All the items ("goods") that an organization has for sale in the normal course of its business.

Inventory Turnover: A ratio that shows how fast inventory is sold, or "turns over."

Joint Costs: These costs are incurred on behalf of the overall operation and therefore cannot be associated with the provision of specific health services. The finance office is a typical example of a joint cost. Also known as indirect cost.

Liabilities: What the organization owes.

Liabilities to Fund Balance Ratio: A solvency ratio used as a quick indicator of debt load. Computed by dividing total liabilities by unrestricted net assets. Also known as Debt to Net Worth Ratio.

LIFO: The Last-In, First-Out (LIFO) inventory costing method recognizes the latest, or last, costs placed into inventory as the first costs moved out into cost of goods sold when a sale occurs.

Liquidity Ratios: Ratios that reflect the ability of the organization to meet its current obligations. Liquidity ratios are measures of short-term sufficiency.

Loan Costs: Those costs necessary to close a loan.

Managed Care: A means of providing healthcare services within a network of healthcare providers. The central concept is coordination of all healthcare services for an individual.

Managerial Accounting: Is generally for inside, or internal, use and thus emphasizes information useful for managerial employees.

Meaningful Use: Providers must show that they are "meaningfully using" their certified EHR technology by meeting thresholds, or minimums, for certain program objectives.

Meaningful User: To be a meaningful user of electronic health records, the provider must be using EHR in a meaningful manner, be connected in a way that allows electronic exchange of health information, and be reporting on measures using EHR.

Medicaid Program: A federal and state matching entitlement program intended to provide medical assistance to eligible needy individuals and families. The program was established under Title XIX of the Social Security Act.

Medicare Program: A federal health insurance program for the aged (and, in certain instances, for the disabled) intended to complement other federal benefits. The program was established under Title XVIII of the Social Security Act.

Menu Objective: EHR Incentive Program criteria that is necessary to achieve meaningful use. Menu objectives provide a choice; thus the provider must meet a certain number of applicable menu objectives, but not all of them. See also Core Objectives.

Mission Statement: A Mission Statement explains the purpose of the organization. It explains "what we are now."

Mixed Cost: Those costs that contain an element of variable cost and an element of fixed cost.

Monetary Unit: A measure of units of currency, such as the dollar. Monetary units should be comparable when reporting financial results.

Mortgage Bonds: Bonds that are backed, or secured, by certain real property.

Municipal Bonds: Long-term obligations that are typically used to finance capital projects.

Net Worth: See Equity.

Noncontrollable Expenses: Outside the manager's power to make decisions, and thus "noncontrollable."

Nonproductive Time: Paid-for time when the employee is not on duty—that is, not producing. Paid-for vacation days and holidays are examples of nonproductive time.

Nonprofit Organization: Indicates the taxable status of the organization. A nonprofit (or voluntary) organization is exempt from paying income taxes.

Not-for-Profit Organization: See Nonprofit Organization.

Numerator: The top part of a fraction. The numerator indicates the total number of parts of the denominator taken. See also Denominator.

Operating Budget: A budget that generally deals with actual short-term revenues and expenses necessary to operate the facility.

Operating Lease: A lease that is considered an operating expense and thus is treated as an expense of current operations. This type of lease does not meet the criteria to be treated as a financial lease.

Operating Margin: A profitability ratio generally expressed as a percentage, the operating margin is a multipurpose measure. It is used for a number of managerial purposes and also sometimes enters into credit analysis. Computed by dividing operating income (loss) by total operating revenues.

Operations Expenses: This type of expense provides service directly related to patient care. Examples of operations expenses are radiology expense and drug expense.

Organization Chart: Indicates the formal lines of communication and reporting and how responsibility is assigned to managers.

Organizational Values: Organizational values express the philosophy of the organization, most often expressed in a Values Statement.

Organizing: Deciding how to use the resources of the organization to most effectively carry out the plans that have been established.

Original Records: Provide evidence that some event has occurred in the healthcare financial system.

Overhead: Refers to the remaining expenses of operation that are necessary to produce the service but that are not directly attributable to that service.

Pareto Analysis: An analytical tool employing the Pareto principle, also known as the 80/20 rule. The Pareto principle states that 80% of an organization's problems are caused by 20% of the possible causes.

Patient Mix: A term indicating the mix of payers; thus, whether the individual is a Medicare patient, a Medicaid patient, a patient covered by private insurance, or a private pay patient varies the patient mix proportions. Patient mix information allows estimated payment levels to be associated with the service utilization assumptions.

Payback Period: The length of time required for the cash coming in from an investment to equal the amount of cash originally spent when the investment was acquired.

Payer Mix: The proportion of revenues realized from different types of payers. A measure often included in the profile of a healthcare organization.

Payment Adjustment: Term used for the downward adjustment of a provider's payment. A payment adjustment is usually viewed as a penalty.

Performance Measures: Measures that compare and quantify performance. Performance measures may be financial, nonfinancial, or a combination of both types.

Period Cost: For purposes of healthcare businesses, period cost is necessary to support the existence of the organization itself, rather than actual delivery of a service. Period costs are matched with revenue on the basis of the period during which the cost is incurred. The term originated with the manufacturing industry.

Planning: Identifying objectives of the organization and identifying the steps required to accomplish the objectives.

Preferred Stock: Stock that has preference over common stock in certain issues such as payment of dividends.

Prescriber: A physician, dentist, or other person who issues prescriptions for drugs for human use, and who is licensed, registered, or otherwise permitted by the United States or the jurisdiction in which he or she practices to do so.

Present Value Analysis: A concept based on the time value of money. The value of a dollar today is more than the value of a dollar in the future.

Private Sector Organizations: Those organizations that are not part of the government.

Procedures: A common method of grouping healthcare expenses for purposes of planning and control. Such a grouping will generally be by Current Procedural Terminology (or CPT) codes, which list descriptive terms and identifying codes for medical services and procedures performed.

Product Cost: For the purposes of healthcare businesses, product cost is necessary to actually deliver the service. The term originated with the manufacturing industry.

Productive Time: Equates to the employee's net hours on duty when performing the functions in his or her job description.

Profit Center: Makes a manager responsible for both the revenue/volume (inflow) side and the expense (outflow) side of a department, division, unit, or program. Also known as a responsibility center.

Profitability Ratios: Ratios that reflect the ability of the organization to operate with an excess of operating revenue over operating expense.

Profit-Oriented Organization: Indicates the taxable status of the organization. A profit-oriented (or proprietary) organization is responsible for paying income taxes.

Profit-Volume (PV) Ratio: The contribution margin (i.e., net revenues less variable costs) expressed as a percentage of net revenue.

Project Management Phases: A format for project management whereby the project is divided into a series of sequential phases.

Proprietary Organization: Indicates the taxable status of the organization. A proprietary (or profit-oriented) organization is responsible for paying income taxes.

Quartiles: A distribution into four classes, each of which contains one-quarter of the whole; any one of the four classes is a quartile.

Quick Ratio: A liquidity ratio considered the most severe test of short-term debt-paying ability (even more severe than the current ratio). Computed by dividing cash and cash equivalents plus net receivables by current liabilities. Also known as the acid-test ratio.

Reporting System: Produces reports of an event's effect in the healthcare financial system.

Responsibility Centers: Makes a manager responsible for both the revenue/volume (inflow) side and the expense (outflow) side of a department, division, unit, or program. Also known as a profit center.

Return on Total Assets: A profitability ratio generally expressed as a percentage, this is a broad measure of profitability in common use. Computed by dividing earnings before interest and taxes, or EBIT, by total assets. This ratio is known by its acronym, EBIT, in credit analysis circles.

Revenue: Actual or expected cash inflows due to the organization's major business. Revenues are amounts earned in the course of doing business. In the case of health care, revenues are mostly earned by rendering services to patients.

Revenue Amount: Refers to how much each payer is expected to pay for the service and/or drug or device.

Revenue Sources: Refers to how many payers will pay for the service and/or drug and device, and in what proportion.

Revenue Type: A designation as to whether, for example, revenue is derived entirely from services or whether part of the revenue is derived from drugs and devices.

Salvage Value: Salvage value, also known as residual value or scrap value, represents any expected cash value of the asset at the end of its useful life.

Semifixed Costs: Those costs that stay fixed for a time when activity levels or volume of operations change; rises will occur, but not in direct proportion.

Semivariable Costs: Those costs that vary when activity levels or volume of operations change, but not in direct proportion. A supervisor's salary is an example of a semivariable cost.

Situational Analysis: Management tool that reviews, assesses, and analyzes the organization's internal operations for strengths and weaknesses and the organization's external environment for opportunities and threats.

Solvency Ratios: Ratios that reflect the ability of the organization to pay the annual interest and principal obligations on its long-term debt. These ratios determine ability to "be solvent."

Space Occupancy: Within the context of a forecast or projection, refers to the overall cost of occupying the space required for the service or procedure. Considered to be an indirect cost.

Staffing: A term that means the assigning of staff to fill scheduled positions.

Statement of Cash Flows: One of the four basic financial statements, this statement reports the current period cash flow by taking the accrual basis statements and converting them to an effective cash flow. This is accomplished by a series of reconciling adjustments that account for the noncash amounts.

Statement of Fund Balance/Net Worth: One of the four basic financial statements, this statement reports the excess of revenue over expenses (or vice versa) for the period as the excess flows into equity (or reduces equity, in the case of a loss for the period).

Statement of Revenue and Expense: One of the four basic financial statements, this statement reports the inflow of revenue and the outflow of expense over a stated period of time. The net result is also reported, either as excess of revenue over expense or, in the case of a loss for the period, excess of expense over revenue.

Static Budget: A budget based on a single level of operations, or volume. After it is approved and finalized, the single level of operations (volume) is never adjusted; thus, the budget is "static" or unchanging.

Stock Warrants: Warrants allow the owner of the warrant to purchase additional shares of stock in the company, generally at a particular price and prior to an expiration date.

Strategic Objective: A strategic objective further defines intended outcomes in order to achieve a goal.

Structured Data: Data that adheres to standards that allow patient information to be easily retrieved and transferred.

Subsidiary Journals: Documents that contain specific sets of transactions and that support the general ledger.

Subsidiary Reports: Reports that support, and thus are subsidiary to, the four major financial statements.

Supplies: Within the context of a forecast or projection, refers to the necessary supplies that are required to perform a procedure or service. Considered to be a direct expense.

Support Services Expenses: This type of expense provides support to both general services expenses and to operations expenses. It is necessary for support, but it is neither directly related to patient care nor is it a service necessary to maintain the patient. Examples of support services are insurance and payroll taxes.

SWOT Analysis: Acronym for a method of situational analysis assessing an organization's strengths-weaknesses-opportunities-threats; thus "SWOT."

Target Operating Income: Allows the manager to determine, or target, how many units must be sold in order to yield a particular operating income.

Three-Variance Method: A method of variance analysis that compares volume variance to use (or quantity) variance and to spending (or price) variance.

Threshold: A minimum number, or percentage, to be met.

Time Value of Money: The present value concept, which is that the value of a dollar today is more than the value of a dollar in the future.

Trend Analysis: The process of comparing and analyzing figures over several time periods. Also known as horizontal analysis.

Trial Balance: A document used to balance the general ledger accounts and to produce financial statements.

Two-Variance Method: A method of variance analysis that compares volume variance to budgeted costs (defined as standard hours for actual production)—thus the "two-variance" method.

Unadjusted Rate of Return: An unsophisticated return on investment method, the answer for which is an estimate containing no precision.

Unexpired Costs: Costs that are not yet used up and will be matched against future revenues.

Useful Life: The useful life of a fixed asset determines the period over which the fixed asset's cost will be spread.

Values Statement: See Organizational Values.

Variable Costs: Those costs that vary in direct proportion to changes in activity levels of volume of operations. Food for meal preparation is an example of variable cost.

Variance Analysis: A variance is the difference between standard and actual prices and quantities. Variance analysis analyzes these differences.

Version 5010 of Transmission Standards: The current version of electronic transmission standards at the time of this writing. See Electronic Transmission Standards.

Vertical Analysis: A process of converting dollar amounts to percentages to put information on the same relative basis. Also known as common sizing.

Vision Statement: The Vision Statement explains "what we want to be." It is a look further into the future.

Voluntary Organization: Indicates the taxable status of the organization. A voluntary (or nonprofit) organization is exempt from paying income taxes.

Examples and Exercises, Supplemental Materials, and Solutions

The following examples and exercises include examples, practice exercises, and assignment exercises. Solutions to the practice exercises are found at the end of this section. Exercises are designated by chapter number.

EXAMPLES AND EXERCISES

CHAPTER 1

Assignment Exercise 1–1

Review the chapter text about types of organizations and examine the list in Exhibit 1–1.

Required

1. Obtain listings of healthcare organizations from the yellow pages of a telephone book.
2. Set up a worksheet listing the classifications of organizations found in Exhibit 1–1.
3. Enter the organizations you found in the yellow pages onto the worksheet.
4. For each organization indicate the type of organization.
5. If some cannot be identified by type, comment on what you would expect them to be; that is, proprietary, voluntary, or government owned.

Assignment Exercise 1–2

Review the chapter text about organization charts. Also examine the organization charts appearing in Figures 1–2 and 1–3.

Required

1. Refer to the Metropolis Health System (MHS) case study appearing in Chapter 28. Read about the various types of services offered by MHS.
2. The MHS organization chart has seven major areas of responsibility, each headed by a senior vice president. Select one of the seven areas and design additional levels

of detail that indicate the managers. If you have considerable detail you may choose one department (such as ambulatory operations) instead of the entire area of responsibility for that senior vice president.

3. Do you believe your design of the detailed organization chart indicates centralized or decentralized lines of authority for decision making? Can you explain your approach in one to two sentences?

CHAPTER 2

Assignment Exercise 2–1: Health System Flowsheets

Review the chapter text about information flow and Figures 2–2 and 2–3.

Required

1. Find an information flowsheet from a healthcare organization. It can be from a published source or from an actual organization.
2. Based on this flowsheet, comment on what the structure of the organization's information system appears to be.
3. If you were a manager (at this organization), would you want to change the structure? If so, why? If not, why not?

Assignment Exercise 2–2: Chart of Accounts

Review the chapter text about the chart of accounts and how it is a map of the company elements. Also review Exhibits 2–1, 2–2, and 2–3.

Required

1. Find an excerpt from a healthcare organization's chart of accounts. It can be from a published source or from an actual organization.
2. Based on this chart of accounts excerpt, comment on what the structure of the organization's reporting system appears to be.
3. If you were a manager (at this organization), would you want to change the system? If so, why? If not, why not?

CHAPTER 3

Example 3A: Assets and Liabilities

Study the chapter text concerning examples of assets and liabilities. Is the difference between short-term and long-term assets and liabilities clear to you?

Practice Exercise 3–I

Place an "X" in the appropriate classification for each balance sheet item listed below.

	Short-Term Asset	*Long-Term Asset*	*Short-Term Liability*	*Long-Term Liability*
Payroll taxes due				
Accounts receivable				
Land				
Mortgage payable (noncurrent)				
Buildings				
Note payable (due in 24 months)				
Inventory				
Accounts payable				
Cash on hand				

Assignment Exercise 3–1: Balance Sheet

Locate a healthcare-related balance sheet. The source of the balance sheet can be internal (within a healthcare facility of some type) or external (from a published article or from a company's annual report, for example). Write your impressions and/or comments about the assets, liabilities, and net worth found on your balance sheet. Would you have preferred more detail in this statement? If so, why?

Assignment Exercise 3–2: Balance Sheet

Locate a second healthcare-related balance sheet. Again, the source of the balance sheet can be either internal or external. Compare the balance sheet you acquired for Assignment Exercise 3-1 with the second balance sheet you have now obtained. What is the same? What is different? Which one do you find more informative? Why?

CHAPTER 4

Example 4A: Contractual Allowances

Contractual allowances represent the difference between the full established rate and the agreed-upon contractual rate that will be paid. An example was given in the text of Chapter 4 by which the hospital's full established rate for a certain procedure is $100, but Giant Health Plan has negotiated a managed care contract whereby the plan pays only $90 for that procedure. The contractual allowance is $10 ($100 less $90 = $10). Assume instead that Near-By Health Plan has negotiated its own managed care contract whereby this plan pays $95 for that procedure. In this case the contractual allowance is $5 ($100 less $95 = $5).

Assignment Exercise 4–1: Contractual Allowances

Physician office revenue for visit code 99214 has a full established rate of $72.00. Of 10 different payers, there are 9 different contracted rates, as follows:

Payer	Contracted Rate
FHP	$35.70
HPHP	58.85
MC	54.90
UND	60.40
CCN	70.20
MO	70.75
CGN	10.00
PRU	54.90
PHCS	50.00
ANA	45.00

Rates for illustration only.

Required

1. Set up a worksheet with four columns: Payer, Full Rate, Contracted Rate, and Contractual Allowance.
2. For each payer, enter the full rate and the contracted rate.
3. For each payer, compute the contractual allowance.

The first payer has been computed below:

Payer	Full Rate	(less)	Contracted Rate	(equals)	Contractual Allowance
FHP	$72.00		$35.70		$36.30

Example 4B: Revenue Sources and Grouping Revenue

Sources of healthcare revenue are often grouped by payer. Thus, services might be grouped as follows:

Revenue from the Medicare Program (payer = Medicare)
Revenue from the Medicaid Program (payer = Medicaid)
Revenue from Blue Cross Blue Shield (payer = Commercial Insurance)
or
Revenue from Blue Cross Blue Shield (payer = Managed Care Contract)

Assignment Exercise 4–2: Revenue Sources and Grouping Revenue

The Metropolis Health System (MHS) has revenue sources from operations, donations, and interest income. The revenue from operations is primarily received for services. MHS groups its revenue first by cost center. Within each cost center the services revenue is then grouped by payer.

Required

1. Set up a worksheet with individual columns across the top for six revenue sources (payers): Medicare, Medicaid, Other Public Programs, Patients, Commercial Insurance, and Managed Care Contracts.
2. Certain situations concerning the Intensive Care Unit and the Laboratory are described below.

   Set up six vertical line items on your worksheet, numbered 1 through 6. Six situations are described below. For each of the six situations, indicate its number (1 through 6) and enter the appropriate cost center (either Intensive Care Unit or Laboratory). Then place an X in the column(s) that represents the correct revenue source(s) for the item. The six situations are as follows:

   (1) ICU stay billed to employee's insurance program.
   (2) Lab test paid for by an individual.
   (3) Pathology work performed for the state.
   (4) ICU stay billed to member's health plan.
   (5) ICU stay billed for Medicare beneficiary.
   (6) Series of allergy tests run for eligible Medicaid beneficiary.

Headings for your worksheet:

	Medicare	Medicaid	Other Public Programs	Patients	Commercial Insurance	Managed Care Contracts
(1)						
(2)						
(3)						
(4)						
(5)						
(6)						

CHAPTER 5

Example 5A: Grouping Expenses by Cost Center

Cost centers are one method of grouping expenses. For example, a nursing home may consider the Admitting department as a cost center. In that case the expenses grouped under the Admitting department cost center may include:

- Administrative and Clerical Salaries
- Admitting Supplies
- Dues
- Periodicals and Books
- Employee Education
- Purchased Maintenance

Practice Exercise 5–I: Grouping Expenses by Cost Center

The Metropolis Health System groups expenses for the Intensive Care Unit into its own cost center. Laboratory expenses and Laundry expenses are likewise grouped into their own cost centers.

Required

1. Set up a worksheet with individual columns across the top for the three cost centers: Intensive Care Unit, Laboratory, and Laundry.
2. Indicate the appropriate cost center for each of the following expenses:
   - Drugs Requisitioned
   - Pathology Supplies
   - Detergents and Bleach
   - Nursing Salaries
   - Clerical Salaries
   - Uniforms (for Laundry Aides)
   - Repairs (parts for microscopes)
     (Hint: One of the expenses will apply to more than one cost center.)

Headings for your worksheet:

Intensive Care Unit	Laboratory	Laundry

Assignment Exercise 5–1: Grouping Expenses by Cost Center

The Metropolis Health System's Rehabilitation and Wellness Center offers outpatient therapy and return-to-work services plus cardiac and pulmonary rehabilitation to get people back to a normal way of living. The Rehabilitation and Wellness Center expenses include the following:

- Nursing Salaries
- Physical Therapist Salaries
- Occupational Therapist Salaries
- Cardiac Rehab Salaries
- Pulmonary Rehab Salaries
- Patient Education Coordinator Salary
- Nursing Supplies
- Physical Therapist Supplies
- Occupational Therapist Supplies
- Cardiac Rehab Supplies

- Pulmonary Rehab Supplies
- Training Supplies
- Clerical Office Supplies
- Employee Education

Required

1. Decide how many cost centers should be used for the above expenses at the Rehabilitation and Wellness Center.
2. Set up a worksheet with individual columns across the top for the cost centers you have chosen.
3. For each of the expenses listed above, indicate to which of your cost centers it should be assigned.

Example 5B

Study the chapter text concerning grouping expenses by diagnoses and procedures. Refer to Exhibits 5–3 and 5–4 (about major diagnostic categories), Exhibit 5–5 (about DRGs and MDCs), and Table 5–1 (about procedure codes) for examples of different ways to group expenses by diagnoses and procedures.

Assignment Exercise 5–2

Required

Find a listing of expenses by diagnosis or by procedure. The source of the list can be internal (within a healthcare facility of some type) or external (such as a published article, report, or survey). Comment upon whether you believe the expense grouping used is appropriate. Would you have grouped the expenses in another way?

CHAPTER 6

Example 6A: Direct and Indirect Costs

Review the chapter text regarding direct and indirect costs. In particular, review the example of ambulance direct costs (Exhibit 6–1) and indirect costs (Exhibit 6–2). Remember that indirect costs are shared and are sometimes called joint costs or common costs. Because such costs are shared they must be allocated. Also, remember that one test of a direct cost is to ask: "If the operating unit (such as a department) did not exist, would this cost not be in existence?"

Practice Exercise 6–I: Identifying Direct and Indirect Costs

Make a worksheet with two columns: Direct Cost and Indirect Cost. Place each of the following items in the appropriate column:

- Managed care marketing expense
- Real estate taxes
- Liability insurance
- Clinic telephone expense

- Utilities (for the entire facility)
- Emergency room medical supplies

Assignment Exercise 6–1: Allocating Indirect Costs

Study Table 6–1, Table 6–2, and review the chapter text describing how the indirect cost is allocated. This assignment will change the allocation bases input for (A) Number of Visits (Volume), (B) Proportion of Direct Costs, and (C) Number of Computers in Service.

Required

1. Compute the costs allocated to cost centers "Clerical Salaries," "Administrative Salaries," and "Computer Services" using the new allocation bases shown below. Use worksheet #1 that replicates the set up in Table 6–2. Total the new results.
   The new allocation bases are:

   A = # Visits (Volume): PT = 9,600/OT = 4,000/ST = 2,400/Total = 16,000
   (16,000 × $3.50 = $56,000)
   B = Proportion of Direct Costs: PT = 60%/OT = 25%/ST = 15%/Total = 100%
   (% × $55,000)
   C = # Computers in Service: PT = 10/OT = 3/ST = 3/Total = 16
   (16 × $5,000 each = $80,000).

2. Using worksheet #2 that replicates the set up in Table 6–1, enter the new direct cost and the new totals for indirect costs resulting from your work. Total the new results.

Practice Exercise 6–II: Responsibility Centers

The Metropolis Health System has one director who supervises the areas of Security, Communications, and Ambulance Services. This director also supervises the medical records relevant to Ambulance Services, the educational training for Security and Ambulance Services personnel, and the human resources for Security, Communications, and Ambulance Services personnel.

Required

Of the duties and services described, all of which are supervised by one director, which areas should be responsibility centers and which areas should be support centers? Draw them in a visual and indicate the reporting requirements.

Assignment Exercise 6–2: Responsibility Centers

Choose among the Case Study in Chapter 27, the clinic in Mini-Case Study 2, or the Metropolis Health System information as contained in its Case Study and the Appendix that contains its financial statements. Designate the responsibility centers and the support centers for the organization selected. Prepare a rationale for the structure you have designed.

CHAPTER 7

Example 7A: Fixed, Variable, and Semivariable Distinction

Review the chapter text for the distinction between fixed, variable, and semivariable costs. Pay particular attention to the accompanying Figures 7–1 through 7–5.

Practice Exercise 7–I: Analyzing Mixed Costs

The Metropolis Health System (MHS) has a system-wide training course for nurse aides. The course requires a packet of materials that MHS calls the training pack. Due to turnover and because the course is system-wide, there is a monthly demand for new packs. In addition, the local community college also obtains the training packs used in their credit courses from MHS.

The education coordinator needs to know how much of the cost is fixed and how much of the cost is variable for these training packs. She decides to use the high–low method of computation.

Required

Using the monthly utilization information presented below, find the fixed and variable portion of costs through the high–low method.

Month	Number of Training Packs	Cost
January	1,000	$6,200
February	200	1,820
March	250	2,350
April	400	3,440
May	700	4,900
June	300	2,730
July	150	1,470
August	100	1,010
September	1,100	7,150
October	300	2,850
November	250	2,300
December	100	1,010

Assignment Exercise 7–1: Analyzing Mixed Costs

The education coordinator decides that the community college packs may be unduly influencing the high–low computation. She decides to rerun the results, omitting the community college volume.

Required

1. Using the monthly utilization information presented here, and omitting the community college training packs, find the fixed and variable portion of costs through the

high–low method. Note that the college only acquires packs in three months of the year: January, May, and September. These dates coincide with the start dates of their semesters and summer school.

2. The reason the education coordinator needs to know how much of the cost is fixed is because she is supposed to collect the appropriate variable cost from the community college for their packs. For her purposes, which computation do you believe is better? Why?

Month	Total Number of Training Packs	Total Cost	Community College Number Packs	Community College Cost
January	1,000	$6,200	200	$1,240
February	200	1,820		
March	250	2,350		
April	400	3,440		
May	700	4,900	300	2,100
June	300	2,730		
July	150	1,470		
August	100	1,010		
September	1,100	7,150	300	1,950
October	300	2,850		
November	250	2,300		
December	100	1,010		

Example 7B: Contribution Margin

Computation of a contribution margin is simplified if the fixed and variable expense has already been determined. Examine Table 7–1, which contains Operating Room fixed and variable costs. We can see that the total costs are $1,217,756. Of this amount, $600,822 is designated as variable cost and $616,934 is designated as fixed ($529,556 + $87,378 = $616,934). For purposes of our example, assume the Operating Room revenue amounts to $1,260,000. The contribution margin is computed as follows:

	Amount
Revenue	$1,260,000
Less Variable Cost	(600,822)
Contribution Margin	$659,178

Thus, $659,178 is available to contribute to fixed costs and to profit. (In this example fixed costs amount to $616,934, so there is an amount left to contribute toward profit.)

Practice Exercise 7–II: Calculating the Contribution Margin

Greenside Clinic has revenue totaling $3,500,000. The clinic has costs totaling $3,450,000. Of this amount, 40% is variable cost and 60% is fixed cost.

Required

Compute the contribution margin for Greenside Clinic.

Assignment Exercise 7–2: Calculating the Contribution Margin

The Mental Health program for the Community Center has just completed its fiscal year end. The program director determines that his program has revenue for the year of $1,210,000. He believes his variable expense amounts to $205,000 and he knows his fixed expense amounts to $1,100,000.

Required

1. Compute the contribution margin for the Community Center Mental Health Program.
2. What does the result tell you about the program?

Example 7-3: Cost-Volume-Profit (CVP) Ratio and Profit-Volume (PV) Ratio

Closely review the examples of ratio calculations in the chapter text. Also note that examples are presented in visuals as well as text.

Practice Exercise 7–3: Calculating the PV Ratio

The profit-volume (PV) ratio is also known as the contribution margin (CM) ratio. Use the same assumptions for the Community Center Mental Health Program. In addition to the contribution margin figures already computed, now compute the PV ratio (also known as the CM ratio).

Assignment Exercise 7–3: Calculating the PV Ratio and the CVP Ratio

Use the same assumptions for the Greenside Clinic. One more assumption will be added: the clinic had 35,000 visits.

Required

1. In addition to the contribution margin figures already computed, now compute the PV ratio (also known as the CM ratio).
2. Add another column to your worksheet and compute the clinic's per-visit revenue and costs.
3. Create a Cost-Volume-Profit chart. Refer to the chapter text along with Figure 7–6.

CHAPTER 8

Assignment Exercise 8–1: FIFO and LIFO Inventory

Study the FIFO and LIFO explanations in the chapter.

Required

> a1. Use the format in Exhibit 8–1 to compute the ending FIFO inventory and the cost of goods sold, assuming $90,000 in sales; beginning inventory 500 units @ $50; purchases of 400 units @ $50; 100 units @ $65; 400 units @ $80.
>
> a2. Also compute the cost of goods sold percentage of sales.
>
> b1. Use the format in Exhibit 8–2 to compute the ending LIFO inventory and the cost of goods sold, using same assumptions.
>
> b2. Also compute the cost of goods sold percentage of sales.
>
> c. Comment on the difference in outcomes.

Assignment Exercise 8–2: Inventory Turnover

Study the "Calculating Inventory Turnover" portion of the chapter closely, whereby the cost of goods sold divided by the average inventory equals the inventory turnover.

Required

Compute two inventory turnover calculations as follows:

1. Use the LIFO information in the previous assignment to first compute the average inventory and then to compute the inventory turnover.
2. Use the FIFO information in the previous assignment to first compute the average inventory and then to compute the inventory turnover.

Example 8A: Depreciation Concept

Assume that Metropolis Health System (MHS) purchased equipment for $200,000 cash on April 1 (the first day of its fiscal year). This equipment has an expected life of 10 years. The salvage value is 10% of cost. No equipment was traded in on this purchase.

Straight-line depreciation is a method that charges an equal amount of depreciation for each year the asset is in service. In the case of this purchase, straight-line depreciation would amount to $18,000 per year for 10 years. This amount is computed as follows:

> Step 1. Compute the cost net of salvage or trade-in value: 200,000 less 10% salvage value or 20,000 equals 180,000.
>
> Step 2. Divide the resulting figure by the expected life (also known as estimated useful life): 180,000 divided by 10 equals 18,000 depreciation per year for 10 years.

Accelerated depreciation represents methods that are speeded up, or accelerated. In other words a greater amount of depreciation is taken earlier in the life of the asset. One example of accelerated depreciation is the double-declining balance method. Unlike straight-line depreciation, trade-in or salvage value is not taken into account until the end of the depreciation schedule. This method uses *book value*, which is the net amount remaining when cumulative previous depreciation is deducted from the asset's cost. The computation is as follows:

> Step 1. Compute the straight-line rate: 1 divided by 10 equals 10%.
>
> Step 2. Now double the rate (as in *double-declining method*): 10% times 2 equals 20%.

Step 3. Compute the first year's depreciation expense: 200,000 times 20% equals 40,000.

Step 4. Compute the carry-forward book value at the beginning of the second year: 200,000 book value beginning Year 1 less Year 1 depreciation of 40,000 equals book value at the beginning of the second year of 160,000.

Step 5. Compute the second year's depreciation expense: 160,000 times 20% equals 32,000.

Step 6. Compute the carry-forward book value at the beginning of the third year: 160,000 book value beginning Year 2 less Year 2 depreciation of 32,000 equals book value at the beginning of the third year of 128,000.

—Continue until the asset's salvage or trade-in value has been reached.

—Do not depreciate beyond the salvage or trade-in value.

Practice Exercise 8–I: Depreciation Concept

Assume that MHS purchased equipment for $600,000 cash on April 1 (the first day of its fiscal year). This equipment has an expected life of 10 years. The salvage value is 10% of cost. No equipment was traded in on this purchase.

Required

1. Compute the straight-line depreciation for this purchase.
2. Compute the double-declining balance depreciation for this purchase.

Assignment Exercise 8–3: Depreciation Concept

Assume that MHS purchased two additional pieces of equipment on April 1 (the first day of its fiscal year), as follows:

1. The laboratory equipment cost $300,000 and has an expected life of 5 years. The salvage value is 5% of cost. No equipment was traded in on this purchase.
2. The radiology equipment cost $800,000 and has an expected life of 7 years. The salvage value is 10% of cost. No equipment was traded in on this purchase.

Required

For both pieces of equipment:

1. Compute the straight-line depreciation.
2. Compute the double-declining balance depreciation.

Example 8B: Depreciation

This example shows straight-line depreciation computed at a five-year useful life with no salvage value. Straight-line depreciation is the method commonly used for financing projections and funding proposals.

Depreciation Expense Computation: Straight Line

Five year useful life; no salvage value

Year #	Annual Depreciation	Remaining Balance
Beginning Balance =		60,000
1	12,000	48,000
2	12,000	36,000
3	12,000	24,000
4	12,000	12,000
5	12,000	-0-

Example 8C: Depreciation

This example shows straight-line depreciation computed at a five-year useful life with a remaining salvage value of $10,000. Note the difference in annual depreciation between Example 8B and Example 8C.

Depreciation Expense Computation: Straight Line

Five year useful life; $10,000 salvage value

Year #	Annual Depreciation	Remaining Balance
Beginning Balance =		60,000
1	10,000	50,000
2	10,000	40,000
3	10,000	30,000
4	10,000	20,000
5	10,000	10,000

Example 8D: Depreciation

This example shows double-declining depreciation computed at a five-year useful life with no salvage value. As is often the case with a five-year life, the double-declining method is used for the first three years and the straight-line method is used for the remaining two years. The double-declining method first computes what the straight-line percentage would be. In this case 100% divided by five years equals 20%. The 20% is then doubled. In this case 20% times 2 equals 40%. Then the 40% is multiplied by the remaining balance to be depreciated. Thus 60,000 times 40% for year one equals 24,000 depreciation, with a remaining balance of 36,000. Then 36,000 times 40% for year two equals 14,400 depreciation, and 36,000 minus 14,400 equals 21,600 remaining balance, and so on.

Now note the difference in annual depreciation between Example 8B, using straight-line for all five years, and Example 8D, using the combined double-declining and straight-line methods.

Depreciation Expense Computation: Double-Declining-Balance

Five year useful life; $10,000 salvage value

Year #	Annual Depreciation	Remaining Balance
Beginning Balance =		60,000
1	24,000*	36,000
2	14,400*	21,600
3	8,640*	12,960
4	6,480**	6,480
5	6,480**	6,480

*double-declining balance depreciation
** straight-line depreciation for remaining two years (12,960 divided by 2 = 6,480/yr)

Practice Exercise 8–II: Depreciation

Compute the straight-line depreciation for each year for equipment with a cost of $50,000, a five-year useful life, and a $5,000 salvage value.

Assignment Exercise 8–4: Depreciation

Set up a purchase scenario of your own and compute the depreciation with and without salvage value.

Assignment Exercise 8–5: Depreciation Computation: Units-of-Service

Study the "Units of Service" portion of the chapter closely.

Required

1. Using the format in Table 8–A-5, compute units of service depreciation using the following assumptions:

    Cost to be depreciated = $50,000
    Salvage value = zero
    Total units of service = 10,000
    Units of service per year: Year 1 = 2,200; Year 2 = 2,100;
       Year 3 = 2,300; Year 4 = 2,200; Year 5 = 200

2. Using the same format, compute units of service depreciation using adjusted assumptions as follows:

    Cost to be depreciated = $50,000
    Salvage value = $5,000
    Total units of service = 10,000
    Units of service per year: Year 1 = 2,200; Year 2 = 2,100;
       Year 3 = 2,300; Year 4 = 2,200; Year 5 = 200

CHAPTER 9

Example 9A

Review the chapter text about annualizing positions. In particular review Exhibit 9–2, which contains the annualizing calculations.

Practice Exercise 9–I: FTEs to Annualize Staffing

The office manager for a physicians' group affiliated with Metropolis Health System (MHS) is working on her budget for next year. She wants to annualize her staffing plan. To do so she needs to convert her staff's net paid days worked to a factor. Their office is open and staffed seven days a week, per their agreement with two managed care plans.

The office manager has the MHS worksheet, which shows 9 holidays, 7 sick days, 15 vacation days, and 3 education days, equaling 34 paid days per year not worked. The physicians' group allows 8 holidays, 5 sick days, and 1 education day. An employee must work one full year to earn 5 vacation days. An employee must have worked full time for three full years before earning 10 annual vacation days. Because the turnover is so high, nobody on staff has earned more than 5 vacation days.

Required

1. Compute net paid days worked for a full-time employee in the physicians' group.
2. Convert net paid days worked to a factor so the office manager can annualize her staffing plan.

Assignment Exercise 9–1: FTEs to Annualize Staffing

The Metropolis Health System managers are also working on their budgets for next year. Each manager must annualize his or her staffing plan, and thus must convert staff net paid days worked to a factor. Each manager has the MHS worksheet, which shows 9 holidays, 7 sick days, 15 vacation days, and 3 education days, equaling 34 paid days per year not worked.

The Laboratory is fully staffed 7 days per week and the 34 paid days per year not worked is applicable for the lab. The Medical Records department is also fully staffed 7 days per week. However, Medical Records is an outsourced department so the employee benefits are somewhat different. The Medical Records employees receive 9 holidays plus 21 personal leave days, which can be used for any purpose.

Required

1. Compute net paid days worked for a full-time employee in the Laboratory and in Medical Records.
2. Convert net paid days worked to a factor for the Laboratory and for Medical Records so these MHS managers can annualize their staffing plans.

Example 9B

Review the chapter text about staffing requirements to fill a position. In particular review Exhibit 9–4, which contains (at the bottom of the exhibit) the staffing calculations. Remember this method uses a basic work week as the standard.

Practice Exercise 9–II: FTEs to Fill a Position

Metropolis Health System (MHS) uses a basic work week of 40 hours throughout the system. Thus, one full-time employee works 40 hours per week. MHS also uses a standard 24-hour scheduling system of three 8-hour shifts. The Admissions manager needs to compute the staffing requirements to fill his departmental positions. He has more than one Admissions office staffed within the system. The West Admissions office typically has two Admissions officers on duty during the day shift, one Admissions officer on duty during the evening shift, and one Admissions officer on duty during the night shift. The day shift also has one clerical person on duty. Staffing is identical for all seven days of the week.

Required

1. Set up a staffing requirements worksheet, using the format in Exhibit 9–4.
2. Compute the number of FTEs required to fill the Admissions officer position and the clerical position at the West Admissions office.

Assignment Exercise 9–2: FTEs to Fill a Position

Metropolis Health System (MHS) uses a basic work week of 40 hours throughout the system. Thus, one full-time employee works 40 hours per week. MHS also uses a standard 24-hour scheduling system of three 8-hour shifts. The Director of Nursing needs to compute the staffing requirements to fill the Operating Room (OR) positions. Since MHS is a trauma center, the OR is staffed 24 hours a day, 7 days a week. At present, staffing is identical for all 7 days of the week, although the Director of Nursing is questioning the efficiency of this method.

The Operating Room department is staffed with two nursing supervisors on the day shift and one nursing supervisor apiece on the evening and night shifts. There are two technicians on the day shift, two technicians on the evening shift, and one technician on the night shift. There are three RNs on the day shift, two RNs on the evening shift, and one RN plus one LPN on the night shift. In addition, there is one aide plus one clerical worker on the day shift only.

Required

1. Set up a staffing requirements worksheet, using the format in Exhibit 9–4.
2. Compute the number of FTEs required to fill the Operating Room staffing positions.

CHAPTER 10

Practice Exercise 10–I: Components of Balance Sheet and Statement of Net Income

Financial statements for Doctors Smith and Brown are provided here. Use the doctors' balance sheet, statement of revenue and expenses, and statement of capital for this assignment.

Required

Identify the following doctors' balance sheet and statement of net income components. List the name of each component and its amount(s) from the appropriate financial statement.

- Current Liabilities
- Total Assets
- Income from Operations
- Accumulated Depreciation
- Total Operating Revenue
- Current Portion of Long-Term Debt
- Interest Income
- Inventories

Assignment Exercise 10–1: Components of Balance Sheet and Statement of Net Income

Refer to the Metropolis Health System (MHS) financial statements contained in Appendix 28-A. Use the MHS comparative balance sheet, statement of revenue and expenses, and statement of fund balance for this assignment.

Required

Identify the following MHS balance sheet components. List the name of each component and its amount(s) from the appropriate MHS financial statement.

- Current Liabilities
- Total Assets
- Income from Operations
- Accumulated Depreciation
- Total Operating Revenue
- Current Portion of Long-Term Debt
- Interest Income
- Inventories

Doctors Smith and Brown:
Statement of Net Income
for the Three Months Ended March 31, 2___

Revenue		
Net patient service revenue	180,000	
Other revenue	-0-	
Total Operating Revenue		180,000
Expenses		
Nursing/PA salaries	16,650	
Clerical salaries	10,150	
Payroll taxes/employee benefits	4,800	
Medical supplies and drugs	15,000	
Professional fees	3,000	
Dues and publications	2,400	
Janitorial service	1,200	
Office supplies	1,500	
Repairs and maintenance	1,200	
Utilities and telephone	6,000	
Depreciation	30,000	
Interest	3,100	
Other	5,000	
Total Expenses		100,000
Income from Operations		80,000
Nonoperating Gains (Losses)		
Interest Income		-0-
Nonoperating Gains, Net		-0-
Net Income		80,000

Doctors Smith and Brown
Balance Sheet
March 31, 2___

Assets
Current Assets

Cash and cash equivalents	25,000	
Patient accounts receivable	40,000	
Inventories—supplies and drugs	5,000	
Total Current Assets		70,000

Property, Plant, and Equipment

Buildings and Improvements	500,000	
Equipment	800,000	
Total	1,300,000	
Less Accumulated Depreciation	(480,000)	
Net Depreciable Assets	820,000	
Land	100,000	
Property, Plant, and Equipment, Net		920,000
Other Assets		10,000
Total Assets		1,000,000

Liabilities and Capital
Current Liabilities

Current maturities of long-term debt	10,000	
Accounts payable and accrued expenses	20,000	
Total Current Liabilities		30,000
Long-Term Debt	180,000	
Less Current Portion of Long-Term Debt	(10,000)	
Net Long-Term Debt		170,000
Total Liabilities		200,000
Capital		800,000
Total Liabilities and Capital		1,000,000

Doctors Smith and Brown
Statement of Changes in Capital
for the Three Months Ended March 31, 2___

Beginning Balance	$720,000
Net Income	80,000
Ending Balance	$800,000

The MHS Balance Sheet

Example 10A: Components of Balance Sheet and Income Statement

The "Accounts Receivable (net)" in Exhibit 10–1 means the accounts receivable figure of $250,000 on the balance sheet is net of the allowance for bad debts. If the allowance for bad debts is raised on the balance sheet, then bad debt expense (a.k.a. provision for doubtful accounts) on the income statement (a.k.a. statement of revenue and expense) also rises. Think of these two accounts as a pair.

Practice Exercise 10–II: Components of Balance Sheet and Income Statement

Refer to Doctors Smith and Brown's balance sheet, where patient accounts receivable is stated at $40,000. Do you think this figure is net of an allowance for bad debts?

Assignment Exercise 10–2: Components of Balance Sheet and Income Statement

Refer to the Metropolis Health System (MHS) balance sheet and statement of revenue and expense in Chapter 28's MHS Case Study. Patient accounts receivable of $7,400,000 is shown as net of $1,300,000 allowance for bad debts (8,700,000 − 1,300,000 = 7,400,000). (1) What percentage of gross accounts receivable is the allowance for bad debts? (2) If the allowance for bad debts is raised to $1,500,000, where does the extra $200,000 go?

Example 10B: Components of Balance Sheet and Income Statement

Refer to Exhibit 10–1 and Exhibit 10–2's Westside Clinic statements. The "Property, Plant, and Equipment (net)" total in Exhibit 10–1 means the property, plant, and equipment figure of $360,000 on the balance sheet is net of the reserve for depreciation. If the reserve for depreciation is raised on the balance sheet, then the depreciation expense on the income statement (a.k.a. statement of revenue and expense) also rises. Think of these two accounts as another pair.

Practice Exercise 10–III: Components of Balance Sheet and Income Statement

Refer to Doctors Smith and Brown's balance sheet, where buildings and equipment are both stated as net (the $820,000 figure), but land is not. Do you recall why this is so?

Assignment Exercise 10–3: Components of Balance Sheet and Income Statement

Refer to the Metropolis Health System (MHS) balance sheet and statement of revenue and expense in Chapter 28's MHS Case Study. Property, plant, and equipment of $19,300,000 is shown as "net," meaning net of the reserve for depreciation. If the $19,300,000 is reduced by $200,000 (meaning the reserve for depreciation has risen), what happens on the income statement?

CHAPTER 11

Example 11A

To better understand how the information for the numerator and the denominator of each calculation is obtained, Figure 11–1 illustrates the process. This figure takes the balance sheet and the statement of revenue and expense that were discussed in the preceding chapter and illustrates the source of each figure in the four liquidity ratios. The multiple computations in days cash on hand and in days receivables are further broken out into a three-step process to better illustrate sources of information.

Practice Exercise 11–I: Liquidity Ratios

Two of the liquidity ratios are illustrated in this practice exercise. Refer to Doctors Smith and Brown's financial statements presented in the preceding exercises for Chapter 10.

Required

1. Set up a worksheet for the current ratio and the quick ratio.
2. Compute the ratios for Doctors Smith and Brown.

Assignment Exercise 11–1: Liquidity Ratios

Refer to the Metropolis Health System (MHS) case study in Chapter 28.

Required

1. Set up a worksheet for the liquidity ratios.
2. Compute the four liquidity ratios using the Chapter 28 MHS financial statements.

Example 11B

To better understand how the information for the numerator and the denominator of each calculation is obtained, Figure 11–2 illustrates the process. This figure takes the balance sheet and the statement of revenue and expense that were discussed in the preceding chapter and illustrates the source of each figure in the two solvency ratios. Any multiple computations are further broken out to better explain sources of information.

Practice Exercise 11–II: Solvency Ratios

Refer to Doctors Smith and Brown's financial statements presented in the preceding exercises for Chapter 10.

Required

1. Set up a worksheet for the solvency ratios.
2. Compute these ratios for Doctors Smith and Brown. To do so, you will need one additional piece of information that is not present on the doctors' statements: their maximum annual debt service is $22,200.

Assignment Exercise 11–2: Solvency Ratios

Refer to the Metropolis Health System (MHS) case study in Chapter 28.

Required

1. Set up a worksheet for the liquidity ratios.
2. Compute the solvency ratios using the Chapter 28 MHS financial statements.

Example 11C

To better understand how the information for the numerator and the denominator of each calculation is obtained, study Figure 11–2. This figure takes the balance sheet and the statement of revenue and expense that were discussed in the preceding chapter and illustrates the source of each figure in the two profitability ratios. Any multiple computations are further broken out to better explain sources of information.

Practice Exercise 11–III: Profitability Ratios

Refer to Doctors Smith and Brown's financial statements presented in the preceding exercises for Chapter 10.

Required

1. Set up a worksheet for the profitability ratios.
2. Compute these ratios for Doctors Smith and Brown. All the necessary information is present on the doctors' statements.
   [Hint: "Operating Income (Loss)" is also known as "Income from Operations."]

Assignment Exercise 11–3: Profitability Ratios

Refer to the Metropolis Health System (MHS) case study in Chapter 28.

Required

1. Set up a worksheet for the liquidity ratios.
2. Compute the profitability ratios using the Chapter 28 MHS financial statements.

CHAPTER 12

Example 12A: Unadjusted Rate of Return

Assumptions

- Average annual net income = $100,000
- Original investment amount = $1,000,000
- Unrecovered asset cost at the end of useful life (salvage value) = $100,000

Calculation using original investment amount:

$$\frac{\$100,000}{\$1,000,000} = 10\% \text{ Unadjusted Rate of Return}$$

Calculation using average investment amount:

Step 1: Compute average investment amount for total unrecovered asset cost.

At beginning of estimated useful life = $1,000,000
At end of estimated useful life   = $ 100,000
                               Sum $1,100,000

Divided by 2 = $550,000 average investment amount

Step 2: Calculate unadjusted rate of return.

$$\frac{\$100,000}{\$550,000} = 18.2\% \text{ Unadjusted Rate of Return}$$

Practice Exercise 12–I: Unadjusted Rate of Return

Assumptions

- Average annual net income = $100,000
- Original investment amount = $500,000
- Unrecovered asset cost at the end of useful life (salvage value) = $50,000

Required

1. Compute the unadjusted rate of return using the original investment amount.
2. Compute the unadjusted rate of return using the average investment method.

Assignment Exercise 12–1: Unadjusted Rate of Return

Metropolis Health Systems' Laboratory Director expects to purchase a new piece of equipment. The assumptions for the transaction are as follows:

- Average annual net income = $70,000
- Original investment amount = $410,000
- Unrecovered asset cost at the end of useful life (salvage value) = $41,000

Required

1. Compute the unadjusted rate of return using the original investment amount.
2. Compute the unadjusted rate of return using the average investment method.

Example 12B: Finding the Future Value (with a Compound Interest Table)

Betty Dylan is Director of Nurses at Metropolis Health System. Her oldest son will be entering college in five years. Today Betty is trying to figure what his college fund will amount to in five more years. (Hint: Compound interest means interest is not only earned on the principal, but also is earned on the previous interest earnings that have been left in the account. Interest is thus compounded.)

The college fund savings account presently has a balance of $9,000 and any interest earned over the next five years will be left in the account. Betty assumes the annual interest rate will be 6%. How much money will be in the account at the end of five more years?

Solution to Example

Step 1. Refer to the Compound Interest Table found in Appendix 12-B at the back of this chapter. Reading across, or horizontally, find the 6% column. Reading down, or vertically, find Year 5. Trace across the Year 5 line item to the 6% column. The factor is 1.338.

Step 2. Multiply the current savings account balance of $9,000 times the factor of 1.338 to find the future value of $12,042. In five years at compound interest of 6% the college fund will have a balance of $12,042.

Practice Exercise 12–II: Finding the Future Value (with a Compound Interest Table)

Assume the college savings fund in the preceding example presently has a balance of $11,000 and any interest earned will be left in the account. Assume the annual interest rate will be 7%.

Required

Compute how much money will be in the account at the end of six more years. (Use the compound interest table in Appendix 12-B.)

Assignment Exercise 12–2: Finding the Future Value (with a Compound Interest Table)

John Whitten is one of the physicians on staff at Metropolis Health System. His practice is six years old. He has set up an office savings account to accumulate the funds to replace equipment in his practice. Today John is trying to figure what his equipment fund will amount to in four more years.

The equipment fund savings account presently has a balance of $63,500 and any interest earned over the next four years will be left in the account. John assumes the annual interest rate will be 5%. How much money will be in the account at the end of four more years?

Required

Compute how much money will be in the account at the end of four more years. (Use the compound interest table found in Appendix 12-B.)

Example 12C: Finding the Present Value (with a Present-Value Table)

Betty Dylan is taking an adult education night course in personal finance at the community college. The class is presently studying retirement planning. Each student is to estimate the amount of funds (in addition to pension plans and social security) they believe will be needed at retirement. Then they are to make a retirement plan.

Betty has estimated she would need $100,000 fifteen years from now. In order to complete her assignment she needs to know the present value of the $100,000. Betty further assumes an interest rate of 6%.

Solution to Example

Step 1. Refer to the Present-Value Table found in Appendix 12-A at the back of this chapter. Reading across, or horizontally, find the 6% column. Reading down, or vertically, find Year 15. Trace across the Year 15 line item to the 6% column. The factor is 0.4173.

Step 2. Multiply $100,000 times the factor of 0.4173 to find the present value of $41,730.

Practice Exercise 12–III: Finding the Present Value (with a Present-Value Table)

Betty isn't finished with her assignment. Now she wants to find the present value of $150,000 accumulated fifteen years from now. She further assumes a better interest rate of 7%.

Required

Compute the present value of $150,000 accumulated fifteen years from now. Assume an interest rate of 7%. (Use the Present-Value Table found in Appendix 12-A at the back of this chapter.)

Assignment Exercise 12–3: Finding the Present Value (with a Present-Value Table)

Part 1—Dr. John Whitten is still figuring out his equipment fund. According to his calculations he needs $250,000 to be accumulated six years from now. John is now trying to find the present value of the $250,000. He continues to assume an interest rate of 5%.

Required

Compute the present value of $250,000 accumulated fifteen years from now. Assume an interest rate of 5%. (Use the Present-Value Table found in Appendix 12-A at the back of this chapter.)

Part 2—John doesn't like the answer he gets. What if he can raise the interest rate to 7%? How much difference would that make?

Required

Compute the present value of $250,000 accumulated fifteen years from now assuming an interest rate of 7%. Compare the difference between this amount and the present value at 5%.

Example 12D: Internal Rate of Return

Review the chapter text to follow the steps set out to compute the internal rate of return.

Practice Exercise 12–IV: Internal Rate of Return

Metropolis Health System (MHS) is considering purchasing a tractor to mow the grounds. It would cost $16,950 and have a 10-year useful life. It will have zero salvage value at the end of 10 years. The head of the MHS grounds crew estimates it would save $3,000 per year. He figures this savings because just one of the present maintenance crew would be driving the tractor, replacing the labor of several men now using small household-type lawn mowers. Compute the internal rate of return for this proposed acquisition.

Assignment Exercise 12–4: Computing an Internal Rate of Return

Dr. Whitten has decided to purchase equipment that has a cost of $60,000 and will produce a pretax net cash inflow of $30,000 per year over its estimated useful life of six years. The equipment will have no salvage value and will be depreciated by the straight-line method. The tax rate is 50%. Determine Dr. Whitten's approximate after-tax internal rate of return.

Example 12E: Payback Period

Review the chapter text and follow the Doctor Green detailed example of payback period computation.

Practice Exercise 12–V: Payback

The MHS Chief Financial Officer is considering a request by the Emergency Room department for purchase of new equipment. It will cost $500,000. There is no trade-in. Its useful life would be 10 years. This type of machine is new to the department but it is estimated that it will result in $84,000 annual revenue and operating costs would be one-quarter of that amount. The CFO wants to find the payback period for this piece of equipment.

Assignment Exercise 12–5: Payback Period

The MHS Chief Financial Officer is considering alternate proposals for the hospital Radiology department. The Director of Radiology has suggested purchasing one of two pieces of equipment. Machine A costs $15,000 and Machine B costs $12,000. Both machines are estimated to reduce radiology operating costs by $5,000 per year.

Required

Which machine should be purchased? Make your payback calculations to provide the answer.

CHAPTER 13

Example 13A: Common Sizing

Common sizing converts numbers to percentages so that comparative analysis can be performed. Reread the chapter text about common sizing and examine the percentages shown in Table 13–1.

Practice Exercise 13–I: Common Sizing

The worksheet below shows the assets of two hospitals.

Required

Perform common sizing for the assets of the two hospitals.

	Same Year for Both Hospitals	
	Hospital A	Hospital B
Current Assets	$ 2,000,000	$ 8,000,000
Property, Plant, & Equipment	7,500,000	30,000,000
Other Assets	500,000	2,000,000
Total Assets	$10,000,000	$40,000,000

Assignment Exercise 13–1: Common Sizing

Refer to the Metropolis Health System (MHS) comparative financial statements contained in Appendix 28-A.

Required

Common size the MHS statement of revenue and expenses.

Example 13B: Trend Analysis

Trend analysis allows comparison of figures over time. Reread the chapter text about trend analysis and examine the difference columns shown in Table 13–3.

Practice Exercise 13–II: Trend Analysis

The worksheet below shows the assets of Hospital A over two years.

Required

Perform trend analysis for the assets of Hospital A.

Hospital A

	Year 1	Year 2
Current Assets	$1,600,000	$ 2,000,000
Property, Plant, & Equipment	6,000,000	7,500,000
Other Assets	400,000	500,000
Total Assets	$8,000,000	$10,000,000

Assignment Exercise 13–2: Trend Analysis

Refer to the Metropolis Health System (MHS) comparative financial statements contained in Appendix 28-A.

Required

Perform trend analysis on the MHS statement of revenue and expenses.

Practice Exercise 13–III: Contractual Allowance

Assumptions:

1. Your unit's gross charges for the period to date amount to $200,000.
2. The uniform gross charge for each procedure in your unit is $100.
3. The unit receives revenue from four major payers. For purposes of this exercise, assume the revenue volume from each represents 25% of the total. (The equal proportion is unrealistic, but serves the purpose for this exercise.)
4. The following contractual payment arrangements are in effect for the current period. The percentage of the gross charge that is currently paid by each payer is as follows:
   Payer 1 = 90%
   Payer 2 = 80%
   Payer 3 = 70%
   Payer 4 = 50%

Q: How many procedures has your unit recorded for the period to date?

Q: Of these, how many procedures are attributed to each payer?

Q: How much is the net revenue per procedure for each payer, and how much is the contractual allowance per procedure for each payer?

Assignment Exercise 13–3

As a follow-up to the previous Practice Exercise, new assumptions are as follows:

1. Your unit's gross charges for the period to date amount to $200,000.
2. The uniform gross charge for each procedure in your unit is $100.

3. The unit receives revenue from four major payers. The number of procedures performed for the period totals 2,000. Of that total, the number of procedures per payer (stated as a percentage) is as follows:
   Payer 1 = 30%
   Payer 2 = 40%
   Payer 3 = 20%
   Payer 4 = 10%
4. The following contractual payment arrangements are in effect for the current period. The percentage of the gross charge that is currently paid by each payer is as follows:
   Payer 1 = 80% [Medicare]
   Payer 2 = 70% [Commercial managed care plans]
   Payer 3 = 50% [Medicaid]
   Payer 4 = 90% [Self-pay]

Q: How many procedures are attributed to each payer?

Q: How much is the net revenue per procedure for each payer, and how much is the contractual allowance per procedure for each payer?

Q: How much is the total net revenue for each payer, and how much is the total contractual allowance for each payer?

Assignment Exercise 13–4.1: Forecast Capacity Levels

Review the information in Exhibit 13–1. The exhibit assumes three chairs and one 40-hour RN, for a realistic capacity level of seven patients infused per day.

Required

Prepare another Infusion Center Capacity Level Forecast as follows:
   Assume the same three infusion chairs, but add another nurse for either four or six hours per day. How would this change the daily capacity level for number of patients infused per day?

Assignment Exercise 13–4.2

Required

Prepare another Infusion Center Capacity Level Forecast as follows:
   Increase the number of infusion chairs to four, and add another nurse for either four or six hours per day. How would this change the daily capacity level for number of patients infused per day?

CHAPTER 14

Assignment Exercise 14–1: Comparable Data in a Graph

Review Figures 14–1 through 14–5. Each of the five figures presents a graph depicting some type of comparative data.

Required

Locate healthcare information that can reasonably be compared. (1) Prepare your comparative data. (2) Using your data, create one or more graphs similar to those found in Figures 14–1 through 14–5.

Assignment Exercise 14–2: Cumulative Inflation Factor for Comparable Data

Review Table 14–3 and the accompanying text.

Assumptions

Two hospitals report their annual projected revenue for five years to the local newspaper for a story on the area's future economic outlook. However, Hospital 1 has applied a cumulative inflation factor of 5% per year while Hospital 2 has not applied any inflation factor. Thus the information is not properly comparable.

	Projected Revenue				
	Year 1	Year 2	Year 3	Year 4	Year 5
Hospital 1	$20,000,000	$22,500,000	$27,500,000	$27,500,000	$30,000,000
Hospital 2	$20,000,000	$21,000,000	$25,000,000	$24,000,000	$26,000,000

Required

Revise Hospital 2's projections by applying a cumulative inflation factor of 5% per year.

Assignment Exercise 14–3

The head of your department is a prominent researcher. A health research foundation has asked him travel to London to give an important speech at a conference. He will then travel to Paris to tour a research facility before returning home. Although his travel expenses are being funded by the foundation, he will still need to take along some personal money. Consequently, he asks you to figure the exchange rates for $500 and for $1,000 in both pounds and euros. He explains that he is trying to judge the spending power of U.S. dollars when converted to the other currencies so he can decide how much personal money to take on the trip.

Required

Locate the current exchange rates for pounds and euros and compute the currency conversion for $500 and for $1,000.

Assignment Exercise 14–4: The Discovery

The Chief Financial Officer at Sample General Hospital has just discovered that the hospital's Chief of the Medical Staff's son Jason, a student at the local community college, is paid $100 per week year-round for grounds maintenance at the hospital's Outpatient Center.

The CFO, no fan of the Chief of Medical Staff, now wants you to prepare a report that compares the relative costs of lawn care at each of three locations: the hospital itself, the outpatient center, and the hospital-affiliated nursing home down the block.

Required

Review the available information for grounds maintenance at the three facilities. Decide how to convert this information into comparable data. Then prepare a report, based on your assumptions, that presents comparable costs of grounds care. Also provide your assessment of what the best future course of action should be.

Relevant Information

So far you have assembled the following information. Now you need to decide how it can be converted into comparable data.

Introduction to the Three Facilities

Sample General Hospital is an older 100-bed hospital. The new Outpatient Center, built last year, is across the street and the Golden Age Nursing Facility is down one block, on the corner. All three facilities are part of the Metropolis Health System. (Appendix 28-A contains some financial details about Sample Hospital.) The hospital is located in the midwestern sunbelt; there is occasional frost in the winter but no snow.

Grounds Maintenance Tasks That Should Be Performed at All Three Sites

- Mowing and edging
- Walk sweeping
- Raking leaves
- Blowing off parking lot
- Flower bed maintenance (where necessary)
- Hedge trimming and minor tree pruning (major tree trimming is performed by a contractor on an as-needed basis and thus should be disregarded)

Figure Ex-1 provides a map that illustrates the layout of the grounds for each facility and their proximity to each other.

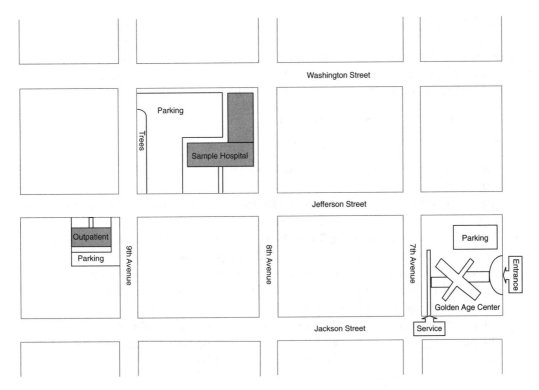

Figure Ex–1 Sample Hospital Map.

Grounds Maintenance Arrangements for the Three Facilities

The current grounds maintenance arrangements vary among the three facilities as follows:

1. Sample General Hospital uses its Maintenance department employees for grounds care. The hospital pays these employees $15 per hour plus 15% employee benefits; it is estimated they spend 1,000 hours per year on grounds maintenance work. Another estimated 120 hours per year are spent on maintaining the lawn care equipment. The employees use a riding lawn mower, edger, and blower, all owned by the hospital. The hospital just bought a new mower for $2,995 less a 10% discount. It is expected that the mower should last for five years.

2. The hospital's Chief of the Medical Staff's son Jason, a student at the local community college, is paid $100 per week year-round for grounds maintenance at the hospital's Outpatient Center. A friend sometimes helps, but when that happens Jason pays him out of his weekly $100. It takes about 1.5 hours to mow, edge, and blow. Jason uses his dad's riding mower and blower, but Jason recently bought his own edger. Jason also buys fertilizer for the grass twice a year.

3. The Nursing Facility contracts with a landscape service on a seasonally adjusted sliding scale. The landscape service is paid $600 per month from April to October (mowing season); $400 per month for February, March, and November; and $200 per month for November, December, and January. The landscape service provides all their own equipment. They also provide fertilizer and provide annuals to plant in the flower beds every quarter.

Sample General Hospital Property Description

The grounds to be maintained are as follows:

- The front lawn is grass in two sections on either side of the front entrance. Each section is about 50' by 60'.
- There is a hedge along the front of the building that is about 50' on either side of the front entrance.
- There are two small matching flower beds on either side of the front entrance.
- Another strip of grass alongside of the building is 30' by 100'.
- A third small strip of grass about 5' by 25' is by the Emergency entrance.
- The walkway dimensions are as follows: about 50' of front walk; about 30' of staff entrance walk, both of which are 5' wide.
- The Emergency Department's paved patient drop-off area is about 25' by 30'.
- The parking lot surface is about 200' by 250'. Along one side are overhanging trees that drop leaves and debris and are a constant sweeping problem. These are the only trees on the hospital site.

Outpatient Center Property Description

The grounds to be maintained are as follows:

- There is a strip of grass at the front of the building that is 12' wide and 65' long, split in the middle by a walkway 5' wide.
- There is a strip of grass at the back of the building between the building and the parking lot that is 5' wide and 50' long
- All the rest of the property is paved.

Nursing Center Property Description

Golden Age Nursing Center occupies one whole block. The grounds have many large trees. Flowerbeds have been planted around the trees as well as along the front walk and entrance. There are also two secured patio areas at the side of the building, screened by hedges, and each has a small bed of annuals. Because of the unique design of the building, grounds maintenance requires considerable handwork such as edging with a weed eater.

CHAPTER 15

Example 15A: Budgeting

A static budget is based on a single level of operations that is never adjusted. Therefore, the static budgeted expense amounts will not change, even though actual volume does change during the year.

The computation of a static budget variance only requires one calculation, as follows:

Actual Results	minus	Static Budget Amount	equals	Static Budget Variance

We can set up the example in the chapter text in this format as follows:

Use patient days as an example of level of volume, or output. Assume that the budget anticipated 40,000 patient days this year at an average of $600 revenue per day, or $2,400,000. Further assume that expenses were budgeted at $560 per patient day, or $22,400,000. The budget would look like this:

	As Budgeted
Revenue	$24,000,000
Expenses	22,400,000
Excess of Revenue over Expenses	$1,600,000

Now assume that only 36,000, or 90%, of the patient days are going to actually be achieved for the year. The average revenue of $600 per day will be achieved for these 36,000 days (thus 36,000 times 600 equals 21,600,000). Further assume that, despite the best efforts of the Chief Financial Officer, the expenses will amount to $22,000,000. The actual results would look like this:

	Actual
Revenue	$21,600,000
Expenses	22,000,000
Excess of Expenses over Revenue	$ (400,000)

The budgeted revenue and expenses still reflect the original expectation of 40,000 patient days; the budget report would look like this:

	Actual	Budget	Static Budget Variance
Revenue	$21,600,000	$24,000,000	$(2,400,000)
Expenses	22,000,000	22,400,000	(400,000)
Excess of Expenses over Revenue	$ (400,000)	$ 1,600,000	$(2,000,000)

Note: The negative actual result of (400,000) combined with the positive budget expectation of 1,600,000 amounts to the negative net variance of (2,000,000).

This example has shown a static budget, geared toward only one level of activity and remaining constant or static.

Practice Exercise 15–I: Budgeting

Budget assumptions for this exercise include both inpatient and outpatient revenue and expense. Assumptions are as follows:

As to the initial budget:

- The budget anticipated 30,000 inpatient days this year at an average of $650 revenue per day.
- Inpatient expenses were budgeted at $600 per patient day.
- The budget anticipated 10,000 outpatient visits this year at an average of $400 revenue per visit.
- Outpatient expenses were budgeted at $380 per visit.

As to the actual results:

- Assume that only 27,000, or 90%, of the inpatient days are going to actually be achieved for the year.
- The average revenue of $650 per day will be achieved for these 270,000 inpatient days.
- The outpatient visits will actually amount to 110%, or 11,000 for the year.
- The average revenue of $400 per visit will be achieved for these 11,000 visits.
- Further assume that, due to the heroic efforts of the Chief Financial Officer, the actual inpatient expenses will amount to $11,600,000 and the actual outpatient expenses will amount to $4,000,000.

Required

1. Set up three worksheets that follow the format of those in Example 15A. However, in each of your worksheets make two lines for revenue; label one as Revenue—Inpatient and the other Revenue—Outpatient. Add a Revenue Subtotal line. Likewise, make two lines for expense; label one as Expense—Inpatient and the other Expense—Outpatient. Add an Expense Subtotal line.
2. Using the new assumptions, complete the first worksheet for "As Budgeted."
3. Using the new assumptions, complete the second worksheet for "Actual."
4. Using the new assumptions, complete the third worksheet for "Static Budget Variance."

Assignment Exercise 15–1: Budgeting

Select an organization: either from the Case Studies in Chapters 27–28 or from one of the Mini-Case Studies in Chapters 29–31.

Required

1. Using the organization selected, create a budget for the next fiscal year. Set out the details of all assumptions you needed in order to build this budget.
2. Use the "Checklist for Building a Budget" (Exhibit 15–2) and critique your own budget.

Assignment Exercise 15–2: Budgeting

Find an existing budget from a published source. Detail should be extensive enough to present a challenge.

Required

1. Using the existing budget, create a new budget for the next fiscal year. Set out the details of all the assumptions you needed in order to build this budget.
2. Use the "Checklist for Building a Budget" (Exhibit 15–2) and critique your own effort.
3. Use the "Checklist for Reviewing a Budget" (Exhibit 15–3) and critique the existing budget.

Assignment Exercise 15–3: Transactions Outside the Operating Budget

Review Figure 15–2 and the accompanying text.

Metropolis Health System (MHS) has received a wellness grant from the charitable arm of an area electronics company. The grant will run for 24 months, beginning at the first of the next fiscal year. Two therapists and two registered nurses will each be spending half of their time working on the wellness grant. All four individuals are full-time employees of MHS. The electronics company has only recently begun to operate the charitable organization that awarded the grant. While they have gained all the legal approvals necessary, they have not yet provided the manuals and instructions for grant transactions that MHS usually receives when grants are awarded. Consequently, guidance about separate accounting is not yet forthcoming from the grantor.

Required

How would you handle this issue on the MHS operating budget for next year?

Assignment Exercise 15–4: Identified Versus Allocated Costs in Budgeting

Review Figure 15–3 and the accompanying text.

Metropolis Health System is preparing for a significant upgrade in both hardware and software for its information systems. As part of the project, the Chief of Information Operations (CIO) has indicated that the Information Systems (IS) department can change the format of the MHS operating budgets and related reports before the operating budget is constructed for the coming fiscal year. The Chief Financial Officer (CFO) has long wanted to modify what costs are identified and what costs are allocated (along with the method of allocation). This is a golden opportunity to do so. To gain ammunition for the change, the CFO is preparing to conduct a survey. The survey will obtain a variety of suggestions for potential changes in allocation methods for the new operating budget report formats. You have been selected as one of the employees who will be surveyed.

Required

You may choose your role for this assignment, as follows:

Refer to the "MHS Executive-Level Organization Chart" (Figure 28–2 in the MHS Case Study). (1) Either (a) choose any type of patient service that would be under the direction of the Senior Vice President of Service Delivery Operations or (b) choose any other function shown on the organization chart. (Your function could be a whole department or a division or unit of that department. For example, you might choose Community Outreach or Human Resources Operations or the Emergency department, etc.) (2) Make up your own organization chart for other employee levels within the function you have chosen. (3) Now make up another chart that indicates the operating budget costs you think would be mostly identifiable for the department or unit or division you have chosen and what other operating budget costs you think would be mostly allocated to it. (You may use Figure 15–3 as a rough guide, but do not let it limit your imagination. Model the detail on your "identifiable versus allocated costs" chart after a real department if you so choose.) Use MHS hospital statistics shown in Exhibit 28–8 of the MHS Case Study as a basis for allocation if these statistics are helpful. If they are not, make a note of what other statistics you would like to have.

Note: As an alternative approach, you may choose a function from the "Nursing Practice and Administration Organization Chart" as shown in Figure 28–1 of the MHS Case Study instead of choosing from the Executive-Level Organization Chart.

CHAPTER 16

Example 16A: Description of Capital Expenditure Proposals Scoring System

Worthwhile Hospital has a total capital expenditure budget for next year of five million dollars. Of this amount, three million is already committed as spending for capital assets that have already been acquired and are in place. The remaining two million dollars is available for new assets and for new projects or programs.

Worthwhile Hospital typically divides the available capital expenditure funds into monies available for inpatient purposes and monies available for outpatient purposes. This year the split is proposed to be 50-50.

The hospital's CFO is also proposing that a scoring system be used to evaluate this year's proposals. She has set up a scoring system that allows a maximum of five points. Thus the low is a score of one point and the high is a score of five points.

In addition to the points earned by a funding proposal, the CFO will allow one "bonus point" for upgrading existing equipment and one "bonus point" for funding expansion of existing programs.

Practice Exercise 16–I: Capital Expenditure Proposals

Jody Smith, the director who supervises the Intensive Care Units, wants to secure as much of the one million dollars available for inpatient purposes as is possible for the ICU. At the same time Ted Jones, the director who supervises the Surgery Unit, also wants to secure as much of the one million dollars available for inpatient purposes as is possible for his Surgery Unit.

Given the CFO's new scoring system, how should Jody go about choosing exactly what to request?

Assignment Exercise 16–1: Capital Expenditure Proposals

Ted Jones, the Surgery Unit Director, is about to choose his strategy for creating a capital expenditure funding proposal for the coming year. Ted's unit needs more room. The Surgery Unit is running at over 90% capacity. In addition, a prominent cardiology surgeon on staff at the hospital wants to create a new cardiac surgery program that would require extensive funding for more space and for new state-of-the-art equipment. The surgeon has been campaigning with the hospital board members.

Required

What should Ted decide to ask for? How should he go about crafting a strategy to justify his request, given the hospital's new scoring system?

CHAPTER 17

Example 17A: Variance Analysis

Our variance analysis example and practice exercise use the flexible budget approach. A flexible budget is one that is created using budgeted revenue and/or budgeted cost amounts. A flexible budget is adjusted, or flexed, to the actual level of output achieved (or perhaps expected to be achieved) during the budget period. A flexible budget thus looks toward a range of activity or volume (versus only one level in the static budget).

Examples of how the variance analysis works are contained in Figure 17–1 (the elements), in Figure 17-2 (the composition), and in Figures 17–3 and 17–4 (the calculations). Study these examples before undertaking the Practice Exercise.

We have restated Exhibit 17–2 in a worksheet format for purposes of this example. The new format appears as follows. (The numbers have not changed.)

Actual Cost	$920,000
Less: Flexible Budget	990,000
Price Variance (favorable)	$ 70,000
Budgeted Cost	$937,500
Less: Flexible Budget	990,000
Quantity Variance (unfavorable)	− $52,500
Net Variance (favorable)	$ 17,500

Assumptions (*refer to Exhibit 17-2*)

	Overhead Cost	divided by	# Therapy Minutes (Activity Level)	equals	Cost per Therapy Minute
Actual	(1) $920,000		(3) 330,000		(5) $2.79
Budgeted	(2) $937,500		(4) 312,500		(6) $3.00

Practice Exercise 17–1

Exhibit 17–2 presents the Variance Analysis for hospital rehab services for the third quarter. For our practice exercise we will duplicate this report for the fourth quarter. We are able to reformat the information in Exhibit 17–2 into a worksheet as follows. The fourth quarter assumptions appear below the worksheet.

Actual Cost	
Less: Flexible Budget	
Price Variance (favorable)	
Budgeted Cost	
Less: Flexible Budget	
Quantity Variance (unfavorable)	
Net Variance (unfavorable)	

Assumptions

	Overhead Cost	divided by	# Therapy Minutes (Activity Level)	equals	Cost per Therapy Minute
Actual	(1) $950,000		(3) 350,000		(5) $2.71
Budgeted	(2) $930,000		(4) 310,000		(6) $3.00

Required

1. Set up a worksheet for the fourth quarter like that shown in Exhibit 17–2 for the third quarter.
2. Insert the Fourth Quarter Input Data (per assumptions given above) on the worksheet.
3. Complete the "Actual Cost," "Flexible Budget," and "Budgeted Cost" sections at the top of the worksheet.
4. Compute the Price Variance and the Quantity Variance in the middle of the worksheet.
5. Indicate whether the Price and the Quantity Variances are favorable or unfavorable for the fourth quarter.

Optional

Can you compute how the $950,000 actual overhead costs and the $930,000 budgeted overhead costs were calculated?

Assignment Exercise 17–1: Variance Analysis

Greenview Hospital operated at 120% of normal capacity in two of its departments during the year. It operated 120% times 20,000 normal capacity direct labor nursing hours in routine services and it operated 120% times 20,000 normal capacity equipment hours in the laboratory. The lab allocates overhead by measuring minutes and hours the equipment is used; thus equipment hours.

Assumptions:

For Routine Services Nursing:

- 20,000 hours × 120% = 24,000 direct labor nursing hours.
- Budgeted Overhead at 24,000 hours = $42,000 fixed plus $6,000 variable = $48,000 total.
- Actual Overhead at 24,000 hours = $42,000 fixed plus $7,000 variable = $49,000 total.
- Applied Overhead for 24,000 hours at $2.35 = $56,400.

For Laboratory:

- 20,000 hours × 120% = 24,000 equipment hours.
- Budgeted Overhead at 24,000 hours = $59,600 fixed plus $11,400 variable = $71,000 total.
- Actual Overhead at 24,000 hours = $59,600 fixed plus $11,600 variable = $71,200 total.
- Applied Overhead for 24,000 hours at $3.455 = $82,920.

Required

1. Set up a worksheet for applied overhead costs and volume variance with a column for Routine Services Nursing and a second column for Laboratory.
2. Set up a worksheet for actual overhead costs and budget variance with a column for Routine Services Nursing and a second column for Laboratory.
3. Set up a worksheet for volume variance and budget variance totaling net variance with a column for Routine Services Nursing and a second column for Laboratory.
4. Insert input data from the Assumptions.
5. Complete computations for all three worksheets.

Example 17B

Review the "Sensitivity Analysis Overview" section and Figure 17–5 in Chapter 17.

Assignment Exercise 17–2: Three-Level Revenue Forecast

Three eye-ear-nose-and-throat physicians decide to hire an experienced audiologist in order to add a new service line to their practice.* They ask the practice manager to prepare a three-level volume forecast as a first step in their decision-making.

Assumptions: for the base level (most likely) revenue forecast, assume $200 per procedure times 4 procedures per day times 5 days equals 20 procedures per week times 50 weeks per year equals 1,000 potential procedures per year.

For the best case revenue forecast, assume an increase in volume of one procedure per day average, for an annual increase of 250 procedures (5 days per week times 50 weeks equals 250). (The best case is if the practice gains a particular managed care contract.)

For the worst case revenue forecast, assume a decrease in volume of 2 procedures per day average, for an annual decrease of 500 procedures. (The worst case is if the practice loses a major payer.)

*Audiologists were designated as "eligible for physician and other prescriber incentives" as discussed elsewhere. Thus the new service line was a logical move.

Required

Using the above assumptions, prepare a three-level forecast similar to the example in Figure 17–5 and document your calculations.

Practice Exercise 17–II

Closely study the chapter text concerning target operating income.
   The necessary inputs for target operating income include the following:

- Desired (target) operating income amount = $20,000
- Unit price for sales = $500
- Variable cost per unit = $300
- Total fixed cost = $10,000

Compute the required revenue to achieve the target operating income and compute a contribution income statement to prove the totals.

Assignment Exercise 17–3: Target Operating Income

Acme Medical Supply Company desires a target operating income amount of $100,000, with assumption inputs as follows:

- Desired (target) operating income amount = $100,000
- Unit price for sales = $80
- Variable cost per unit = $60
- Total fixed cost = $60,000

Compute the required revenue to achieve the target operating income and compute a contribution income statement to prove the totals.

CHAPTER 18

Assignment Exercise 18–1: Estimate of Loss

You are the practice manager for a four-physician office. You arrive on Monday morning to find the entire office suite flooded from overhead sprinklers that malfunctioned over the weekend. Water stands ankle-deep everywhere. The computers are fried and the contents of all the filing cabinets are soaked. Your own office, where most of the records were stored, has the worst damage.

The practice carries valuable papers insurance coverage for an amount up to $250,000. It is your responsibility to prepare an estimate of the financial loss so that a claim can be filed with the insurance company. How would you go about it? What would your summary of the losses look like?

Assignment Exercise 18–2: Estimate of Replacement Cost

The landlord carries contents insurance that should cover the damage to the furnishings, equipment, and to the computers, and the insurance company adjuster will come tomorrow to assess the furnishings and equipment damage. However, your boss is sure that the insurance settlement will not cover replacement costs. Consequently, you have been instructed to prepare an estimate of what has been lost and/or damaged plus an estimate of what the replacement cost might be. How would you go about it? What would your summary of these losses look like?

Assignment Exercise 18–3: Benchmarking

Review the chapter text about benchmarking.

Required

1. Select an organization: either from the Case Studies in Chapters 27–28 or from one of the Mini-Case Studies in Chapters 29–31.
2. Prepare a list of measures that could be benchmarked for this organization. Comment on why these items are important for benchmarking purposes.
3. Find another example of benchmarking for a healthcare organization. The example can be an organization report or it can be taken from a published source such as a journal article.

Assignment Exercise 18–4: Pareto Rule

Review the chapter text about the Pareto rule and examine Figure 18–4. Note that the text says Pareto diagrams are often drawn to reflect before and after results.

Assume that Figure 18–4 is the before diagram for the Billing department. Further assume that the after results are as follows:

Activity	Activity Code	Number
Process Denied Bills	PDB	12
Review with Supervisor	RWS	10
Locate Documentation	LD	6
Copy Documentation	CD	5
		33

Required

1. Redo the Pareto diagram with the after results. (Use Figure 18-4 as a guide.)
2. Comment on the before and after results for the Billing department.

Assignment Exercise 18–5: Quartiles

Review the chapter text about quartiles and study Table 18–1, which indicates results in quartiles.

Required

1. Locate healthcare information (such as bed days, number of visits, payment amounts, etc.) that contains a list of no less than twelve numerical amounts.
2. Divide the list you have found into quartiles.
3. Enter your results on a worksheet with the highest quartile first and the lowest quartile last. Include an explanation of your computations.

CHAPTER 19

Assignment Exercise 19–1

Review the information about public companies and stock exchanges in the Chapter 19 text.

Required

Obtain a copy of the *Wall Street Journal*. Locate the "Stock Tables" section of the *Journal*. Review the column headings in the tables and locate the names of various stock exchanges that are included in the findings. See if you can find the abbreviated names and the stock exchange symbols for healthcare companies that are publicly held.

Alternatively, explore the websites of three or four publicly held healthcare organizations. Somewhere on the website they should identify their stock exchange symbol. Then go onto a web-based stock exchange listing of the market for the day, locate the symbols, and determine their current stock prices according to the listing.

CHAPTER 20

Example 20A: Loan Amortization

This example illustrates the initial monthly payments of a loan with a principal balance of $50,000, an interest rate of 10%, and a payment period of 3 years or 36 months.
Loan Amortization Schedule
Principal borrowed: $50,000
Total payments: 36
Annual interest rate 10.00% (monthly rate = 0.8333%)

Payment #	Total Payment	Principal Portion of Payment	Interest Expense Portion of Payment	Remaining Principal Balance
			Beginning balance =	$50,000.00
1	$1,613.36	$1,196.69	$416.67	$48,403.31
2	1,613.36	1,206.67	406.69	47,596.64
3	1,613.36	1,216.72	396.64	46,379.92
4	1,613.36	1,226.86	386.50	45,153.06
5	1,613.36	1,237.08	376.28	43,915.98
6	1,613.36	1,247.39	365.97	42,668.58

Practice Exercise 20–I: Loan Amortization

This exercise illustrates a different principal amount than Example 20A, but computed at the same monthly interest rate and the same number of payments.

Required

Compute the first 6 months of a loan amortization schedule with a principal balance of $60,000, an interest rate of 10%, and a payment period of 3 years or 36 months.
Loan Amortization Schedule
Principal borrowed: $60,000
Total payments: 36
Annual interest rate 10.00% (monthly rate = 0.8333%)

Payment #	Total Payment	Principal Portion of Payment	Interest Expense Portion of Payment	Remaining Principal Balance
			Beginning balance =	$60,000.00
1				
2				
3				
4				
5				
6				

Assignment Exercise 20–1: Financial Statement Capital Structures

Required

Find three different financial statements that have varying capital structures. Write a paragraph about each that explains the debt-equity relationship and that computes the percentage of debt and the percentage of equity represented.

Also note whether the percentage of annual interest on debt is revealed in the notes to the financial statements. If so, do you believe the interest rate is fair and equitable? Why?

CHAPTER 21

Practice Exercise 21–I: Cost of Leasing

A cost of leasing table is reproduced below.

Required

Using the appropriate table from the Chapter 12 Appendices, record the present-value factor at 6% for each year and compute the present-value cost of leasing.

Cost of Leasing: Suburban Clinic—Comparative Present Value

Not-for-Profit Cost of Leasing:	Year 0	Year 1	Year 2	Year 3	Year 4	Year 5
Net Cash Flow	(11,000)	(11,000)	(11,000)	(11,000)	(11,000)	—
Present-value factor (at 6%)						
Present-value answer =						
Present-value cost of leasing =						

Assignment Exercise 21–1: Cost of Owning and Cost of Leasing

Cost of owning and cost of leasing tables are reproduced below.

Required

Using the appropriate table from the Chapter 12 Appendices, record the present-value factor at 10% for each year and compute the present-value cost of owning and the present value of leasing. Which alternative is more desirable at this interest rate? Do you think your answer would change if the interest rate was 6% instead of 10%?

Cost of Owning: Anywhere Clinic—Comparative Present Value

For-Profit Cost of Owning:	Year 0	Year 1	Year 2	Year 3	Year 4	Year 5
Net Cash Flow	(48,750)	2,500	2,500	2,500	2,500	5,000
Present-value factor						
Present-value answers =						
Present-value cost of owning =						

Cost of Leasing: Anywhere Clinic—Comparative Present Value

Line #	For-Profit Cost of Leasing:	Year 0	Year 1	Year 2	Year 3	Year 4	Year 5
19	Net Cash Flow	(8,250)	(8,250)	(8,250)	(8,250)	(8,250)	—
20	Present-value factor						
21	Present-value answers =						
22	Present-value cost of leasing =						

Assignment Exercise 21–2

Great Docs, a three-physician practice with two office sites, is considering whether to buy or lease a new computer system. Currently they own a low-tech (and low-cost) information system. The new system will have to meet all government specifications for an electronic health record system and will also have to connect the two office sites. It will be considerably more sophisticated than the current hardware and software and thus will require training for office staff, clinical staff, and the physicians. Everyone agrees there will be a learning curve in order to reach the system's full potential.

Doctor Smith, the majority owner of the practice, wants to buy a medical records system from Sam's Club. He argues that the package is supposed to electronically prescribe, track billings, set appointments, and keep records, so it should meet their needs. The cost of the first installed system is supposed to be $25,000, plus $10,000 for each additional system. The doctors are not sure if this means $25,000 for one office site plus $10,000 for the (connected) second office site for a total of $35,000, or if this means $25,000 for the first installed system plus $10,000 each for three more doctors, for a total of $55,000. There is also supposed to be $4,000 to $5,000 in maintenance costs each year as part of the purchased package. Doctor Smith proposes to pay 20% down and obtain a five-year installment loan from the local bank for the remaining 80% at an interest rate of 8%.

Doctor Jones, the youngest of the three physicians, has been recently added to the practice. A computer nerd, he wants to lease a complete system from the small company his college roommate began last year. While he has received a quote of $20,000 for the entire system including first year maintenance, it does not meet the government requirements for an electronic health record system. Consequently, the other two doctors have outvoted Doctor Jones and this system will not be seriously considered.

Doctor Brown, the usual peace-maker between Doctor Smith and Doctor Jones, wants to lease a system. He argues that leasing will place the responsibility for upgrades and maintenance upon the lessor company, and that removing the responsibilities of ownership is advantageous. He has received a quote of $20,000 per year for a five-year lease that includes hardware and software for both offices, that meets the government requirements for an electronic health record system, and that includes training, maintenance, and upgrades.

Required

Summarize the costs to the practice of owning a system (per Doctor Smith) versus leasing (per Doctor Brown). Include a computation of comparative present value. (Refer to Assignment 21-1 for setting up a comparative present-value table.)

Assignment Exercise 21–3

Metropolis Health System has to do something about their ambulance situation. They have to (1) buy a new ambulance, (2) lease a new one, or (3) renovate an existing ambulance that MHS already owns. Rob Lackey, the Assistant Controller, has been asked to gather pertinent information in order to make a decision. So far Rob has found these facts:

1. It will cost at least $250,000 to purchase a new ambulance, although the cost varies widely depending upon the quantity and sophistication of the emergency equipment contained on the vehicle.

2. In order to renovate the existing vehicle, it will cost at least $100,000 to purchase and install a new "box." (In other words, a new emergency-equipped body is installed on the existing chassis.) Rob has found this existing ambulance has an odometer reading of 80,000 miles. The vehicle will also need a new fuel pump and new tires, but he believes these items would be recorded as repair and maintenance operating expenses and thus would not be included in his calculations.

3. Lease terms for ambulances also vary widely, but so far Rob believes a cost of $60,000 per year is a ballpark figure.

Required

How much more information should Rob have before he begins to make any calculations? Make a list. Which alternative do you believe would be best? Give your reasons.

CHAPTER 22

Assignment Exercise 22–1

This group project assignment concerns situational analysis.

Create a hypothetical organization, complete with an IT department and financial, clinical, and administrative staff levels. This IT department is tasked with adopting and implementing EHR.

Required

Step 1. Using your hypothetical organization's personnel, assign a variety of scores to a Scoring Summary Sheet such as that shown in Exhibit 22–A-1 in the chapter Appendix.

Step 2. Summarize the scores and place the net scores in a SWOT matrix such as the one shown in Figure 22–6.

Step 3. Create a report to the organization's CEO that summarizes the (good or bad) results.

Optional Additional Assignment

Required

Locate several healthcare organizations' mission, value, and vision statements. Use public sources with no privacy concerns.

Then fit the statements you have discovered into the chapter's categories of recognizing a special status or focus within the statements; financial emphasis within the statements; and/or relaying the message.

CHAPTER 23

Example 23A: Assumptions

Types of assumptions required for the financial portion of a business plan typically include answers to the following questions:

- What types of revenue?
- How many services will be offered to produce the revenue (by month)?
- How much labor will be required (FTEs)?
- What will the labor cost?
- How many and what type of supplies, drugs, and/or devices will be required to offer the service?
- What will the supplies, drugs, and/or devices cost?
- How much space will be required?
- What will the required space occupancy cost?
- Is special equipment required?
- If so, how much will it cost?
- Is staff training required to use the special equipment?
- If so, how much time is required, and what will it cost?

Practice Exercise 23–I: Assumptions

Refer to the proposal to add a retail pharmacy in the mini-case study in Chapter 29.

Required

Identify how many of the assumption items listed in the example above can be found in the retail pharmacy proposal worksheets.

Assignment Exercise 23–1: Business Plan

Refer to the proposal to add a retail pharmacy in the mini-case study in Chapter 29.

Required

Build a business plan for this proposal. Prepare the service description using your consumer knowledge of a retail pharmacy (if necessary). Of course this retail pharmacy will be located within the hospital, but its purpose is to dispense prescriptions to carry off-site and use at home. Thus, it operates pretty much like the neighborhood retail pharmacy that you use yourself.

Use the information provided in Chapter 29 to prepare the financial section of the business plan. Use your imagination to create the marketing segment and the organization segment.

CHAPTER 24

Assignment Exercise 24–1

This chapter discusses how the private sector has contributed to the adoption and implementation electronic health records (EHR) and provides two examples.

Required

Locate one or more additional examples of instances where the private sector has led the way in demonstrating how electronic health records can be successfully conceived and implemented.

Put your examples in the form of a report.

Assignment Exercise 24–2

Recollect one of your own personal encounters with electronic health records.

Required

Report, in writing, about an encounter you or one of your family members has had with electronic health records. In so doing, do not overstep privacy concerns and boundaries. Include whether you believe the encounter was successful and why. If not, describe the reasons why it was unsuccessful.

CHAPTER 25

Assignment Exercise 25–1: Physician Incentive Payments and Costs Under the HITECH Act

Refer to the description of physician incentives under the HITECH Act within the chapter text. See also the maximum incentive payments an eligible professional can receive (Figure 25–1). Also review the definition of physicians who are "meaningful electronic health records users" (and thus eligible for payment under this program).

Required

Locate additional information about electronic health records systems that are being sold to physicians based on their qualification under the HITECH Incentive Program. Attempt to determine what the net cost of hardware, software, and installation would be for an average physician practice. Compare this cost with the payments that an eligible physician who is a meaningful electronic health records user would receive over a five-year period. Determine the approximate net technology cost to the physician after such incentive payments.

As an extension of this assignment you might also determine what start-up costs other than the technology costs may be incurred by the physician.

Assignment Exercise 25–2

This chapter defines meaningful use and meaningful user.

Required

Locate the "meaningful EHR users" listed on the CMS website. Review the listings to locate organizations that are in your geographic area.

Assignment Exercise 25–3

Meaningful use training is an important aspect of EHR adoption.

Required

Locate advertising that offers training related to meaningful use and/or meaningful users. What level or type of professional do they target? What does the advertising promise?

CHAPTER 26

Practice Exercise 26–I

The Productivity Loss section of this chapter describes how the dollar amount of such loss was computed after determining that it took coders an extra 1.7 minutes per claim in the first month of ICD-10 transition.

   Assume a hospital's coders are dealing with 1,500 claims within a certain period. What would the dollar amount of productivity loss be if the coders took an extra two minutes (instead of 1.7 minutes) per claim?

Assignment Exercise 26–1: Information About the ICD-10-CM and ICD-10-PCS Transition

Required

Locate some articles and/or government websites that describe the ICD-10-CM and ICD-10-PCS Diagnosis Codes and tools for their implementation over a period of years. Write a summary of whether the materials you have found fully explain the breadth and depth of the transition challenge for managers who must live through the transition.

Assignment Exercise 26–2: Hospital Conversion to ICD-10

Try to locate sufficient detail about a healthcare organization—enough that you can perform a make-believe SWOT analysis about a conversion of electronic systems to ICD-10 as required. Write a description of the organization's background, including its information system. (Add imaginary details if you need to.) This description will then lead into the ICD-10 conversion's situation analysis. Perform the make-believe SWOT analysis, using the four-part format (internal Strengths and Weaknesses and external Opportunities and Threats).

   As an alternative approach, you can use the Sample General Hospital information in Appendix 28-A as a starting point and use your personal experience and observations to fill out the rest of the details you would need in order to commence a make-believe SWOT analysis for this hospital's ICD-10 conversion.

Assignment Exercise 26–3: Hospital Costs to Implement

Refer to the Scenario for a Midwestern Community Hospital, located in Appendix 26-A.

Required

Part 1—Within this scenario the productivity loss for the six-month learning period is calculated to be $1,233. Beginning with month 1 at $353 ($1.41 times 250 equals $353), compute the cost of productivity loss for the remaining five months as explained in the scenario, to total an overall amount of $1,233. Be prepared to show and explain your computations.

Part 2—Later in the scenario, CMS states that the hospital's total cost amounts to $303,990. Study the explanation and summarize the totals of each type of cost discussed. When you are finished your total should amount to $303,990. Be prepared to show and explain how you arrived at this total.

SUPPLEMENTARY MATERIALS: THE MECHANICS OF PERCENTAGE COMPUTATIONS

The Reason for This Explanation: Author's Note

I had just finished presenting a day-long finance seminar when the vice president of a bank who had been attending pulled me aside. After looking around to make sure no one was listening, he asked me to show him how to calculate a percentage.

As I didn't know him or anyone from the town he lived and worked in, he wasn't embarrassed to ask me. So we believe if the vice president of a bank can ask about how to figure a percentage, then that calculation deserves to be described within this Appendix, as follows.

The Fraction's Parts: Numerator and Denominator

Reminder: A fraction has two parts—the numerator is the top number and the denominator is the bottom number. Or, to be more precise, the numerator is the part of a fraction that is above the line and signifies the number of parts of the denominator taken.[1]

The denominator is the part of a fraction that is below the line and signifies division and that in fractions with 1 as the numerator indicates into how many parts the unit is divided.[2]

First Calculate the Fraction (Including the Decimal)

To calculate a fraction, the bottom number (denominator) is divided into the top number (numerator). For example, if the numerator is 90 and the denominator is 100, divide 100 into 90. The resulting answer is 0.90. (Note that the decimal point is to the left of the 0.90 answer.)

Next Convert the Fraction to a Percentage

To obtain the percentage, we need to convert the fraction. To do so, move the decimal two places to the right. Now the answer is 90, and the percentage answer is 90%.

Summary

We know that your computer or tablet will perform this computation automatically, but situations may still arise when you may need to calculate by hand. It's a good thing to know.

Notes

1. *Merriam Webster's Collegiate Dictionary*, 10th ed., s.v. "Numerator".
2. *Merriam Webster's Collegiate Dictionary*, 10th ed., s.v. "Denominator".

SOLUTIONS TO PRACTICE EXERCISES

SOLUTION TO PRACTICE EXERCISE 3–I

Short-term assets: cash on hand; accounts receivable; inventory
Long-term assets: land; buildings
Short-term liabilities: payroll taxes due; accounts payable
Long-term liabilities: mortgage payable (noncurrent); note payable (due in 24 months)

SOLUTION TO PRACTICE EXERCISE 5–I

	Intensive Care Unit	*Laboratory*	*Laundry*
Drugs requisitioned	X		
Pathology supplies		X	
Detergents and bleach			X
Nursing salaries	X		
Clerical salaries	X	X	X
Uniforms (for laundry aides)			X
Repairs (parts for microscopes)		X	

Note: If no clerical salaries are assigned to Laundry, this is an acceptable alternative solution.

SOLUTION TO PRACTICE EXERCISE 6–I

	Direct Cost	*Indirect Cost*
Managed care marketing expense	X	
Real estate taxes		X
Liability insurance		X
Clinic telephone expense	X	
Utilities (for the entire facility)		X
Emergency room medical supplies	X	

SOLUTION TO PRACTICE EXERCISE 6–II

In real life the solution to this exercise will depend upon factors unique to the particular organization. The following solution is a generic one.

	Responsibility Center	*Support Center*
Security	X	
Communications	X	
Ambulance services	X	
Medical records		X
Educational resources		X
Human resources		X

Reporting: Each responsibility center has a manager. All report to the director.

SOLUTION TO PRACTICE EXERCISE 7–I

Step 1. Find the highest volume of 1,100 packs at a cost of $7,150 in September and the lowest volume of 100 packs at a cost of $1,010 in August.

Step 2. Compute the variable rate per pack as:

	# of Packs	*Training Pack Cost*
Highest volume	1,100	$7,150
Lowest volume	100	1,010
Difference	1,000	$6,140

Step 3. Divide the difference in cost ($6,140) by the difference in # of packs (1,000) to arrive at the variable cost rate:

$6,140 divided by 1,000 packs = $6.14 per pack

Step 4. Compute the fixed overhead rate as follows:

At the highest level:

Total cost	$7,150
Less: Variable portion [1,100 packs × $6.14]	(6,754)
Fixed Portion of Cost	$ 396

At the lowest level:

Total cost	$1,010
Less: Variable portion [100 packs × $6.14]	(614)
Fixed Portion of Cost	$ 396

Proof totals: $396 fixed portion at both levels.

SOLUTION TO PRACTICE EXERCISE 7–II

Step 1. Divide costs into variable and fixed portions. In this case $3,450,000 times 40% equals $1,380,000 variable cost and $3,450,000 times 60% equals $2,070,000 fixed cost.

Step 2. Compute the contribution margin:

	Amount
Revenue	$3,500,000
Less variable cost	(1,380,000)
Contribution margin	$2,120,000
Less fixed cost	2,070,000
Operating income	$ 50,000

SOLUTION TO PRACTICE EXERCISE 7–III

	Amount	%	
Revenue	$1,210,000	100.00	
Less variable cost	(205,000)	16.94	
Contribution margin	$1,005,000	83.06	= PV or CM Ratio
Less fixed cost	(1,100,000)	90.91	
Operating loss	$(95,000)	7.85	

SOLUTION TO PRACTICE EXERCISE 8–I

1. Straight-line depreciation would amount to $54,000 per year for 10 years. This amount is computed as follows:

   Step 1. Compute the cost net of salvage or trade-in value: 600,000 less 10% salvage value or 60,000 equals 540,000.

   Step 2. Divide the resulting figure by the expected life (also known as estimated useful life): 540,000 divided by 10 equals 54,000 depreciation per year for 10 years.

2. Double-declining depreciation is computed as follows:

   Step 1. Compute the straight-line rate: 1 divided by 10 equals 10%.

   Step 2. Now double the rate (as in "double-declining method"): 10% times 2 equals 20%.

   Step 3. Compute the first year's depreciation expense: 600,000 times 20% = 120,000.

   Step 4. Compute the carry-forward book value at the beginning of the second year: 600,000 book value beginning year 1 less year 1 depreciation of 120,000 equals book value at beginning of the second year of 480,000.

   Step 5. Compute the second year's depreciation expense: 480,000 times 20% = 96,000.

Step 6. Compute the carry-forward book value at the beginning of the third year: 480,000 book value beginning year 2 less year 2 depreciation of 96,000 equals book value at beginning of the third year of 384,000.

Continue until the asset's salvage or trade-in value has been reached.

Book Value at Beginning of Year	Depreciation Expense	Book Value at End of Year
600,000	600,000 × 20% = 120,000	600,000 − 120,000 = 480,000
480,000	480,000 × 20% = 96,000	480,000 − 96,000 = 384,000
384,000	384,000 × 20% = 76,800	384,000 − 76,800 = 307,200
307,200	307,200 × 20% = 61,440	307,200 − 61,440 = 245,760
245,760	245,760 × 20% = 49,152	245,760 − 49,152 = 196,608
196,608	196,608 × 20% = 39,322	196,608 − 39,322 = 157,286
157,286	157,286 × 20% = 31,457	157,286 − 31,457 = 125,829
125,829	125,829 × 20% = 25,166	125,829 − 25,166 = 100,663
100,663	100,663 × 20% = 20,132	100,663 − 20,132 = 80,531
80,531	80,561 at 10th year	80,561 − 20,561 = 60,000

Balance remaining at end of 10th year represents the salvage or trade-in value.

Note: Under the double-declining balance method, book value never reaches zero. Therefore, a company typically adopts the straight-line method at the point where straight line would exceed the double-declining balance.

SOLUTION TO PRACTICE EXERCISE 8–II

Straight-line depreciation would amount to $9,000 per year for five years. This amount is computed as follows:

Step 1. Compute the cost of salvage or trade-in value: 50,000 less 10% salvage value or 5,000 equals 45,000.

Step 2. Divide the resulting figure by the expected life (also known as the estimated useful life): 45,000 divided by 5 equals 9,000 depreciation per year for 5 years.

SOLUTION TO PRACTICE EXERCISE 9–I

1. Compute Net Paid Days Worked

Total days in business year	364
Less two days off per week	104
# Paid days per year	260

Less paid days not worked

Holidays	8	
Sick days	5	
Education day	1	
Vacation days	5	
		19
Net paid days worked		241

2. Convert Net Paid Days Worked to a Factor

Total days in business year divided by net paid days worked equals factor

$$364/241 = 1.510373$$

SOLUTION TO PRACTICE EXERCISE 9–II

	Shift 1 Day	Shift 2 Evening	Shift 3 Night	=	24-Hour Scheduling Total
Position: Admissions officer	2	1	1		four 8-hour shifts
FTEs—to cover position					
7 days/week equals	2.8	1.4	1.4		5.6 FTEs
Position: Clerical	1	0	0		one 8-hour shift
FTEs—to cover position					
7 days/week equals	1.4	0	0		1.4 FTEs

SOLUTION TO PRACTICE EXERCISE 10–I

Current Liabilities	30,000
Total Assets	1,000,000
Income from Operations	80,000
Accumulated Depreciation	480,000
Total Operating Revenue	180,000
Current Portion of Long-Term Debt	10,000
Interest Income	-0-
Inventories	5,000

SOLUTION TO PRACTICE EXERCISE 10–II

No, Doctors Smith and Brown's patient accounts receivable does not appear to be net of an allowance for bad debts, because we cannot find an equivalent bad debt expense on their statement of net income. Do you think the doctors should have an allowance for bad debts on their statement? Why do you think they do not?

SOLUTION TO PRACTICE EXERCISE 10–III

As mentioned in the chapter text, land is not stated at "net" because land is never depreciated.

SOLUTION TO PRACTICE EXERCISE 11–I

Current Ratio

The current ratio is represented as Current Ratio equals Current Assets divided by Current Liabilities. This ratio is considered to be a measure of short-term debt-paying ability. However, it must be carefully interpreted.

Current Ratio Computation

$$\frac{\text{Current Assets}}{\text{Current Liabilities}} = \frac{\$70,000}{\$30,000} = 2.33 \text{ to } 1$$

Quick Ratio

The quick ratio is represented as Quick Ratio equals Cash and Short-Term Investments plus Net Receivables, divided by Current Liabilities. This ratio is considered to be an even more severe test of short-term debt-paying ability (even more severe than the current ratio). The quick ratio is also known as the acid-test ratio, for obvious reasons.

$$\frac{\text{Cash and Short-Term Investments} + \text{Net Receivables}}{\text{Current Liabilities}} = \frac{\$65,000}{30,000} = 2.167 \text{ to } 1$$

SOLUTION TO PRACTICE EXERCISE 11–II

Solvency Ratios

Debt Service Coverage Ratio (DSCR)

The Debt Service Coverage Ratio (DSCR) is represented as change in unrestricted net assets (net income) plus interest, depreciation, and amortization, divided by maximum annual debt service. This ratio is universally used in credit analysis.

$$\frac{\substack{\text{Change in Unrestricted Net Assets (net income)} \\ \text{plus Interest, Depreciation, Amortization}}}{\text{Maximum Annual Debt Service}} = \frac{\$113,100}{\$22,200} = 5.1$$

Note: $80,000 + $3,100 + $30,000 = $113,100.

Liabilities to Fund Balance (or Debt to Net Worth)

The liabilities to fund balance or net worth computation is represented as total liabilities divided by unrestricted net assets (fund balances or net worth) equals total debt divided by tangible net worth. This figure is a quick indicator of debt load.

$$\frac{\text{Total Liabilities}}{\text{Unrestricted (Fund Balance)}} = \frac{\$200,000}{\$800,000} = 2.5$$

SOLUTION TO PRACTICE EXERCISE 11–III

Profitability Ratios

Operating Margin

The operating margin, which is generally expressed as a percentage, is represented as operating income (loss) divided by total operating revenues. This ratio is used for a number of managerial purposes and also sometimes enters into credit analysis. It is therefore a multi-purpose measure.

$$\frac{\text{Operating Income (Loss)}}{\text{Total Operating Revenues}} = \frac{\$80,000}{\$180,000} = 44.4\%$$

Return on Total Assets

The return on total assets is represented as earnings before interest and taxes (EBIT) divided by total assets. This is a broad measure in common use.

$$\frac{\text{EBIT (Earnings before Interest and Taxes)}}{\text{Total Assets}} = \frac{\$83,100}{\$1,000,000} = 8.3\%$$

Note: $\$80,000 + \$3,100 = \$83,100$.

SOLUTION TO PRACTICE EXERCISE 12–I: UNADJUSTED RATE OF RETURN

1. Calculation using original investment amount:

$$\frac{\$100,000}{\$500,000} = 20\% \text{ Unadjusted Rate of Return}$$

2. Calculation using average investment amount:
   Step 1. Compute average investment amount for total unrecovered asset cost:

At beginning of estimated useful life	= $500,000
At end of estimated useful life	= $ 50,000
Sum	$550,000

   Divided by 2 = $275,000 average investment amount

Step 2. Calculate unadjusted rate of return:

$$\frac{\$100,000}{\$275,000} = 36.4\% \text{ Unadjusted Rate of Return}$$

SOLUTION TO PRACTICE EXERCISE 12–II: FINDING THE FUTURE VALUE (WITH A COMPOUND INTEREST TABLE)

Step 1. Refer to the Compound Interest Table found in Appendix 12-B at the back of this chapter. Reading across, or horizontally, find the 7% column. Reading down, or vertically, find Year 6. Trace across the Year 6 line item to the 7% column. The factor is 1.501.

Step 2. Multiply the current savings account balance of $11,000 times the factor of 1.501 to find the future value of $16,511. In six years at compound interest of 7%, the college fund will have a balance of $16,511.

SOLUTION TO PRACTICE EXERCISE 12–III: FINDING THE PRESENT VALUE

Step 1. Refer to the Present-Value Table found in Appendix 12-A at the back of this chapter. Reading across, or horizontally, find the 7% column. Reading down, or vertically, find Year 15. Trace across the Year 15 line item to the 7% column. The factor is 0.3624.

Step 2. Multiply $150,000 times the factor of 0.3624 to find the present value of $54,360.

SOLUTION TO PRACTICE EXERCISE 12–IV

Assemble the assumptions in an orderly manner:

Assumption 1: Initial cost of the investment = $16,950.
Assumption 2: Estimated annual net cash inflow the investment will generate = $3,000.
Assumption 3: Useful life of the asset = 10 years.

Perform calculation:

Step 1. Divide the initial cost of the investment ($16,950) by the estimated annual net cash inflow it will generate ($3,000). The answer is a ratio amounting to 5.650.

Step 2. Now use the abbreviated look-up table for the Present Value of an Annuity of $1. Find the line item for the number of periods that matches the useful life of the asset (10 years in this case).

Step 3. Look across the 10-year line on the table and find the column that approximates the ratio of 5.650 (as computed in Step 1). That column contains the interest rate representing the rate of return. In this case the rate of return is 12%.

SOLUTION TO PRACTICE EXERCISE 12–V

Assemble assumptions in an orderly manner:

Assumption 1: Purchase price of the equipment = $500,000.
Assumption 2: Useful life of the equipment = 10 years.
Assumption 3: Revenue the machine will generate per year = $84,000.
Assumption 4: Direct operating costs associated with earning the revenue = $21,000.
Assumption 5: Depreciation expense per year (computed as purchase price per assumption 1 divided by useful life per assumption 2) = $50,000.

Perform computation:

Step 1. Find the machine's expected net income after taxes:

Revenue (Assumption 3)	$84,000
Less	
Direct operating costs (Assumption 4)	$21,000
Depreciation (Assumption 5)	50,000
	71,000
Net income	$13,000

Note: No income taxes for this hospital.

Step 2. Find the net annual cash inflow the machine is expected to generate (in other words, convert the net income to a cash basis).

Net income	$13,000
Add back depreciation (a noncash expenditure)	50,000
Annual net cash inflow after taxes	$63,000

Step 3. Compute the payback period:

$$\frac{\text{Investment}}{\text{Net Annual Cash Inflow}} = \frac{\$500,000\ \text{Machine Cost*}}{\$63,000} = 7.9\ \text{Year Payback Period}$$

*Assumption 1 above.
**Per Step 2 above.

The machine will pay back its investment under these assumptions in 7.9 years.

SOLUTION TO PRACTICE EXERCISE 13–I

Common sizing for the assets of the two hospitals appears on the worksheet below. Note that their gross numbers are very different, yet the proportionate relationships of the percentages (20%, 75%, and 5%) are the same for both hospitals.

| | Same Year for Both Hospitals | | | |
	Hospital A		Hospital B	
Current assets	$ 2,000,000	20%	$ 8,000,000	20%
Property, plant, and equipment	7,500,000	75%	30,000,000	75%
Other assets	500,000	5%	2,000,000	5%
Total assets	$10,000,000	100%	$40,000,000	100%

SOLUTION TO PRACTICE EXERCISE 13–II

| | Hospital A | | |
	Year 1	Year 2	Difference	
Current assets	$1,600,000	$ 2,000,000	$ 400,000	25%
Property, plant, and equipment	6,000,000	7,500,000	1,500,000	25%
Other assets	400,000	500,000	100,000	25%
Total assets	$8,000,000	$10,000,000	$2,000,000	—

Note: The worksheet below shows Hospital A with both common sizing and trend analysis:

| | Hospital A | | | | | |
	Year 1		Year 2		Difference	
Current assets	$1,600,000	20%	$ 2,000,000	20%	$ 400,000	25%
Property, plant, and equipment	6,000,000	75%	7,500,000	75%	1,500,000	25%
Other assets	400,000	5%	500,000	5%	100,000	25%
Total assets	$8,000,000	100%	$10,000,000	100%	$2,000,000	—

SOLUTION TO PRACTICE EXERCISE 13–III

Q: How many procedures has your unit recorded for the period to date?

Solution: The unit has recorded 2,000 procedures ($200,000 divided by $100 apiece equals 2,000 procedures).

Q: Of these, how many procedures are attributed to each payer?

Solution: At 25% of the volume per payer, each payer accounts for 500 procedures (2,000 times 25% equals 500 procedures). Proof total: 500 procedures apiece times four payers equals 2,000 procedures.

Q: How much is the net revenue per procedure for each payer, and how much is the contractual allowance per procedure for each payer?

Solution: The computation is as follows:

Payer #	Gross Charges	% Paid by Each Payer	Net Revenue per Procedure	Contractual Allowance per Procedure
1	$100.00	90%	$90.00	$10.00
2	$100.00	80%	$80.00	$20.00
3	$100.00	70%	$70.00	$30.00
4	$100.00	50%	$50.00	$50.00

SOLUTION TO PRACTICE EXERCISE 15–I

Your initial budget assumptions were as follows:

Assume the budget anticipated 30,000 inpatient days this year at an average of $650 revenue per day, or $19,500,000. Further assume that inpatient expenses were budgeted at $600 per patient day, or $18,000,000. Also assume the budget anticipated 10,000 outpatient visits this year at an average of $400 revenue per visit, or $4,000,000. Further assume that outpatient expenses were budgeted at $380 per visit, or $3,800,000. The budget worksheet would look like this:

	As Budgeted
Revenue—Inpatient	$19,500,000
Revenue—Outpatient	4,000,000
Subtotal	$23,500,000
Expenses—Inpatient	$18,000,000
Expenses—Outpatient	3,800,000
Subtotal	$21,800,000
Excess of revenue over expenses	$1,700,000

Now assume that only 27,000, or 90%, of the patient days are going to actually be achieved for the year. The average revenue of $650 per day will be achieved for these 27,000 days (thus 27,000 times 650 equals 17,550,000). Also assume that outpatient visits will actually amount to 110%, or 11,000 for the year. The average revenue of $400 per visit will be achieved for these 11,000 visits (thus 11,000 times 400 equals 4,400,000). Further assume that, due to the heroic efforts of the Chief Financial Officer, the actual inpatient expenses will amount to $11,600,000 and the actual outpatient expenses will amount to $4,000,000. The actual results would look like this:

	Actual
Revenue—Inpatient	$17,550,000
Revenue—Outpatient	4,400,000
Subtotal	$21,950,000
Expenses—Inpatient	16,100,000
Expenses—Outpatient	4,000,000
Subtotal	$20,100,000
Excess of revenue over expenses	$1,850,000

Since the budgeted revenues and expenses still reflect the original expectations of 30,000 inpatient days and 10,000 outpatient visits, the budget report would look like this:

	Actual	Budget	Static Budget Variance
Revenue—Inpatient	$17,550,000	$19,500,000	$(1,950,000)
Revenue—Outpatient	4,400,000	4,000,000	400,000
Subtotal	$21,950,000	$23,500,000	$(1,550,000)
Expenses—Inpatient	$16,100,000	$18,000,000	$(1,900,000)
Expenses—Outpatient	4,000,000	3,800,000	200,000
Subtotal	$20,100,000	$21,800,000	$(1,700,000)
Excess of revenue over expenses	$ 1,850,000	$ 1,700,000	$ 150,000

Note: The negative effect of the $1,550,000 net drop in revenue is offset by the greater effect of the $1,700,000 net drop in expenses, resulting in a positive net effect of $150,000.

PRACTICE EXERCISE 16–I

Because there is no one right answer, students will approach this exercise in different ways.

SOLUTION TO PRACTICE EXERCISE 17–1

Required Solution to Practice Exercise 17–1

The Price Variance is $100,000 (favorable).
The Quantity Variance is $120,000 (unfavorable).
The Net Variance is $20,000 (unfavorable).

Actual Cost	$950,000
Less: Flexible Budget	1,050,000
Price Variance (favorable)	$100,000
Budgeted Cost	$930,000
Less: Flexible Budget	1,050,000
Quantity Variance (unfavorable)	− $120,500
Net Variance (favorable)	− $ 20,000

Assumptions

	Overhead Cost	divided by	# Therapy Minutes (Activity Level)	equals	Cost per Therapy Minute
Actual	(1) $950,000		(3) 350,000		(5) $2.71
Budgeted	(2) $930,000		(4) 310,000		(6) $3.00

Optional Solution to Practice Exercise 17–I

The $950,000 actual overhead cost represents 350,000 therapy minutes times $2.71 per therapy minute.

The $930,000 budgeted overhead cost represents 310,000 therapy minutes times $3.00 per therapy minute.

SOLUTION TO PRACTICE EXERCISE 17–II

The required revenue to achieve a target operating income of $20,000 amounts to revenue of $75,000.

The contribution income statement to prove the formula results is as follows:

Revenue $500/unit x 150 units =	$75,000
Variable costs $300/unit x 150 units =	45,000
Contribution margin	$30,000
Fixed costs	10,000
Desire (Target) Operating Income =	$20,000

SOLUTION TO PRACTICE EXERCISE 20–I

With beginning principal of $60,000, the monthly payment is $1,936.03 and the remaining principal balance at the end of six payments is $51,202.30.

SOLUTION TO PRACTICE EXERCISE 21–I

The present-value cost of leasing for Suburban Clinic amounts to $49,116.

SOLUTION TO PRACTICE EXERCISE 23–I

All of the assumption items listed in Example 23A are present in the retail pharmacy mini-case study in Chapter 29.

SOLUTION TO PRACTICE EXERCISE 26–I

$50 per hour divided by 60 minutes equals $0.8333; thus 2 minutes equals $1.6667. If a hospital's coders are dealing with 1,500 claims, then the dollar amount of productivity loss is $2,499 (1.6667 per claim times 1,500 claims equals $2,499).

Index

Note: Page numbers followed by *f* or *t* indicate material in figures or tables, respectively.